AF871552

PERI-IMPLANTITIS
From Diagnosis to Treatment

I. K. Karoussis
N. P. Lang

PERI-IMPLANTITIS

From Diagnosis to Treatment

In collaboration with P. Ntokou

QUINTESSENCE PUBLISHING

Berlin | Chicago | Tokyo
Barcelona | London | Milan | Mexico City | Paris | Prague | Seoul | Warsaw
Beijing | Istanbul | Sao Paulo | Zagreb

One book, one tree: In support of reforestation worldwide and to address the climate crisis, for every book sold Quintessence Publishing will plant a tree (https://onetreeplanted.org/).

A CIP record for this book is available from the British Library.

QUINTESSENCE PUBLISHING DEUTSCHLAND

Quintessenz Verlags-GmbH
Ifenpfad 2–4
12107 Berlin, Germany
www.quintessence-publishing.com

Quintessence Publishing Co Ltd
Grafton Road, New Malden
Surrey KT3 3AB, United Kingdom
www.quintessence-publishing.com

Copyright © 2024 Quintessenz Verlags-GmbH

All rights reserved. This book or any part thereof may not be reproduced, stored in a retrieval system, or transmitted in any form or by any means, electronic, mechanical, photocopying, or otherwise, without prior written permission of the publisher.

Editing and reproduction: Quintessenz Verlags-GmbH, Berlin, Germany
Layout and production: Janina Kuhn, Quintessenz Verlags-GmbH, Berlin, Germany

ISBN 978-1-78698-145-5
Printed and bound in Croatia

Foreword

This book provides a comprehensive overview of the key aspects of diagnosis and treatment of peri-implantitis. The illustrative chapters include many case examples describing situations readers may encounter in their everyday practice, providing practical insights into the management of these complications. The chapters address a range of treatment approaches from non-surgical to surgical management, resective and regenerative treatment, and procedures for peri-implant soft tissue augmentation.

Both authors are renowned for their extensive experience in the fields of implant dentistry, periodontology, and management of peri-implantitis, with Professor Lang having developed the first comprehensive treatment protocol for peri-implantitis known as Cumulative Interceptive Supportive Therapy (CIST), which forms the basis for the contemporary treatment approaches outlined in the book.

The comprehensive approach includes chapters covering the etiology, diagnosis, prevalence, and risk factors for peri-implantitis as well as decision-making steps for treatment planning and practical steps for treatment. The book concludes with key steps for prevention and supportive peri-implant treatment. This informative and illustrative book provides a practical and useful guide for all oral health professionals who practice in the field of implant dentistry.

Lisa J. A. Heitz-Mayfield
Perth, Western Australia, August 2024
Editor-in-Chief
Clinical Oral Implants Research

To our families, with love
and gratitude

Introduction

Peri-implantitis: from diagnosis to treatment is a monograph that aims to present, in a structured and detailed manner, the sum of all available information regarding peri-implant tissue pathology, as well as the knowledge and "secrets" clinicians should be aware so that they can successfully approach the treatment of peri-implant diseases. The tremendously high number of implants placed in millions of patients globally makes knowledge of the treatment of pathologic situations that concern them necessary. In the past, peri-implant diseases were a subject of study for many clinicians and researchers to clarify the etiology and factors that predispose to peri-implantitis or worsen its progress, as well as ways to treat it.

Now that the use of implants has been established in daily clinical practice, it is clear that on occasions, once the highly anticipated osseointegration has been achieved, soft tissue inflammation and gradual bone loss around the implants, which were already functional, may occur at different times. These initial observations caused scientific debate, with some researchers even disputing the existence of peri-implantitis. Later on, many scientists regarded peri-implantitis as a problem that only affected rough implants or implants placed transmucosally. However, since the early 1990s, many researchers have investigated the issue carefully and recognized and named the diseases that affect peri-implant tissues, thus initiating a growing and ongoing interest in and knowledge of the factors that contribute to the establishment and progress of peri-implant diseases, while also seeking more effective therapies. Unfortunately, it soon became clear that treating implants as if they were teeth and treating peri-implant diseases using the same therapies used for periodontal diseases did not achieve satisfactory results.

Even though studies, conferences, and scientific research have reported on specific issues that concern peri-implantitis, there is a significant lack of concentrated knowledge and information about the subject presented through the pages of a book; at a global level, very few published efforts have solely focused on this subject. Thus, to this day, many clinicians apply what they believe is correct, often using tools and techniques that are not adequately documented. This is understandable to a certain extent because clinical application precedes statistical evaluation through research. Moreover, it is not uncommon for some of the interventions used to cause more problems than the ones they are aiming to solve.

Diagnosis and treatment of peri-implantitis are very demanding. This book is a natural by-product of the engagement with implantology through the prism and philosophy of periodontology, but also of the need to gather and assess existing knowledge. The continuous stream of information available via the international literature has been combined with the clinical experience acquired from our courses run at the Periodontology Clinics of the Universities of Athens and Bern, but mainly from treating many patients with peri-implantitis; these have been entrusted to us by many colleagues and patients to whom we owe our warm thanks.

This book is mainly aimed at dental practitioners involved in implantology, either through general dentistry or as a clinical specialization, as well as dental students who want to deepen their knowledge of how to prevent, diagnose, and treat peri-implantitis. Relevant information is provided in a detailed form, guided by necessary and available scientific documentation, offering conclusions gained from the critical evaluation of scientific research. The text is accompanied by a plethora of images that complement, support, and help to interpret scientific knowledge, while also offering a step-by-step methodology; they also complement the techniques presented, depending on the specific indications for each technique. Some of the images have been provided by colleagues or the Departments of Periodontology of the Dental Schools in Athens and Bern.

Schematic illustration, where necessary, helps the reader to understand the pathologic indications for and the application of certain techniques, which are presented in detail via carefully chosen images.

We express our respect and thanks to all those who have played an important role in the creation of this book. We offer our never-ending gratitude to our families and all our teachers, without exception, for their love and support.

Our most heartfelt thanks go to our colleague Dr Panagiota Ntokou; her contribution to the writing of several of the chapters was not only valuable but also plentiful, and her collaboration is rightfully recognized and honored on the book's cover.

We offer warm thanks to Dr Spyridon Silvestros, Assistant Professor at the National and Kapodistrian University of Athens (NKUA), for his collaboration in the writing of Chapter 12.

For the exceptional quality of the illustrations and sketches, we thank Mrs Zoe Karoussi-Patsilinakou.

We thank Dr Kyriaki Kyriakidou for her scientific collaboration and for photographing many laboratory essays used in the book.

We also thank Drs Leonidas Podaropoulos and Paolo Trisi, and Associate Professor Demos Kalyvas, for allowing us to reproduce the histologic images in Fig 1-5a, b, 1-6, 2-1, 2-12, 2-22, and 7-2; Dr Ioannis Fandrides and Professor Triantafyllos Papadopoulos for Fig 1-7a, b, 1-8, 1-9a, b, 1-10a, b, 1-11, 1-12a, b, 2-14a, b, 2-15, 2-17a, b, 2-18, 2-19a, b, and 2-20; and Dr Eustathia Tsetsenekou for allowing us to reproduce the histologic images in Fig 2-7, 2-10a, b, and 2-11a–d.

We thank Dr George Vilos, Oral and Maxillofacial Surgeon, for allowing us to reproduce the images in Fig 6-6, 9-14a–d, 9-16a–e, and 15-8a–f; Dr Nikolaos Nikitakis, Professor of Oral Medicine, for Fig 9-15; Dr Demitrios Vlahodimitropoulos, Associate Professor of Medicine, for Fig 9-17; the Department of Periodontology at NKUA for Fig 9-25a, b, 9-26a–f, and 13-11a–f, and Dr Andreas Gkogkos for Fig 13-11g, h.

We want this book to be a source of information and clinical guidance with regard to the approach dental practitioners must learn and apply to better treat patients who already have or are due to receive implants to rehabilitate complete or partial edentulism.

Ioannis K. Karoussis
Professor of Periodontology

Niklaus P. Lang
Professor of Periodontology

Authors

Prof Ioannis K. Karoussis, DDS, MS, Dr med dent

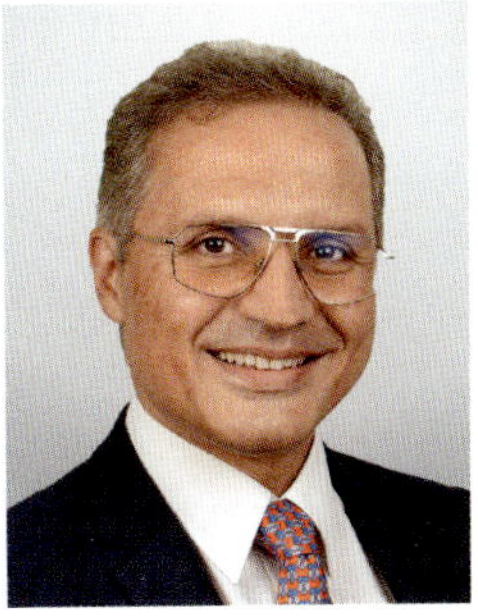

Professor Ioannis K. Karoussis graduated from the Dental School of Athens, Greece, where he also achieved his Master's degree in Oral Biology. He specialized in Periodontology and Implantology at the Universities of Athens, Greece and Bern, Switzerland, where he also completed his doctoral thesis. He has served as coordinator of the Postgraduate clinic of Periodontology at the University of Athens, as Editor of the Journal "Odontostomatological Progress" and President of the Hellenic Society for Odontostomatological Research. His private practice in Athens specializes in periodontics and implant dentistry. He has received awards for his research on peri-implantitis and has authored more than 100 papers in peer-reviewed journals as well as four textbooks in the Greek language.

Prof em Niklaus P. Lang, DMD, MS, PhD, Dr odont hc

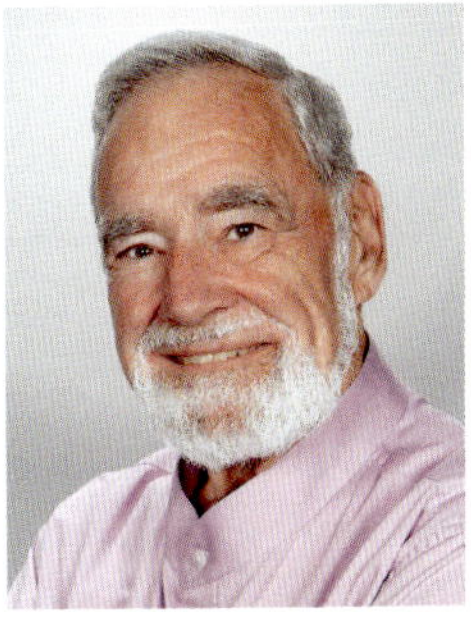

Professor Niklaus P. Lang is the author of more than 730 publications. He holds four honorary doctorates and honorary membership of 20 national and international associations. In 1968, he was awarded the Swiss Dental Association's renowned Prix Louis Metzger, and in 1992, he received the IADR's Basic Science in Periodontal Disease Award. He is a past president of the ITI and the Swiss Society for Periodontology (SSP) and was Editor-in-Chief of the journal "Clinical Oral Implants Research" until 2016. He is active in clinical research related to implant dentistry, periodontology, etiology and pathogenesis of peri-implant infections, risk evaluation, wound healing, and oral microbiology. From 2008 to 2012, he built up the curriculum in implant dentistry at the University of Hong Kong after having headed the Department of Periodontology and Fixed Prosthodontics at the University of Bern, Switzerland from 1978 to 2008.

Contents

1 Anatomy of Periodontal and Peri-Implant Tissues

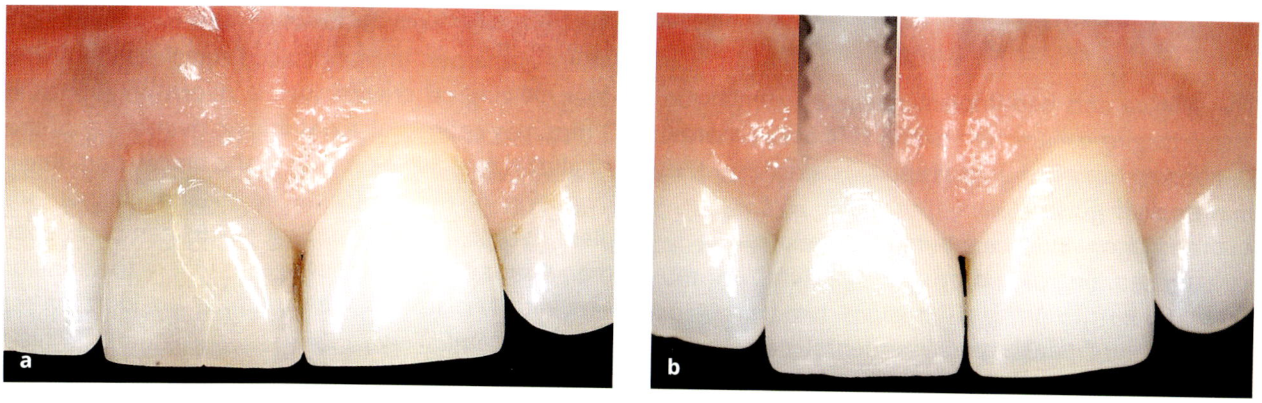

Figs 1-1a, b **(a)** Tooth 11 with a vertical root fracture, warranting its extraction. **(b)** An implant has been placed to replace tooth 11. The peri-implant mucosa shows no esthetic or functional differences compared to the gingiva of the adjacent teeth.

The clinical and histologic imaging of the tissues surrounding teeth and implants present many similarities but also some differences. To better understand the pathology of tissues, the prerequisite is an in-depth knowledge of and familiarization of the clinician with the physiology and anatomy of periodontal and peri-implant tissues.

Periodontal tissues consist of the gingiva, the periodontal membrane, the root cementum, and the alveolar bone. If a tooth is lost, the term "gingiva" is no longer used as an anatomic term and is replaced by the term "peri-implant mucosa". Thus, peri-implant tissues consist of the peri-implant mucosa and the alveolar bone.

The gingiva surround the neck of the tooth and constitute the coronal portion of the oral mucosa. The peri-implant mucosa is the continuation of the oral mucosa toward the crest of the alveolar ridge and surrounds the neck of the implants. The gingiva and peri-implant mucosa have many functional, anatomic, and immunologic similarities. In a healthy mouth, both the gingiva and the peri-implant mucosa are usually a light pink color and are covered with a keratinized epithelium externally (Figs 1-1a, b).[1,2]

The gingiva serve as a barrier against microbes, thus protecting the underlying tissue, and also play a significant role in sensation, phonetics, and esthetics. Both structures constitute the limit between the external environment and the internal organism. Whether a submerged, transmucosal, or non-submerged healing protocol is applied, soft tissue adhesion and protection of osseointegration function in the same way.

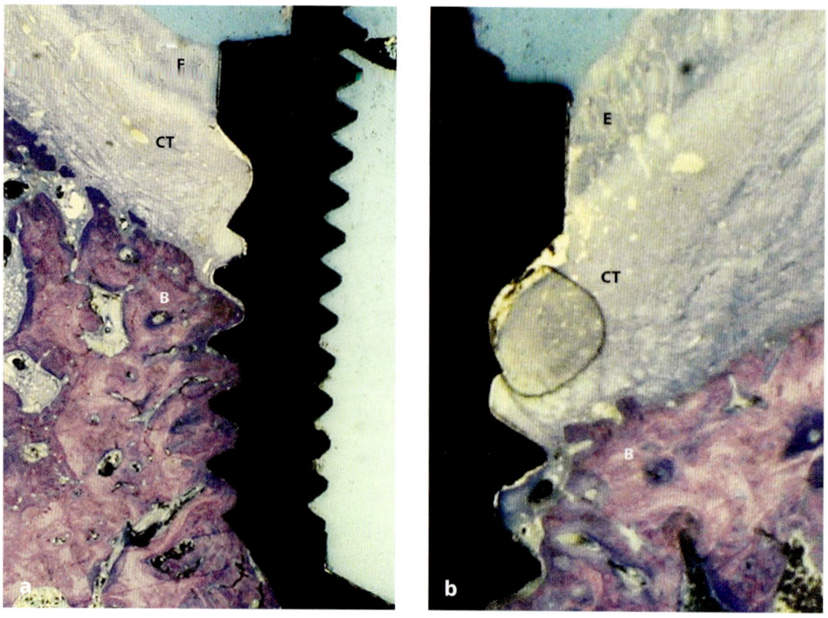

Figs 1-5a, b Histologic images derived from an animal (dog), where the peri-implant tissues are shown. B, bone; CT, connective tissue; E, epithelium. The circular formation shown in **(b)** is an artifact. Apart from the bone, peri-implant soft tissues seem to adhere to the implant, creating a natural barrier against bacterial invasion. The epithelium and implant surface or the surface of the implant restoration separate the peri-implant crevice (courtesy of Drs L. Podaropoulos, P. Trisi, and D. Kalyvas).

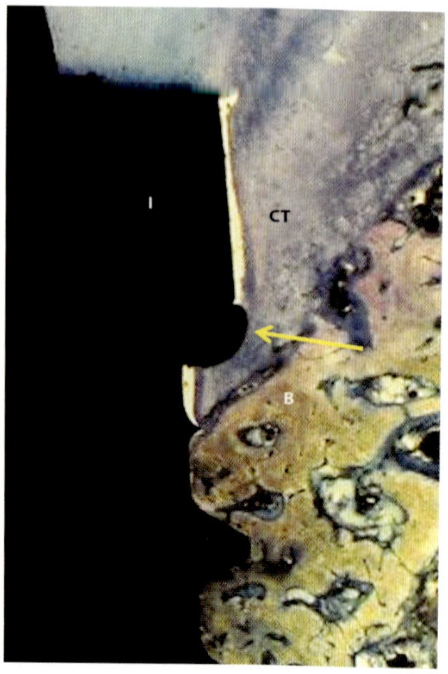

Fig 1-6 Histologic sample derived from an animal (dog), where a titanium implant and its interaction with the adjacent peri-implant tissues can be observed, long after its placement. B, bone; CT, connective tissue; I, implant. The yellow arrow indicates the direct contact of the connective tissue with the implant surface (courtesy of Drs L. Podaropoulos, P. Trisi, and D. Kalyvas).

tron microscopy. However, the supracrestal fibers beneath the junctional epithelium may not have the same orientation in natural teeth.

1.3 Connective tissues

The connective tissues of the gingiva and peri-implant mucosa are the largest part of the soft tissues (attached, free, and interdental) and occupy the space between the epithelium and the alveolar ridge (Fig 1-6). They consist of collagen (60%), oxytalan, reticular and elastic fibers, as well as fibroblasts (5%), the extracellular matrix, blood vessels (35%), and nerves. Connective tissue adjoins the epithelium via the intervention of the basal membrane.

Types I and III collagen fibers, known as gingival fibers, are arranged in a dense mesh and are distinguished according to their primary (dentogingival, alveolo-gingival, dentoperiosteal, circular, transeptal) and secondary orientation (interdental papillary, transgingival, semicircular).

Experimental studies have shown that connective tissue fibers are arranged laminarly to the implant surface. It has been suggested that the orientation of peri-implant connective tissue collagen fibers depends on the existence of keratinized mucosa and the surface roughness of the implant. When the zone of keratinized attached peri-implant mucosa is inadequate, connective tissue fibers are parallel to the implant surface, whereas fibers have a more vertically oriented direction to the implant when there is an abundance of attached keratinized mucosa. Moreover, when adjacent to a rough surface, collagen fibers may present a functional orientation. Scanning electron microscopy of the mesophase between connective tissue and non-submerged implants suggests that some connective tissue fibers are vertically oriented toward the implant surface. Moreover, they come into contact with a glycosaminoglycan layer that covers the implant surface.[11] In addition, rough implant surfaces promote the adhesion of epithelial cells and fibroblasts. However, they also favor the accumulation of microorganisms (Figs 1-7a, b to 1-12a, b).[12,13]

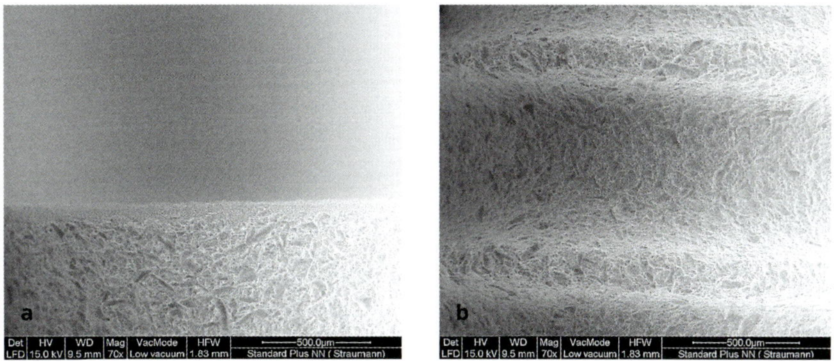

Figs 1-7a, b Micrographs (×70). **(a)** A Straumann implant; specifically, its smooth transmucosal part and its rough part, which must be covered with bone, are shown. **(b)** Part of the rough surface showing two threads and the space between them. The surface was sandblasted with 250- to 500-µm Al_2O_3 grains and acid-etched with HCl + H_2SO_4 at 130°C for 5 minutes (courtesy of Drs T. Papadopoulos and I. Fandridis).

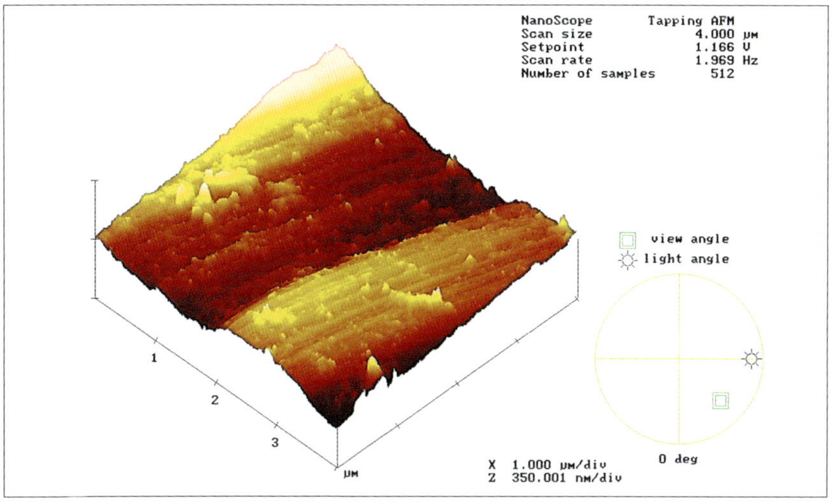

Fig 1-8 Atomic force microscopy reveals the very low roughness of the smooth Straumann surface, which promotes the adhesion of epithelial cells through hemidesmosomes (courtesy of Drs T. Papadopoulos and I. Fandridis).

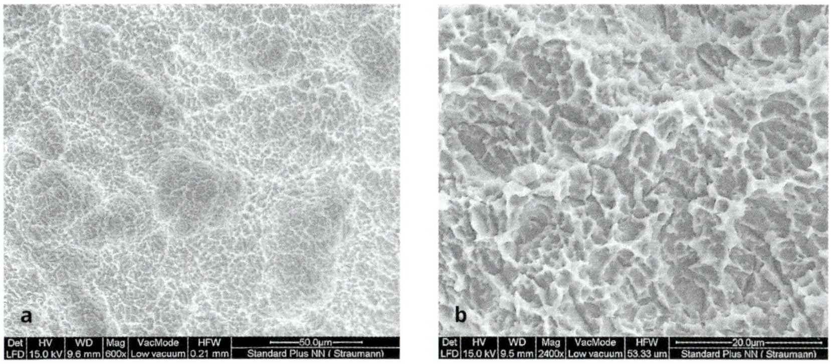

Figs 1-9a, b Scanning electron micrographs. **(a)** The rough surface of the Straumann implant is presented at ×600 magnification. **(b)** The same surface is presented at ×2,400 magnification. The rough surface promotes adhesion and the proliferation of osteoblasts (courtesy of Drs T. Papadopoulos and I. Fandridis).

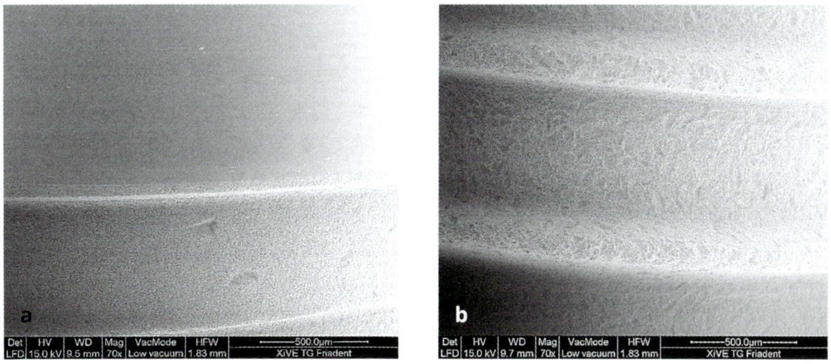

Figs 1-10a, b Scanning electron micrographs (×70). The Xive implant (Dentsply Sirona, Charlotte, NC, USA) is shown. **(a)** The smooth part of the implant, and its rough part that must be placed in the bone, can be seen. **(b)** Part of the surface containing two threads and the space in between them can be observed. The rough surface was airborne-particle abraded with Al_2O_3 grains and chemically acid-etched (courtesy of Drs T. Papadopoulos and I. Fandridis).

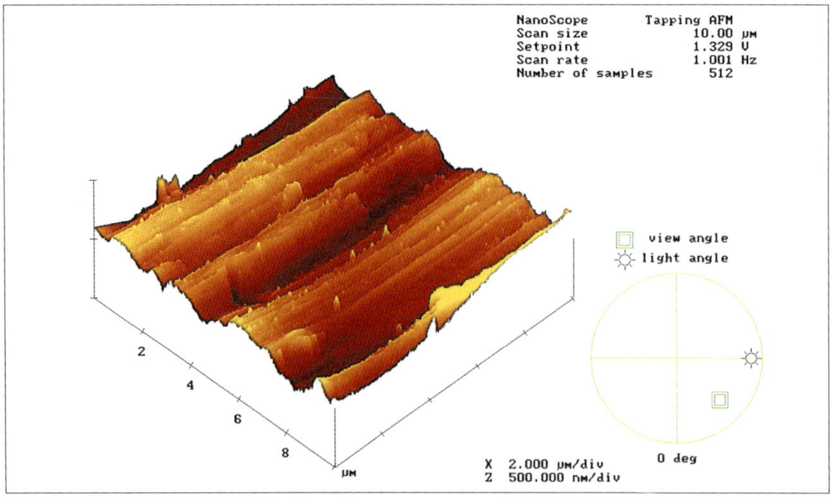

Fig 1-11 Atomic force microscopy revealed the low roughness of the smooth surface of the Xive implant, which promotes the adhesion of epithelial cells through hemidesmosomes (courtesy of Drs T. Papadopoulos and I. Fandridis).

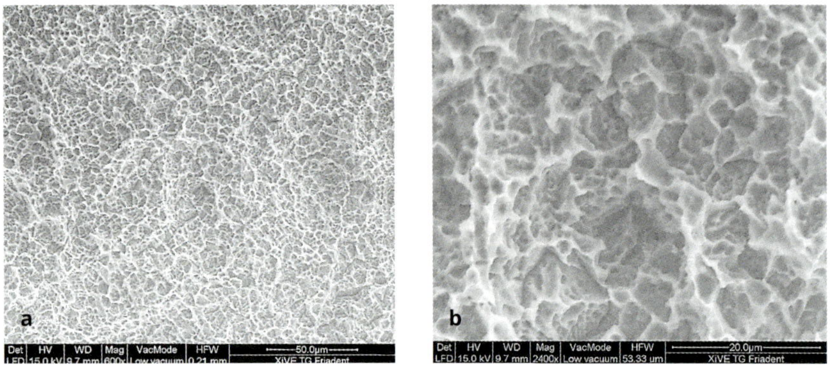

Figs 1-12a, b Scanning electron micrographs. **(a)** The rough surface of the Xive implant is presented at ×600 magnification. **(b)** The same surface is presented at ×2,400 magnification. The rough surface promoted the proliferation and maturation of osteoblasts (courtesy of Drs T. Papadopoulos and I. Fandridis).

Connective tissue around implants has two zones: an internal and an external zone. The internal zone has a thickness of 50 to 100µm thickness and 67% of its mass consists of collagen fibers and 32% consists of fibroblasts, while blood vessels are essentially absent (0.3%), thus resembling scar tissue.

In the external zone, which is 60 µm thick, more collagen fibers and fewer fibroblasts may be observed (85% and 11%, respectively, compared to 3% for vascular structures).

Apart from fibroblasts, the connective tissues of the gingiva and peri-implant mucosa contain inflammatory cells (multinuclear cells, lymphocytes, macrophages, mast cells, and basophilic and eosinophilic granulocytes).

Because they constitute about 65% of connective tissue cells and are arranged between fibers, that is, they are parallel to collagen fibers, fibroblasts are the most abundant group of cells (Figs 1-13 to 1-15).[14,15]

Nevertheless, the connective tissue of the peri-implant mucosa has fewer cellular elements and more collagen compared to the connective tissue around teeth. Immunohistochemical methods showed fundamental differences between healthy peri-implant and periodontal tissues. Types V and VI collagen are distributed differently, while types I, III, IV, and VII, as well as fibronectin, have similar distributions.[16]

1.4 Vascularization

Gingival connective tissue shows rich vascularization, which is mediated by the blood vessels of the periodontal membrane, the blood vessels of the oral mucosa, and vessels that extend through the periosteum. These vessels form an afferent arterial and efferent venous network, which are interlaced in two rich vascular meshes, one below the oral and junctional epithelium and one below the attached epithelium, known as the hypoepithelial vascular mesh. Specialized cells expressing adhesive molecules (such as endothelial-leukocyte adhesion molecule 1 [ELAM-1] and ICAM-1) facilitate the transport of leukocytes.[17]

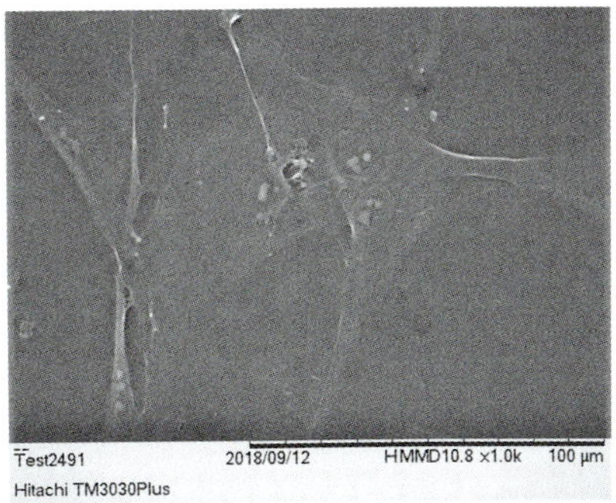

Fig 1-13 Micrograph (×1,000) of human gingival fibroblasts cultured for 24 hours on β-tricalcium phosphate surfaces.

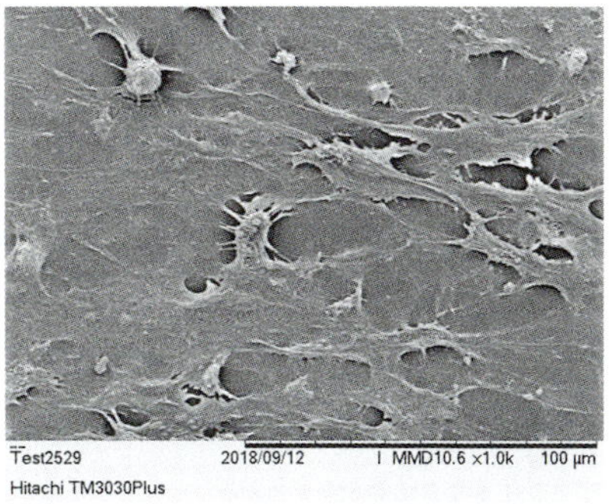

Fig 1-14 Micrograph (×1,000) of human gingival fibroblasts cultured for 72 hours on β-tricalcium phosphate surfaces, after irradiation with an 810-nm diode laser.

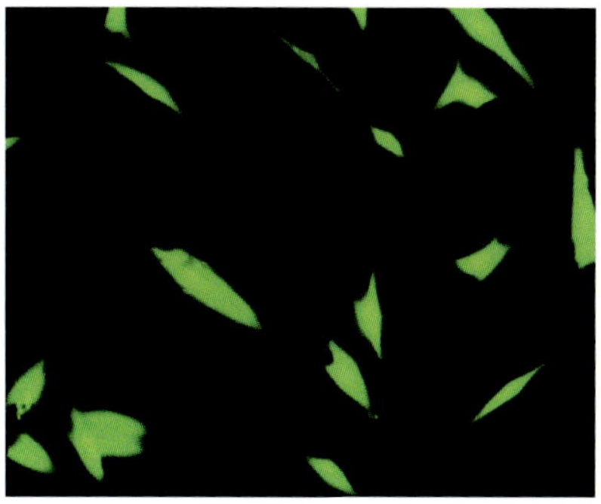

Fig 1-15 Fluorescence microscopy image (×20) of human gingival fibroblasts cultured on β-tricalcium phosphate surfaces for 24 hours. Their characteristic elongated morphology can be seen.

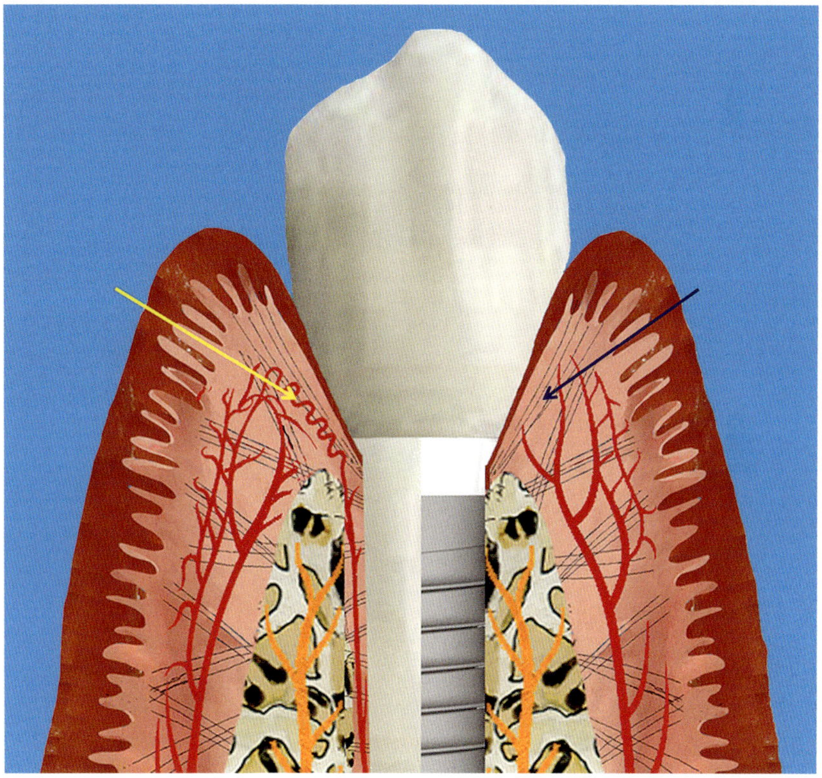

Fig 1-16 Schematic illustration of periodontal and peri-implant tissues demonstrating vascularization.

In peri-implant tissues, there is no periodontal membrane; hence, vascularization originating from it is absent. Thus, the peri-implant mucosa is solely supplied by vessels that emerge from the periosteum. As a result, the tissue below the attached epithelium of implants has reduced vascularization. The lack of a collateral circulation reduces the response of the peri-implant mucosa to inflammation and predisposes to faster peri-implant bone destruction (Fig 1-16).[18]

At implants, both subepithelial vascular mesh and periodontal membrane are missing as the titanium surface is in direct structural and functional contact with the surrounding bone. Moreover, Sharpey fibers that usually insert into the root cementum are absent, and supracrestal connective tissue fibers course parallel to the implant surface.

Lymphatic drainage of the gingiva and peri-implant mucosa is similar, although lymphatic capillaries are missing in the latter. Nerve supply of the

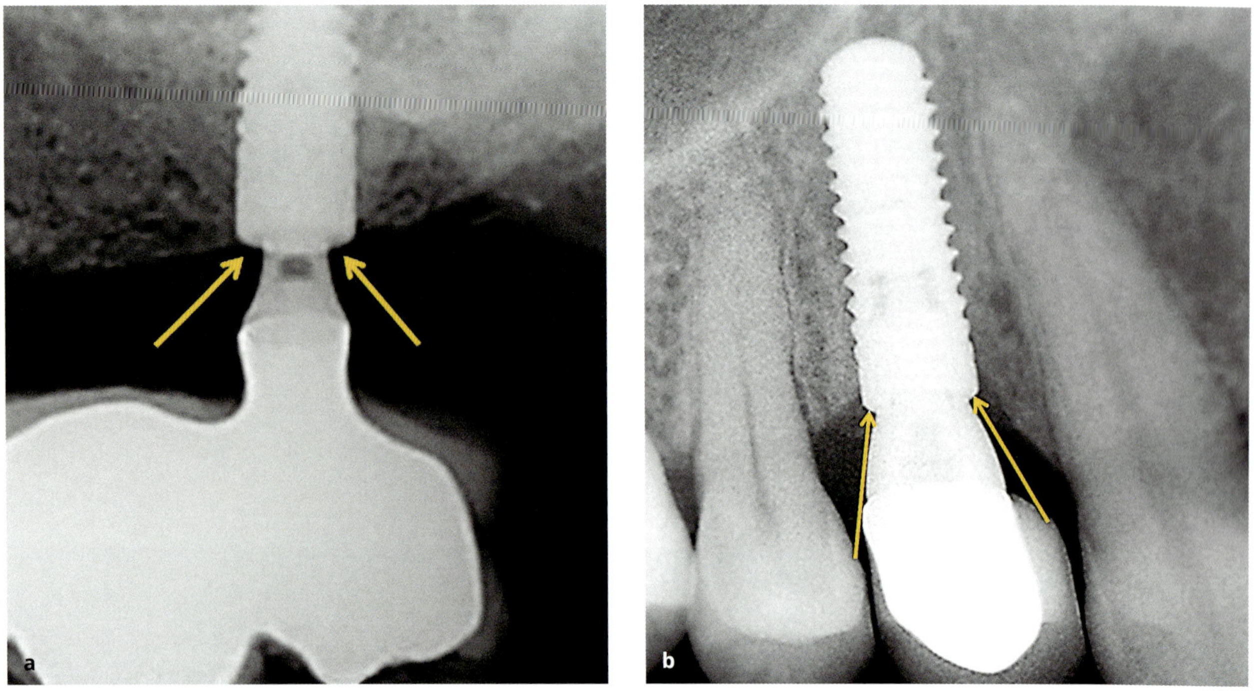

Figs 1-17a, b In cases where platform switching has been selected, the implant abutment leaves a significant width of the implant neck uncovered for the soft tissues to adhere to (yellow arrows). Thus, there is no need to proceed to bone resorption to give enough height for soft tissue adhesion.

gingiva and peri-implant mucosa is achieved with the sensory terminal branches of the second and third branches of the trigeminal nerve. Free nerve endings, responsible for pain and pressure, Meissner corpuscles, responsible for touch, Krause bulboid corpuscles (thermal receptors), as well as sympathetic and parasympathetic fibers, are responsible for vascular nerve supply.[19]

The lack of a periodontal membrane implies a significant absence of proprioperception and pressure sensing, which should be considered when designing implant restorations; the excessive application of pressure, during functional and parafunctional movements, may lead to technical complications. The sensation of pressure from the nerve endings of the osseous tissue is ten times smaller than that of the periodontal membrane.[20,21]

1.5 Biologic width around teeth and implants

Regarding biologic width, the following term has been suggested: "supracrestal tissue attachment" or "supracrestal attached tissues". This is defined as the distance between the most coronal termination of the junctional epithelium to the crest of the alveolar ridge. Its mean length is approximately 3 to 4 mm; it contains the width of the junctional epithelium and of the supracrestal connective tissue fibers that insert into the root cementum as Sharpey fibers. The soft tissue zone that attaches to the implant consists of approximately 2 mm junctional epithelium and 1 to 2 mm connective tissue, that is, a 3- to 4-mm width of soft tissue corresponds to the biologic width around teeth. Biologic width around submerged and non-submerged implants is similar regardless of functional loading.[22]

Due to non-submerged healing or after implant exposure of submerged healing, soft tissue attachment is established circumferentially to the implant neck. The stability of biologic width of soft tissues around implants has also been shown in animal studies. After the extraction of all premolars in the mandible, implants and healing abutments were placed. The mucosa on one side was thinned, while that of the opposing side remained untouched and was therefore left thicker. After 6 months and completion of the healing process, the attachment zone of the soft tissues around both sides was 3.3 to 3.8 mm wide, consisting of 2.0 to 2.1 mm junctional epithelium and 1.3 to 1.8 mm connective tissue. At the site where the mucosa had initially been thinned, bone resorption of the alveolar ridge was noted to ensure the necessary 3to 4 mm soft tissue attachment.[23]

Finally, there was greater bone loss at the buccal site of the alveolar ridge compared to the lingual and palatal sites. Bone resorption to establish biologic width leads to deepening of the peri-implant crevice and is probably related to peri-implant inflammation. To contain bone resorption after connection of the implant abutment, platform switching has been recommended, that is, placement of a healing abutment with a smaller diameter than that of the cervical part of the implant (Figs 1-17a, b).[24] This method, however, poses one significant problem during the maintenance phase: it makes it impossible to evaluate differences between measurements of the depth of the peri-implant sulcus.

References

1. Nanci A, Bosshardt DD. Structure of periodontal tissues in health and disease. Periodontol 2000 2006;40:11–28.
2. Abrahamsson I, Berglundh T, Moon IS, Lindhe J. Peri-implant tissues at submerged and non-submerged titanium implants. J Clin Periodontol 1999;9:600–607.
3. Parpaiola A, Cecchinato D, Toia M, Bressan E, Speroni S, Lindhe J. Dimensions of the healthy gingiva and peri-implant mucosa. Clin Oral Implants Res 2015;26:657–662.
4. Weber HP, Buser D, Donath K, et al. Comparisons of healed tissues adjacent to submerged and non-submerged unloaded titanium dental implants. A histometric study in beagle dogs. Clin Oral Implants Res 1996;7: 11–19.
5. Berglundh T, Lindhe J, Ericsson I, Marinello CP, Liljenberg B, Thomsen P. The soft tissue barrier at implants and teeth. Clin Oral Implants Res 1991;2:81–90.
6. Tonetti MS, Gerber L, Lang NP. Vascular adhesion molecules and initial development of inflammation in clinically healthy human keratinized mucosa around teeth and osseointegrated implants. J Periodontal Res 1994;29: 386–392.
7. Schmid B, Spicher I, Schmid J, Lang NP. Plasminogen activator in human gingival tissue adjacent to dental implants. Clin Oral Implants Res 1992;3:85–89.
8. Glavind L, Zander HA. Dynamics of dental epithelium during tooth eruption. J Dent Res 1970;49:549–555.
9. Lindhe J, Berglundh T. The interface between the mucosa and the implant. Periodontol 2000 1998;17:47–54.
10. Abrahamsson I, Berglundh T, Wennström J, Lindhe J. The peri-implant hard and soft tissues at different implant systems. A comparative study in the dog. Clin Oral Implants Res 1996;7:212–219.
11. Buser D, Weber HP, Donath K, Fiorellini JP, Paquette DW, Williams RC. Soft tissue reactions to non-submerged unloaded titanium implants in beagle dogs. J Periodontol 1992;63:225–235.
12. Schroeder A, van der Zypen E, Stich H, Sutter F. The reactions of bone, connective tissue, and epithelium to endosteal implants with titanium-sprayed surfaces. J Maxillofac Surg 1981;9:15–25.
13. Abrahamsson I, Berglundh T, Glantz PO, Lindhe J. The mucosal attachment at different abutments. An experimental study in dogs. J Clin Periodontol 1998;25:721–727.
14. Cochran DL, Hermann JS, Schenk RK, Higginbottom FL, Buser D. Biologic width around titanium implants. A histometric analysis of the implanto-gingival junction around unloaded and loaded nonsubmerged implants in the canine mandible. J Periodontol 1997;68:186–198.
15. Moon IS, Berglundh T, Abrahamsson I, Linder E, Lindhe J. The barrier between the keratinized mucosa and the dental implant. An experimental study in the dog. J Clin Periodontol 1999;26:658–663.
16. Romanos GE, Schröter-Kermani C, Weingart D, Strub JR. Health human periodontal versus peri-implant gingival tissues: an immunohistochemical differentiation of the extracellular matrix. Int J Oral Maxillofac Implants 1995;10:750–758.
17. Egelberg J. The blood vessels of the dento-gingival junction. J Periodontal Res 1966;1:163–179.
18. Berglundh T, Lindhe J, Jonsson K, Ericsson I. The topography of the vascular systems in the periodontal and peri-implant tissues in the dog. J Clin Periodontol 1994;21:89–93.
19. Marchetti C, Poggi P, Reguzzoni M, Cornaglia AI, Baena YR. Lymphatic vessel system in gingival peri-implant tissues in humans. J Periodontal Res 1999;34:229–231.
20. Hämmerle CH, Wagner T, Brägger U, et al. Threshold of tactile sensitivity perceived with dental endosseous implants and natural teeth. Clin Oral Implants Res 1995;6:83–90.
21. Lindhe J, Berglundh T, Ericsson I, Liljenberg B, Marinello C. Experimental breakdown of peri-implant and periodontal tissues. A study in the beagle dog. Clin Oral Implants Res 1992;3:9–16.
22. Tarnow D, Hochman M, Chu S, Fletcher P. A new definition of attached gingiva around teeth and implants in healthy and diseased sites. Int J Periodontics Restorative Dent 2021;41:43–49.
23. Berglundh T, Lindhe J. Dimension of the peri-implant mucosa. Biological width revisited. J Clin Periodontol 1996;23:971–973.
24. Gupta S, Sabharwal R, Nazeer J, Taneja L, Choudhury BK, Sahu S. Platform switching technique and crestal bone loss around the dental implants: a systematic review. Ann Afr Med 2019;18:1–6.

2 Peri-Implant Tissue Healing after Implant Placement

2.1 Osseointegration

The term "osseointegration" is used to describe the direct structural and functional connection between living bone and the surface of a load-bearing artificial implant without intervening soft tissues, as can be observed under the microscope.[1] The term implies that elements foreign to the organism will be accepted by it and this integration will not be affected after their extended function over time (Fig 2-1).

The initial prerequisite for a foreign body to be integrated within the human organism is to not activate the immune response, causing a foreign body reaction after its placement. Biocompatible materials that satisfy this prerequisite are titanium and ceramic materials. Thus far, titanium alloys have proven to be the optimal choice due to their high resistance to corrosion and superior mechanical properties.[2] The TiO_2 and TiO_3 oxides form crystalline structures that rest on the implant surface and make it biologically inert. They are formed within 0.001 seconds after exposure of titanium to air, biologic fluids, water, or electrolytes.

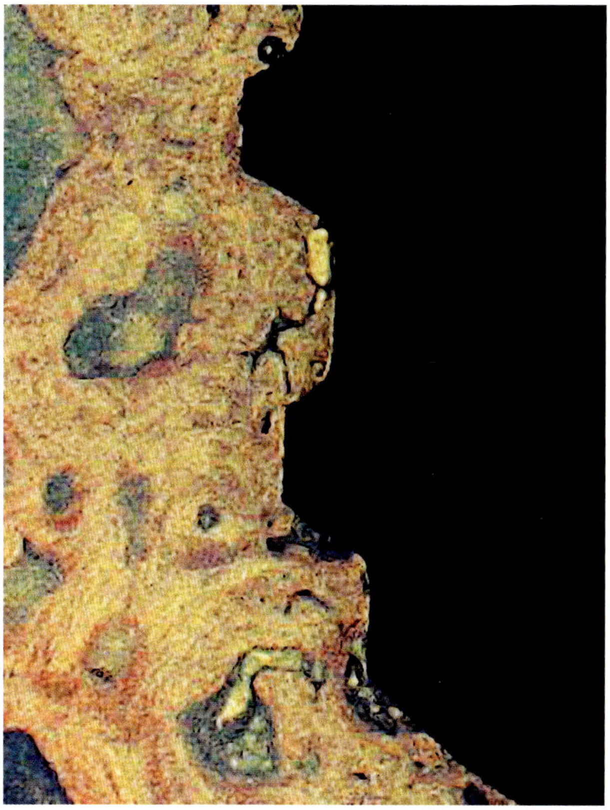

Fig 2-1 Detail of a histologic analysis derived from the maxilla of a dog, where mature osseous tissue in direct structural and functional contact with an implant may be observed. The implant had accepted functional loading for a significant amount of time before the animal was sacrificed (courtesy of Mr L. Podaropoulos, and Drs P. Trisi and D. Kalyvas).

2.2 From bed preparation to osseointegration

During implant placement in an edentulous area, trauma is caused to the underlying bone that is drilled to prepare the bed that will host the implant. In the bone, specifically at the borders of the canal that is prepared, a limited necrotic zone is formed, while bone fragments remain at the preparation site.

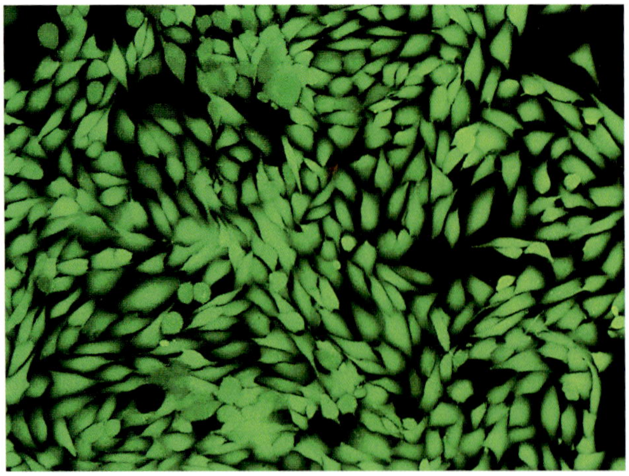

Fig 2-2 Image from fluorescence microscopy (×20 magnification) of immature osteoblasts, MG63, cultured for 48 hours after being irradiated with low-level laser energy to promote cell proliferation, using an Nd:YAG laser (1,064 nm).

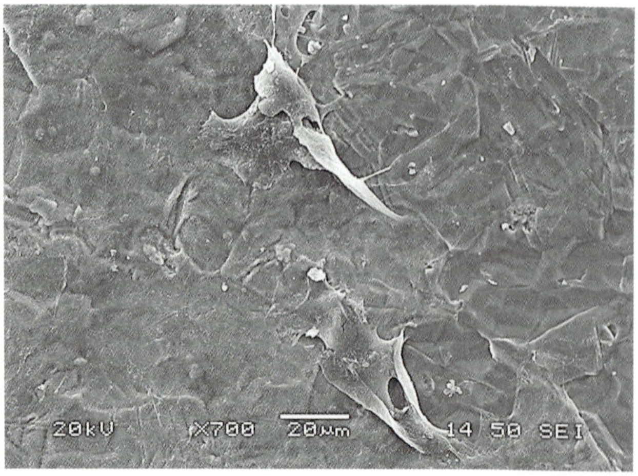

Fig 2-3 Micrograph (×700 magnification) of immature osteoblasts cultured on smooth titanium surfaces for 7 days.

This trauma triggers the healing mechanism. A series of events follow that ultimately lead to the formation of new osseous tissue.

To achieve primary stability, the preparation is made so that its perimeter is slightly smaller than that of the implant. The implant is then inserted so that its threads are 0.5 to 1.0 mm below the borderline of the bed preparation. The pressure applied to screw the implant in crushes the blood vessels, leading to hemorrhage and the formation of a blood clot between the bone and the implant surface.[3] Osteoblasts, cells capable of forming new osseous tissue, are crucial for the healing process. Osteoclasts, multinuclear cells derived from blood monocytes that induce bone resorption, and osteocytes, which participate in osteolytic processes, are also essential. In addition, undifferentiated mesenchymal cells play a key role because they are multipotent and, depending on the stimulus, may differentiate into pre-osteoblasts and later osteoblasts (Figs 2-2 and 2-3).

Occasionally, however, these cells may differentiate into fibroblasts, making osseointegration impossible. For optimal cell function and to trigger the onset of the healing process, sufficient blood supply to the area and formation of new microcirculation are necessary. The speed at which new vessels are created differs significantly between cortical and trabecular bone. For the latter, this process proceeds at a rate of 0.5 mm per day; this is slower for cortical bone, proceeding at 0.05 mm per day. The blood clot created matures over the first few days after surgery and is gradually replaced with granulation tissue replete with neutrophils and monocytes, while white blood cells simultaneously remove necrotic elements at the site. Newly formed vessels begin to organize into granulation tissue.[4]

Three stages of osseointegration have been identified:[5]

- woven bone formation;
- parallel fiber and lamellar bone deposition;
- bone remodeling.

A brief description of the series of events from the day of implant insertion to the development of osseointegration follows.[5]

On the first day after implant placement, its stability may be solely attributed to the mechanical retention achieved by the threadlike (spiral) shape of the implant or pressed fit or friction fit and depends on the size and density of the threads, the precision in bed preparation, and bone type (cortical or trabecular). At this stage, the implant–bone contact, which reaches 35% when observed histomorphometrically, does not constitute osseointegration. The implant surface is mainly in contact with parts of the cortical and trabecular bone that were detached during preparation, with a blood clot or, at the peak of the threads, with condensed trabecular bone due to the screwing process. Multinuclear giant cells and macrophages may also be apparent.

Three days after implant placement, there is significant migration of mesenchymal cells and macro-

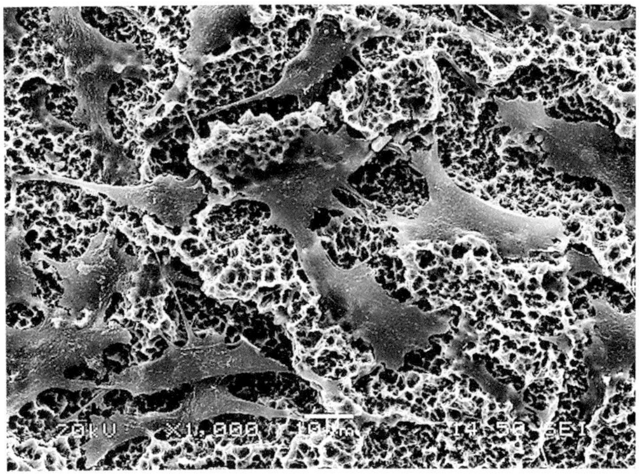

Fig 2-4 Micrograph (×1,000 magnification) showing a strong contact between the body and filopodia of the osteoblasts and the titanium surface 7 days after culturing. An irregular shape of the cells may observed.

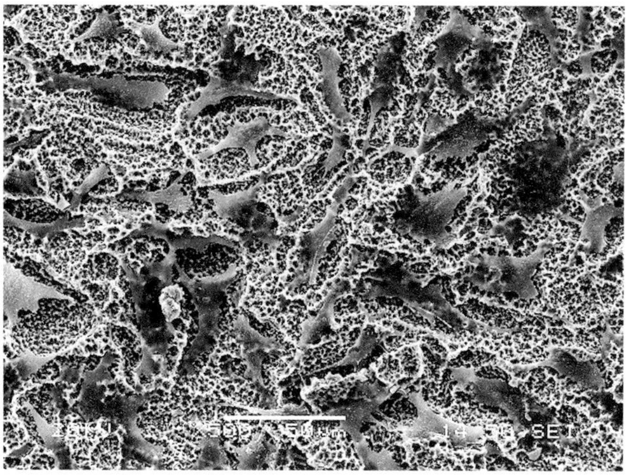

Fig 2-5 Micrograph (×500 magnification) of immature osteoblasts cultured on a rough titanium surface (sandblasted, acid-etched, Straumann) for 7 days. The irregular shape of the cells is evident, as well as the contact between the body and filopodia of the cells with the titanium surface.

phages from the bone marrow to the blood clot between the bone and the implant. The bone–implant contact proportion is stable but this is still due to mechanical retention. There is also development of granulation tissue and the first newly formed capillary vessels. Moreover, collagen fibers may be observed.

Seven days later, production of woven bone can be observed. Woven bone has a similar orientation to that of collagen fibers, that is, perpendicular to the implant surface, and may be used as a matrix to produce osteoid clones from osteoblasts. As time passes, the formed bone occupies the space around the implant threads, increasing the bone–implant contact to around 50% of the implant surface. This newly formed woven bone is circumferentially arranged into a dense net of blood vessels, which had already been established at the peri-implant area, and is characterized by many irregularly shaped osteoblasts (Fig 2-4).

Gradual shaping of a network takes place, which consists of formations that look like sticks and plates. This network expands into the surrounding space at a relatively rapid pace. Woven bone is deposited at a remarkable rate of 30 to 50 µm per day. In contrast to mature osseous tissue, the concentration of inorganic elements is initially low. The fibers of the matrix are randomly ordered and resistance to mechanical strain is low. In areas where there is a lack of implant–bone contact, a layer of multinuclear giant cells may be found, which is retained even though the number of giant cells gradually decreases.

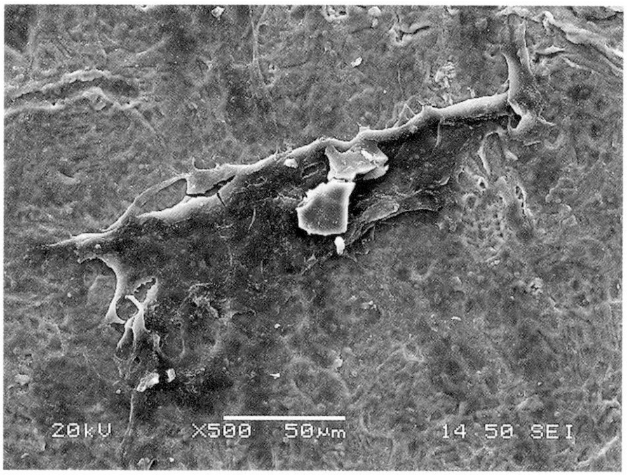

Fig 2-6 Micrograph (×500 magnification) of immature osteoblasts cultured on a smooth titanium surface for 7 days. The irregular shape of the cells may be noted, as well as the relatively weak contact of the cell body and filopodia with the titanium surface, compared to the contact on a rough surface.

From this point onward, all events are significantly affected by the type of implant surface and whether or not this surface has been processed so that its biologic behavior promotes the acceleration of osseointegration (Figs 2-5 and 2-6).

In general, during the first 14 days, woven bone begins to be replaced by lamellar or parallel fiber bone through the osteoclastic process. Mature lamellar bone is characterized by high resistance to mechanical strain (Fig 2-7).

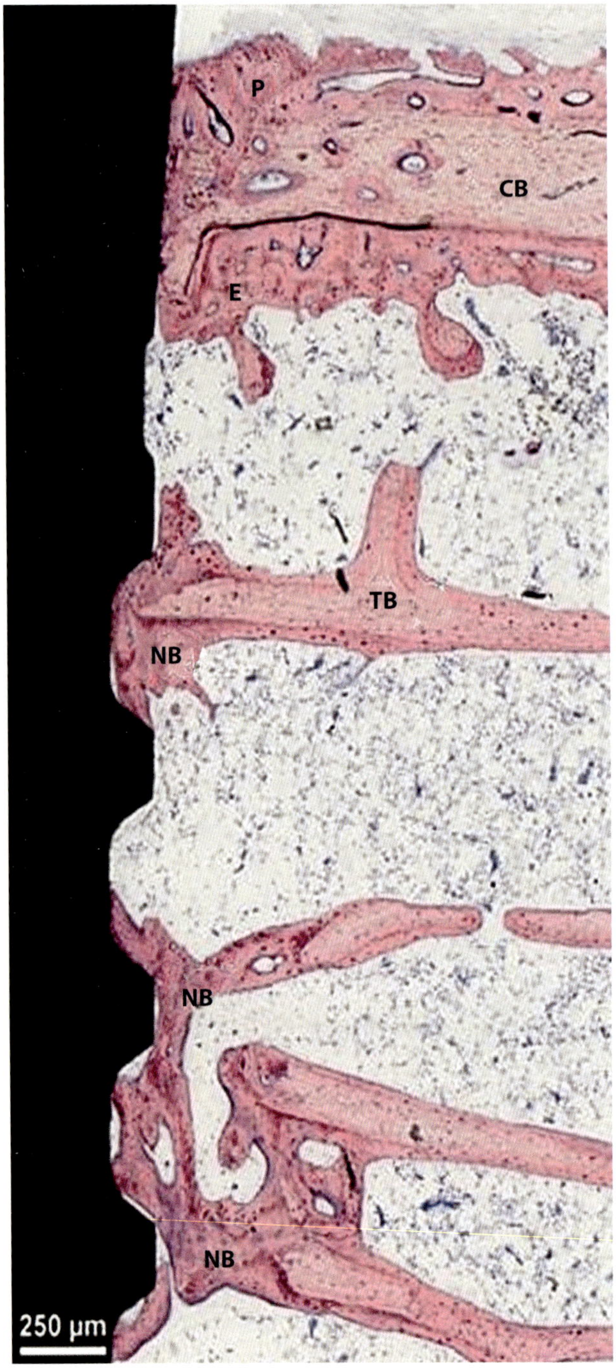

Fig 2-7 The preexisting bone can be divided into cortical (CB) and trabecular (TB). The newly formed bone (NB), which is the result of processes that take place after implantation, may be divided into endosseous (E) and periosteal (P). Levai Laczko staining (Fig 23, page 82 of the thesis by Tsetsenekou[6] reproduced with permission from the author).

As mentioned, the rate of deposition of this type of osseous tissue depends on the type of implant surface and how it is treated. For implants with low roughness, a production rate of 1.0 to 1.5 μm per day has been reported and complete osseointegration is achieved in 22 to 24 weeks. Even though replacement of woven bone in smooth implants may last up to 6 months in the maxilla, improvement of the implant surface characteristics may reduce the time required for complete osseointegration. Research has shown that the time needed is 6 weeks for implants with sandblasted, large-grit, and acid-etched (SLA) surfaces; this may be reduced to 3 weeks for implants with nano-modified implant surfaces (SLActive, sandblasted, large-grit, and acid-etched plus chemically activated) (Figs 2-8 to 2-10a). Once the process is completed (the length of time differs depending on the characteristics of the surface of the implant), the rate of implant–bone contact reaches 70%, corresponding to true osseointegration. The effect of the roughness of the implant surface on osseointegration will be analyzed further in this chapter.

2.3 Bone remodeling

The third and final stage of osseointegration is the lifelong process of bone remodeling (bone resorption followed by bone deposition), which corresponds to changes in functional loading applied to the implant. Remodeling begins at around the third month after implant placement. It is characterized by an initial period of increasing osteoclast activity that lasts for several weeks and gradually decreases, while remaining in function throughout the life of the patient. Bone remodeling is extremely important not only to maintain osseointegration, but also to preserve the functional integrity of the whole skeleton. Through the replacement of woven bone with mature, lamellar bone, the quality of the osseous tissue is improved (Fig 2-10b).

The peri-implant bone endures fatigue due to constant loading. Despite bone remodeling, the accumulation of damage caused by constant loading, may in rare instances lead to aseptic necrosis. During initial bone deposition, primary osteons are formed; during bone remodeling, secondary osteons are created. Initially, there is bone resorption through osteoclasts that results in a cylindrical canal, with an

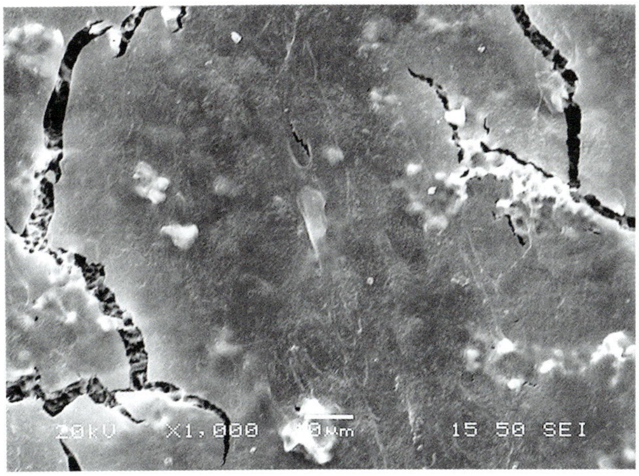

Fig 2-8 Micrograph (×1,000 magnification) of osteoblasts cultured on rough titanium surfaces (sandblasted, acid-etched, Straumann) for 3 weeks. A dense layer of osteoids on the rough surface may be observed.

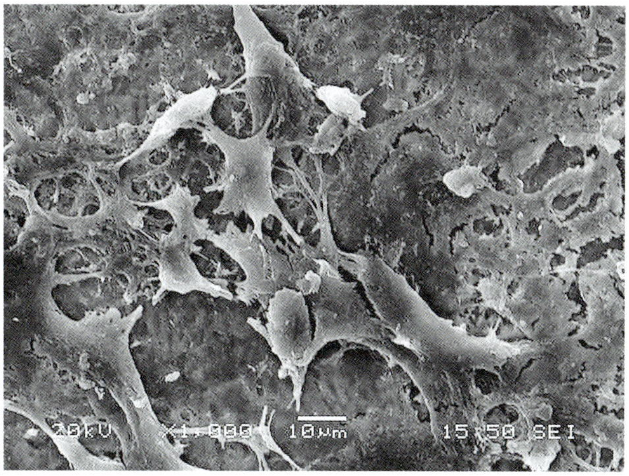

Fig 2-9 Micrograph (×1,000 magnification) of osteoblasts cultured on smooth titanium surfaces for 3 weeks. Cell proliferation is significant on a smooth surface yet it does not result in the formation of a dense layer of osteoids, as is the case on rough surfaces.

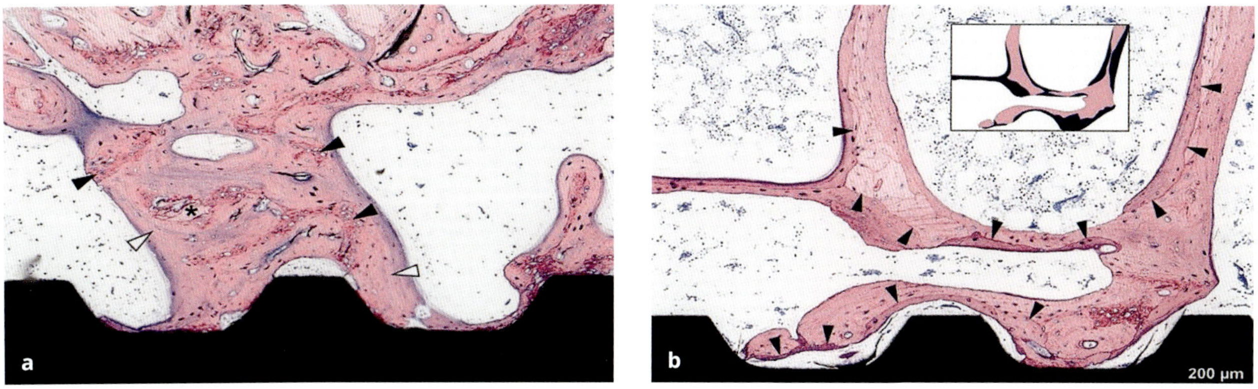

Figs 2-10a, b Quality and synthesis of peri-implant osseous tissue. **(a)** After 6 weeks, the osseous tissue at the area of the mesophase consists of a mesh of woven (black arrows) and lamellar (white arrows) bone. **(b)** After 12 weeks, a significant proportion of this complex bone was replaced with lamellar bone (dark blue areas) amid the procedure of bone remodeling. Inversion lines marked with black arrows indicate the remodeling process (Lavai Laczko staining) **(b)** (Fig 27, page 86 of the thesis by Tsetsenekou[6]; reproduced with permission from the author).

osteon diameter of 150 to 200 µm. The canal is gradually filled with newly formed bone that is deposited by osteoblasts. The bone is deposited in the form of concentric rings. Formation of a new osteon takes up to 2 to 4 months. This process is similar to that of trabecular bone, where osteoclasts gather and leave a corrosive cavity behind that is filled with lamellar bone at approximately 2 weeks. Interestingly, the rate of physiologic remodeling around a functional implant is two to ten times greater than that noted in other areas of the body (Figs 2-11 and 2-12).[7]

2.4 The influence of implant surface configuration on osseointegration

A series of in vitro studies conducted in the 1980s that examined a plethora of factors affecting the success of implant therapy concluded that surface topography had a statistically significant effect on the process of osseointegration. The reason for this was

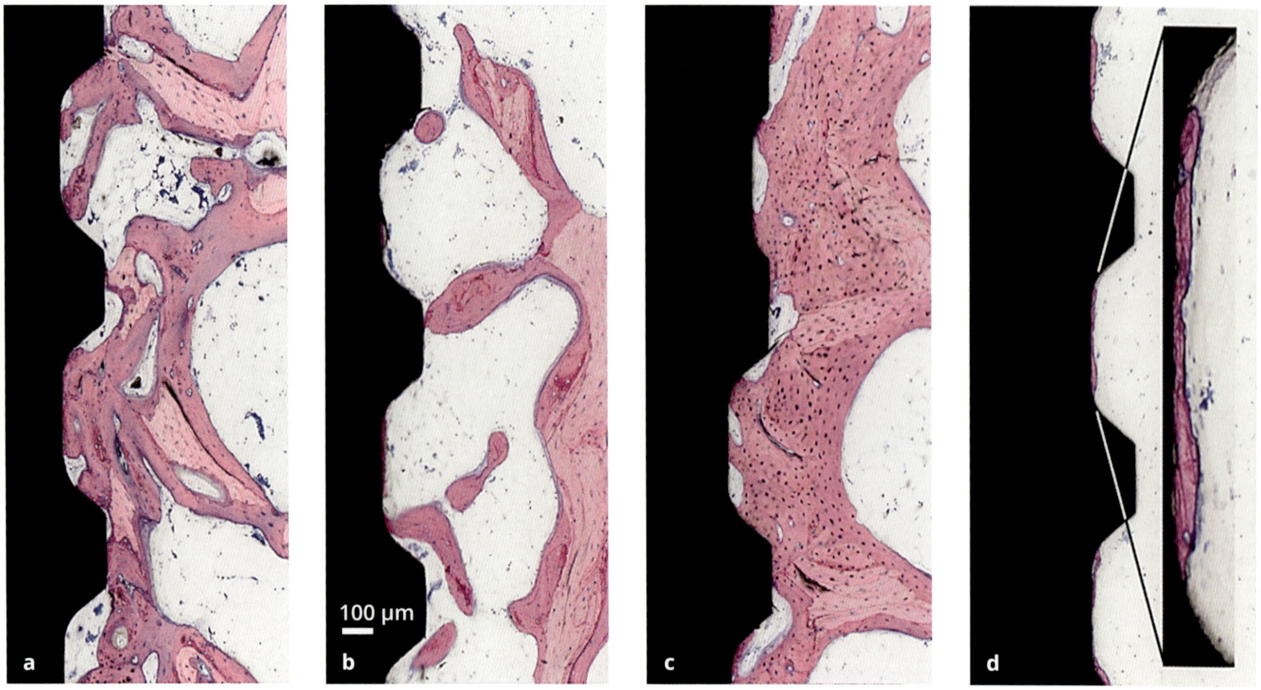

Figs 2-11a–d Different types of bone formation in the bone–implant mesophase. **(a)** The newly formed tissue extends from the preexisting one and covers the implant and adjacent trabeculae. **(b)** Annular forms of new osseous tissue. **(c)** New bone is deposited in wide layers. **(d)** Strips of woven bone (Levai Laczko staining) (Fig 24, page 84 of the thesis by Tsetsenekou[6]; reproduced with permission from the author).

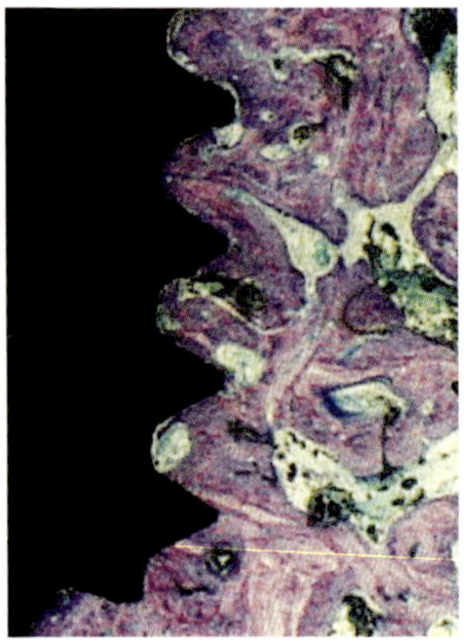

Fig 2-12 Histologic image depicting the direct contact of lamellar bone with the implant surface, which undergoes functional loading with great force (courtesy of Drs L. Podaropoulos, P. Trisi, and D. Kalyvas).

that the nature of a biomaterial, as well as its physical and chemical properties, influence the formation of steady adhesion of the bone to the implant.

Mechanical treatment of a titanium surface (machined surface) and anodic oxidization produce relatively smooth surfaces (Figs 2-13a, b to 2-15).

Surface roughness may be achieved with subtractive, prosthetic, or coating methods. Subtractive methods include treatment with a strong acid or laser, and abrasion with TiO_2 or Al_2O_3 particles of various diameters (such as SLA), whereas prosthetic methods consist of titanium plasma spraying (TPS) and hydroxyapatite coating (Figs 2-16a, b to 2-20).

Histologically, the initial contact between the bone and implant covered with TPS may be achieved just a week after placement. On the other hand, the initial bone contact with an implant with a smooth surface has been observed 3 weeks after placement. In most cases, formation of a blood clot was noted in a tight formation around the microrough surface of TPS implants, which has been attributed to the better retention of the fibrin mesh created during the blood clotting. The connection between the fibrin mesh and the implant surface is a decisive event; it is used as a scaffold for osteoprogenitor cells to migrate toward the implant. For this connection to be stable, primary stability of the implant during its mechanical retention in the implant bed must first be achieved; uncontrolled force application that could lead to its early failure must be avoided (Figs 2-21a–d).

In the years that followed, several in vivo studies compared the rate of bone–implant contact (Fig 2-22) between smooth surfaces and surfaces treated to become rougher. Histologic evaluation was performed between 3 weeks and 1 year and showed more rapid deposition of new bone on roughened surfaces com-

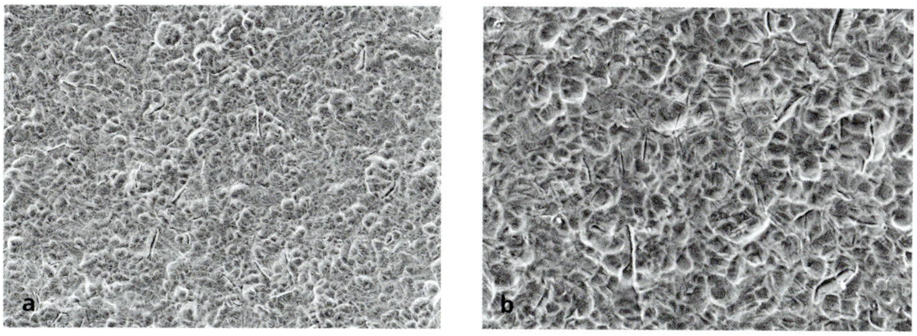

Figs 2-13a, b Polished titanium surface. **(a)** ×500 magnification. **(b)** ×1,000 magnification.

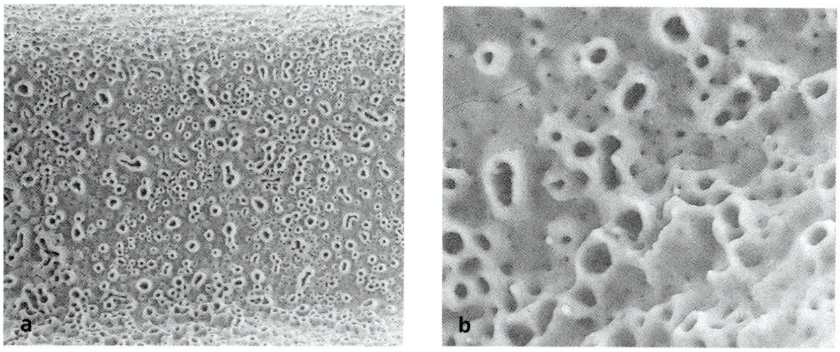

Figs 2-14a, b Scanning electron micrographs. **(a)** Rough surface that has undergone anodic oxidization (Nobel Biocare) at ×600 magnification. **(b)** The same micrograph at ×2,400 magnification (courtesy of Drs T. Papadopoulos and I. Fandrides).

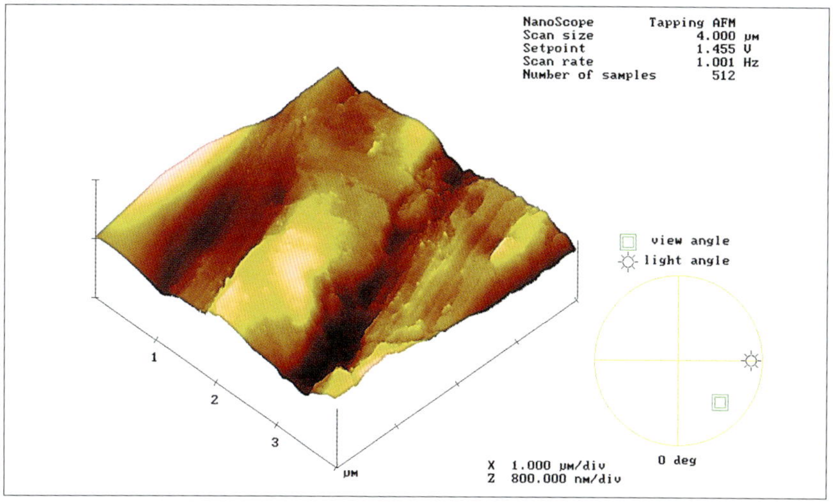

Fig 2-15 Application of atomic force microscopy revealed the low roughness of a smooth surface (Nobel Biocare), which promotes the adhesion of epithelial cells through hemidesmosomes (courtesy of Drs T. Papadopoulos and I. Fandrides).

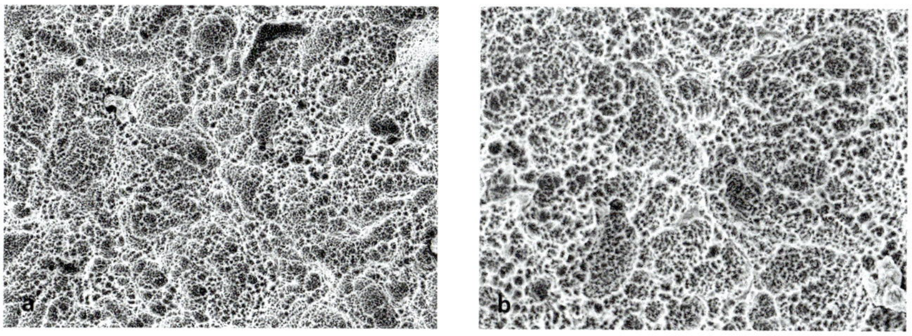

Figs 2-16a, b Titanium surface that has undergone treatment with airborne-particle abrasion and acids (Straumann) as can be seen in the micrographs. **(a)** ×500 magnification. **(b)** ×1,000 magnification.

pared to smooth surfaces, leading to an increased rate of bone–implant contact for these surfaces. Specifically, after 6 weeks of healing, the highest rate of bone–implant contact was noted around implants with an SLA surface (50% to 60%) and those with an hydroxyapatite coating (60% to 70%). In descending order, large-grit airborne-particle abraded surfaces follow (30% to 40%), as well as surfaces that under-

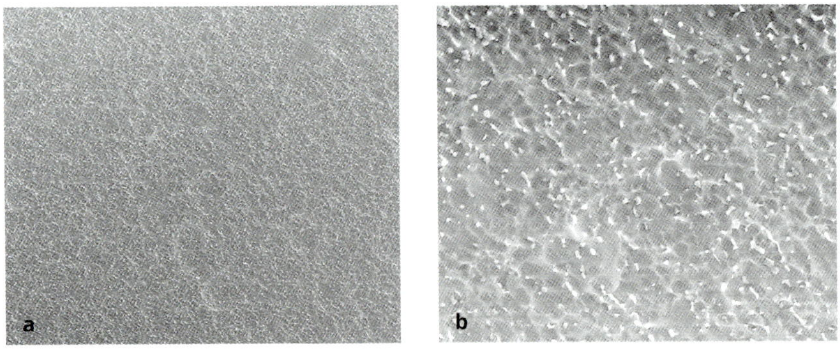

Figs 2-17a, b Micrographs. **(a)** Rough surface that has undergone airborne-particle abrasion with AL_2O_3 grains and chemical etching (MIS) at ×600 magnification. **(b)** the same micrograph at ×2,400 magnification (courtesy of Drs T. Papadopoulos and I. Fandrides).

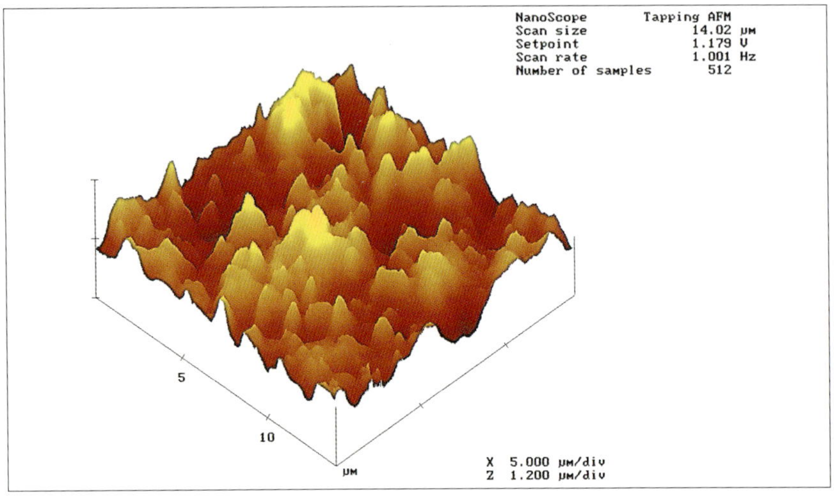

Fig 2-18 Application of atomic force microscopy revealed the roughness of a rough surface (MIS, Misgav, Israel) (courtesy of Drs T. Papadopoulos and I. Fandrides).

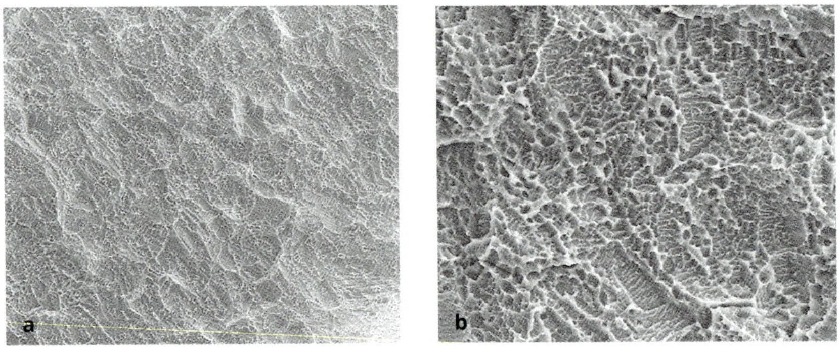

Figs 2-19a, b Micrographs. **(a)** Rough surface that has undergone chemical etching with 15% hydrofluoric acid and H_2SO_4/HCl (6:1) at 60°C to 80°C for 3 to 10 minutes (3i) at ×600 magnification. **(b)** The same micrograph at ×2,400 magnification (courtesy of Drs T. Papadopoulos and I. Fandrides).

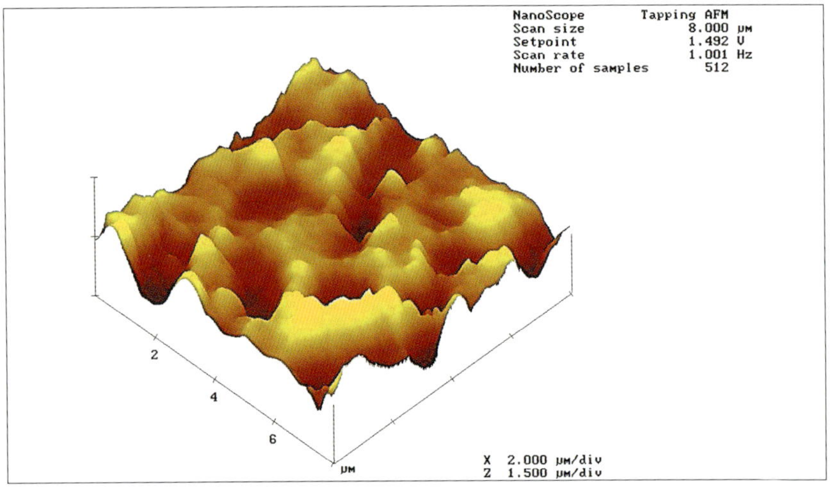

Fig 2-20 Application of atomic force microscopy revealed the roughness of a rough 3i surface (courtesy of Drs T. Papadopoulos and I. Fandrides).

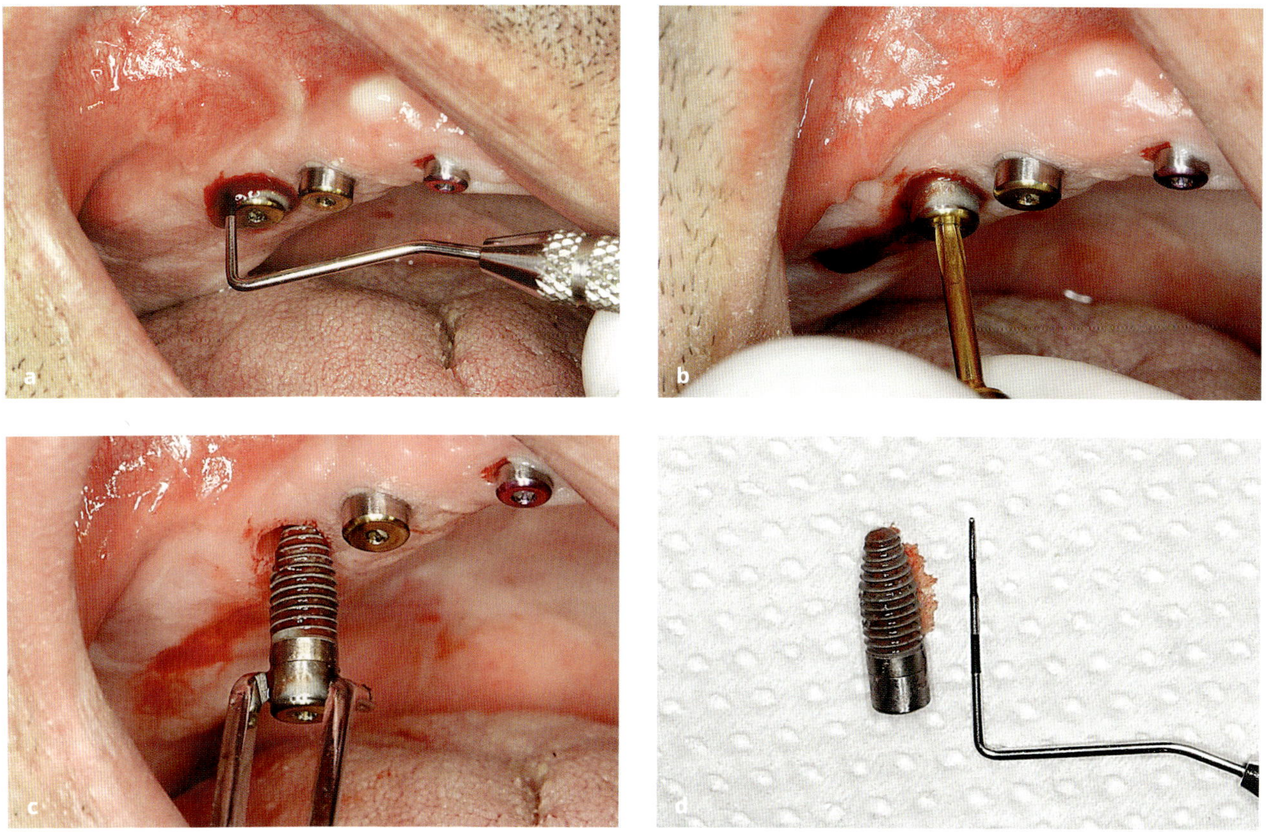

Figs 2-21a–d The loss of this implant was attributed to the failure of osseointegration due to excessive application of force from a complete denture provisional prosthesis.

go airborne-particle abrasion with medium-sized grits, and, finally, machined surfaces (20% to 25%). Implants coated with hydroxyapatite (HA) often show signs of resorption or detachment of their external coat.[7] Notably, surfaces that have undergone treatment with airborne-particle abrasion and acids became hydrophilic, and show improved bone–implant contact. This is achieved by the role of the modified SLA surface in cellular differentiation and production of growth factors. Modification of the SLA surface is achieved with treatment in a nitrogen environment (N_2); the implant is stored in a package that contains an isotonic solution. Thus, the surface is hydrated and the hydroxyl group connections are increased. Only small quantities of hydrogen carbonates and carbon remain on the surface. These implants may be loaded just 3 weeks after placement.[9-17]

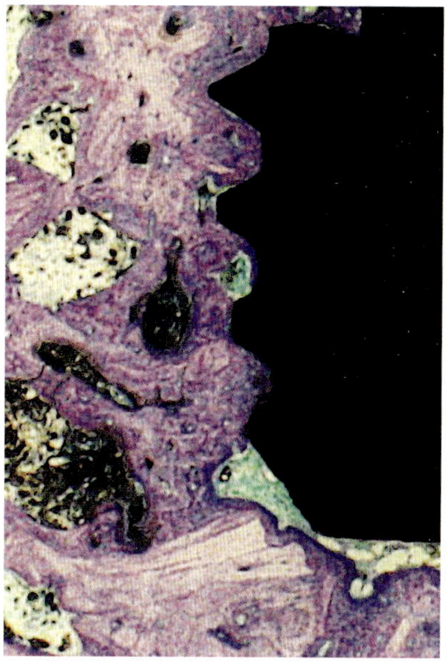

Fig 2-22 The percentage of contact between osseous tissue (not trabeculae) in linear measurements along the implant surface was used to express the quality of osseointegration (bone–implant contact). In this case, a high percentage of bone–implant contact has been achieved (courtesy of Drs L. Podaropoulos, P. Trisi, and D. Kalyvas).

A comparison of implants with treated versus smooth surfaces, with regard to the torque removal force, showed that treated surfaces require greater forces to be loosened from the bone. Those studies were performed in guinea pigs and in bone with a different density than human bone. However, the greatest torque removal forces were achieved for TPS or SLA surfaces.[18]

At the cellular level, the reaction of peri-implant tissues is influenced by the topography of each surface, not only at the level of metabolic activity, but also as far as adhesion to it is concerned. In vitro experiments on TPS or SLA surfaces versus smooth surfaces have shown that osteoblast-like cells in contact with rough surfaces produce up to four times more prostaglandin E2 and tumor growth factor β1. This increased production of biologic mediators suggests that rougher surfaces may lead to alterations in cellular activity and consequently affect healing of the peri-implant bone. Equivalent conclusions have been reached for hormones such as osteocalcin and enzymes such as alkaline phosphatase.[19,20]

Moreover, apart from an increase in metabolic activity, surface topography affects the shape and arrangement of cells. In vitro studies have shown that the length, orientation, and adhesion level of osteoblasts is defined, to a great extent, by the texture of the surface they adhere to. In addition, an increase in osseous tissue production has been noted, with orientation corresponding to the microstructure of the surface. Specifically, osteoblast adhesion is better in rough titanium surfaces, where a greater degree of extracellular matrix and higher salination are present.[21,22]

In conclusion, all interactions between peri-implant tissues and rough surfaces favorably influence the osseointegration process through the faster deposition of new bone, wider bone–implant contact, and greater removal torque.

A catalytic role in the achievement of osseointegration is played by adhesion of plasma proteins to the titanium surface, even though the exact process during trauma healing that leads to bone–implant contact is not yet clear. An additional element thought to play a crucial role is the neoangiogenesis created by the capillary vessels in the area. These cells, as undifferentiated mesenchymal cells, generate osteoblast precursor cells, which in turn lead to increased production of osteoblasts. This eventually leads to a positive effect on osseointegration.

References

1. Brånemark PI, Adell R, Breine U, Hansson BO, Lindström J, Ohlsson A. Intra-osseous anchorage of dental prostheses. I. Experimental studies. Scand J Plast Reconstr Surg 1969;3:81–100.
2. Steinemann S. The properties of titanium. In: Schroeder A, Sutter E, Buser D, Krekeler G (ed). Oral implantology. Basics, ITI Dental Implant System, ed 2. New York: Thieme Medical Publishers, 1996;37–59.
3. Javed F, Ahmed HB, Crespi R, Romanos GE. Role of primary stability for successful osseointegration of dental implants: factors of influence and evaluation. Interv Med Appl Sci 2013;5:162–167.
4. Davies JE. Understanding peri-implant endosseous healing. J Dent Educ 2003;67:932–949.
5. Schenk RK, Buser D. Osseointegration: a reality. Periodontol 2000 1998;17:22–35.
6. Tsetsenekou E. Histological and histomorphometrical evaluation of the osseointegration of nanotreated dental implants in New Zealand Rabbits under alendronate therapy. PhD Thesis, Athens, 2011.
7. Chappard D. Bone modeling and remodeling during osseointegration [in French]. Rev Stomatol Chir Maxillofac Chir Orale 2013;114:159–165.
8. Buser D, Shenk RK, Steinemann S, Fiorellini JP, Fox CH, Stich H. Influence of surface characteristics on bone integration of titanium implants. A histomorphometric study in miniature pigs. J Biomed Mater Res 1991;25:889–902.
9. Carr AB, Beds DW, Larsen PE. Reverse-torque failure of screw-shaped implants in baboons after 6 months of healing. Int J Oral Maxillofac Implants 1997;12:598–603.
10. Claes L, Hutzschenreuter P, Pohler O. The dependence of the removal torque of a leg screw surface and implantation time [in German]. Arch Orthop Unfallchir 1976;85:155–159.
11. Cochran DL, Schenk RK, Lussi A, Higginbottom FL, Buser D. Bone response to unloaded and loaded titanium implants with a sandblasted and acid-etched surface: a histometric study in the canine mandible. J Biomed Mater Res 1998;40:1–11.
12. Gotfredsen K, Nimb L, Hjörting-Hansen E, Jensen JS, Holmén A. Histomorphometric and removal torque analysis for smooth and TiO2-blasted titanium implants. An experimental study on dogs. Clin Oral Implants Res 1992;3:77–84.
13. Gotfredsen K, Wennerberg A, Johansson C, Skovgaard LT, Hjørting-Hansen E. Anchorage of TiO2-blasted, HA-coated, and machined implants: an experimental study with rabbits. J Biomed Mater Res 1995;29:1223–1231.
14. Bosshardt DD, Chappuis V, Buser D. Osseointegration of titanium, titanium alloy and zirconia dental implants: current knowledge and open questions. Periodontol 2000 2017;73:22–40.

15. Stafford GL. Review found little difference between sandblasted and acid-etched (SLA) dental implants and modified surface (SLActive) implants. Evid Based Dent 2014;15:87–88.
16. Smeets R, Stadlinger B, Schwarz F, et al. Impact of dental implant surface modifications on osseointegration. Biomed Res Int 2016;2016:6285620.
17. Carlsson L, Röstlund T, Albrektsson B, Albrektsson T. Removal torques for polished and rough titanium implants. Int J Oral Maxillofac Implants 1988;3:21–24.
18. Buser D, Nydegger T, Oxland T, et al. Interface shear strength of titanium implants with a sandblasted and acid-etched surface: a biomechanical study in the maxilla of miniature pigs. J Biomed Mater Res 1999;45: 75–83.
19. Lincks J, Boyan BD, Blanchard CR, et al. Response of MG63 osteoblast-like cells to titanium and titanium alloy is dependent on surface roughness and composition. Biomaterials 1998;19:2219–2232.
20. Martin JY, Schwartz Z, Hummert TW, et al. Effect of titanium surface roughness on proliferation, differentiation, and protein synthesis of human osteoblast-like cells (MG63). J Biomed Master Res 1995;29:389–401.
21. Lagonegro P, Trevisi G, Nasi L, et al. Osteoblasts preferentially adhere to peaks on micro-structured titanium. Dent Mater J 2018;37:278–285.
22. de Oliveira GJPL, Aroni MAT, Pinotti FE, Marcantonio E Jr, Marcantonio RAC. Low-level laser therapy (LLLT) in sites grafted with osteoconductive bone substitutes improves osseointegration. Lasers Med Sci 2020;35:1519–1529.

3 Classification of Peri-Implant Diseases

The classification of peri-implant diseases and defects is necessary for communication between clinics not only regarding diagnosis and prognosis, but also for a better understanding of the etiological factors involved. In addition, establishing the correct diagnosis helps the clinician to provide the appropriate treatment. Since the early 1990s, experts around the world have agreed to distinguish between two disease entities that affect peri-implant tissues, namely peri-implant mucositis and peri-implantitis. Additional denominators were proposed at the World Workshop on the Classification of Periodontal and Peri-Implant Diseases and Conditions in 2017. The description of health in particular was added:

- **Healthy peri-implant tissues** are characterized clinically and histologically by the absence of signs of inflammation. No bleeding on light probing is observed, even in cases of implants with reduced residual bone support (Figs 3-1 to 3-4a, b).
- **Peri-implant mucositis** is a reversible disease that has a microbial etiology; it is characterized by visible signs of inflammation and bleeding on probing (BOP). The disease is similar to gingivitis for natural dentition (Fig 3-5). Peri-implant mucositis can be treated by removing the main causative factor, namely the microbial biofilm, previously known as dental plaque. According to the 2017 classification, it is a reversible form of inflammation that occurs in the peri-implant mucosa after functional loading.[1] However, inflammation of the soft peri-implant tissues may be induced immediately by placing the implant using a single-phase protocol or uncovering if it was placed using a two-stage protocol. Because inflammation is limited to the soft tissues and is not a condition involving early implant failure, its topography and etiology classify it as peri-implant mucositis. Therefore, it

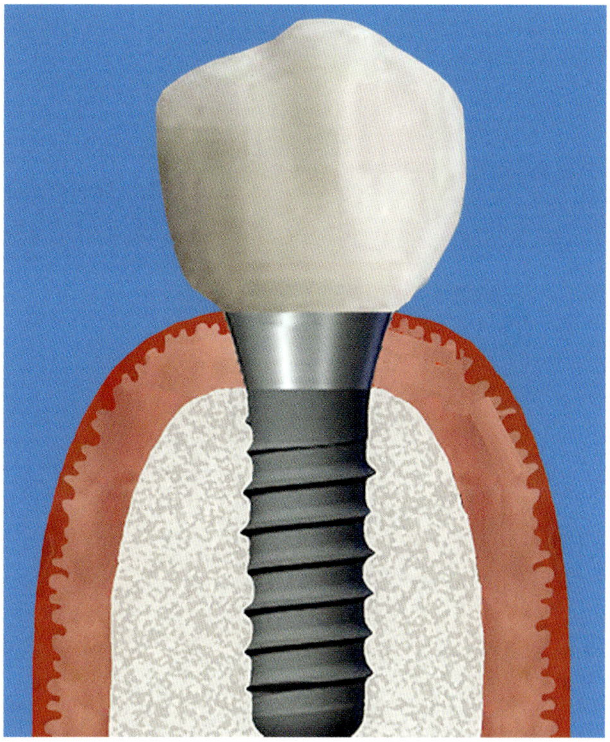

Fig 3-1 Schematic representation of healthy peri-implant tissues. No inflammation or bone loss is observed.

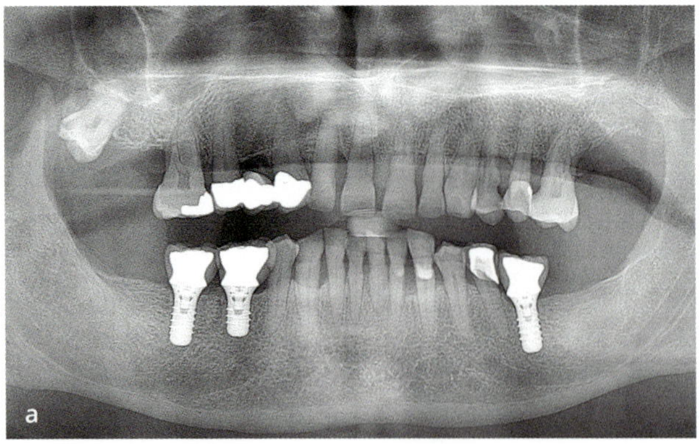

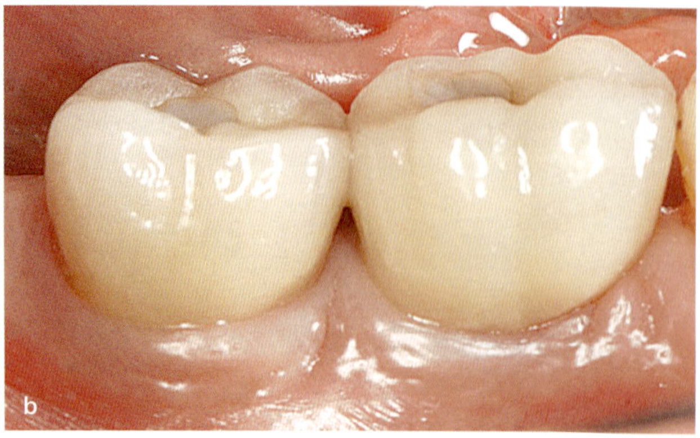

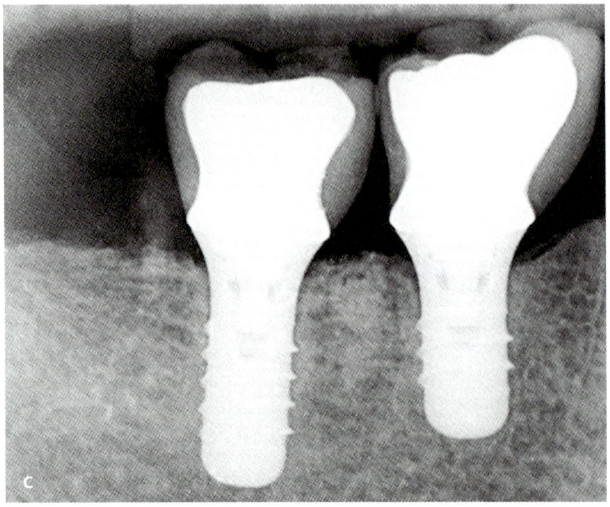

Figs 3-2a–c (a) Radiographic image of a patient after implant placement. **(b and c)** Clinical and radiographic images of healthy peri-implant tissues 6 years after placement of the implant-supported crowns. Note the absence of BOP, pockets, and bone loss.

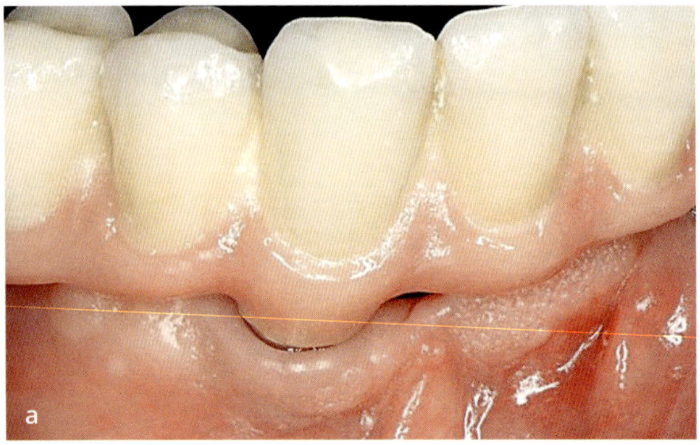

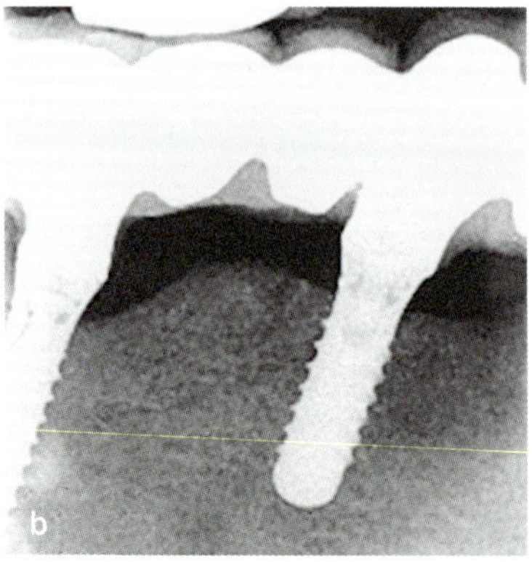

Figs 3-3a, b Clinical and radiographic images of healthy peri-implant tissues 8 years after implant placement. Note the absence of inflammation on probing, pockets, and bone loss.

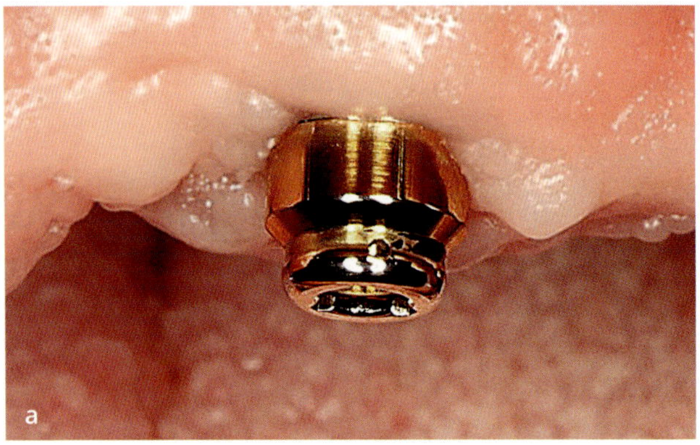

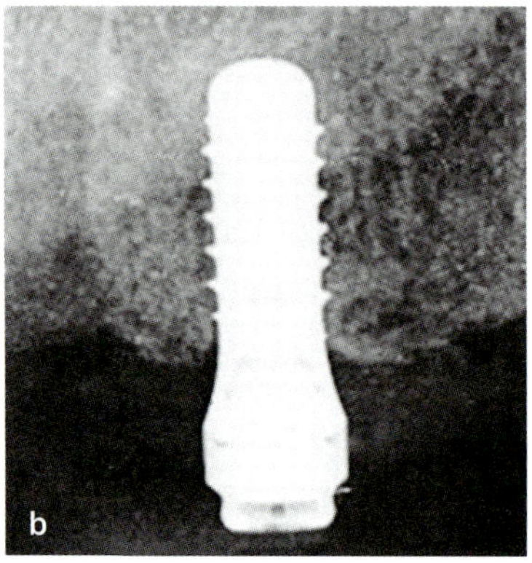

Figs 3-4a, b Clinical and radiographic images of healthy peri-implant tissues 7 years after incorporation of the denture. Note the absence of signs of inflammation and bone destruction.

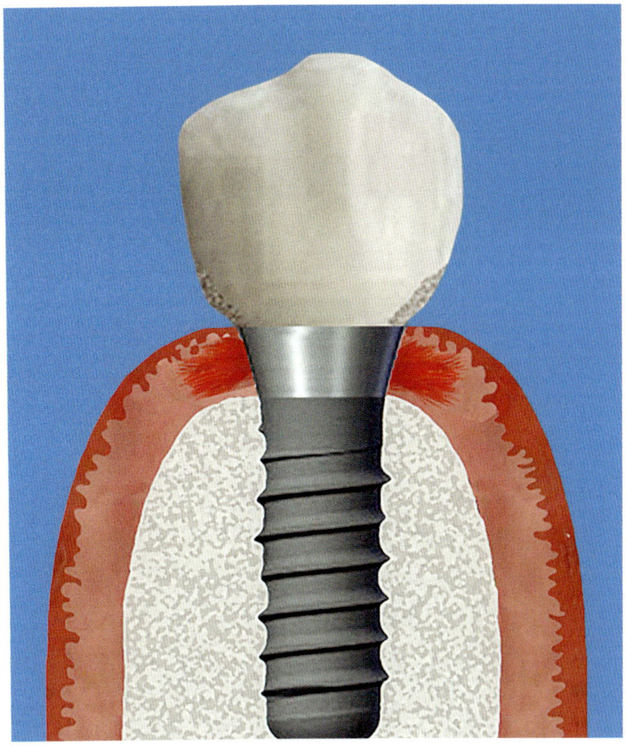

Fig 3-5 Schematic representation of peri-implant mucositis. Inflammation is limited to the peri-implant mucosa. There is no bone loss, while microbial biofilm is detected.

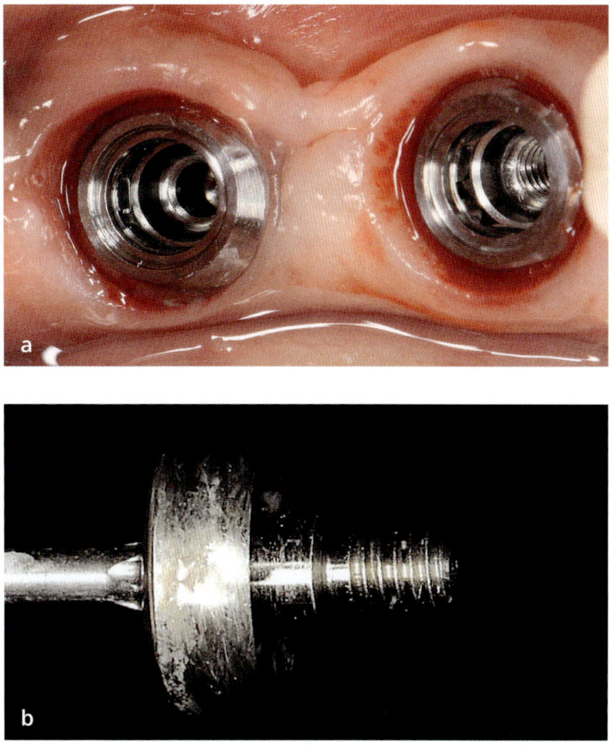

Figs 3-6a, b (a) Peri-implant mucositis can be established immediately after implant placement or uncovering if a single-phase or two-phase placement protocol is applied, respectively. In this case, inflammation was observed 6 weeks after implant placement. (b) Significant microbial deposits can be observed on the cover screw.

is more appropriate to include the following in the term peri-implant mucositis:

- Reversible inflammation that occurs in the peri-implant mucosa before functional loading that is due to the accumulation of the biofilm around the transmucosal healing screw (Figs 3-6a, b),[2,3] as well as reversible inflammation that occurs in the peri-implant mucosa after functional loading.

- **Peri-implantitis** represents a disease of the peri-implant tissues; it has a microbial etiology, which is accompanied by both inflammation of the peri-implant mucosa and destruction of the supporting bone of an implant. Peri-implantitis is directly related to the presence of biofilm but also to the patient's history of periodontitis and, if not treated effectively, may progress rapidly.[4]

Significant differences are observed between peri-implant mucositis and peri-implantitis, both clinically and histologically; in peri-implant mucositis, inflammation is limited to the soft peri-implant tissues (Figs 3-7a, b to 3-9a, b), whereas peri-implantitis causes irreversible damage to the supporting bone (Figs 3-10 to 3-12a–d).[5]

To detect even minor bone loss, it is necessary to keep a record of radiographic images of the implant at various stages, beginning immediately after placement, as illustrated in Chapter 7. Hence, it may be necessary to ascertain whether a radiographic image of a small amount of bone loss is due to bone remodeling, due to the connection of implant and transmucosal abutments, or if it is true bone loss due to peri-implantitis.[6] If peri-implantitis is untreated or poorly treated, it may progress rapidly (Figs 3-13a, b and 3-14a, b).[4]

As there is no defined peri-implant sulcus depth that indicates the transition from peri-implant mucositis to peri-implantitis, a record of the peri-implant sulcus depth measurements should be kept at various times, such as after prosthetic restoration and after the first year in function. It is important to note that probing depth ≥ 4 mm does not necessarily suggest the existence of a pocket.[7]

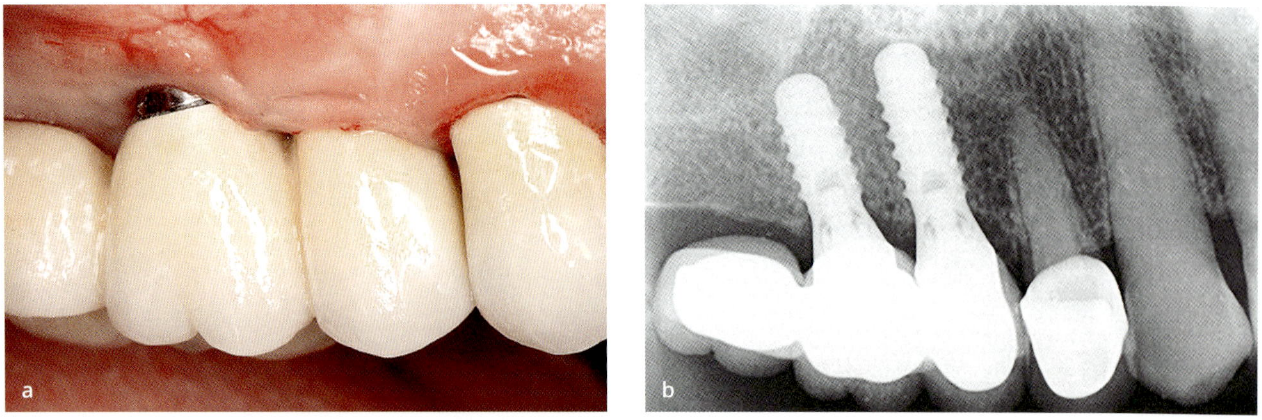

Figs 3-7a, b Clinical and radiographic images of peri-implant mucositis. Visible signs of inflammation, such as red, swollen, and bleeding soft tissues can be observed, while no bone loss is detected radiographically.

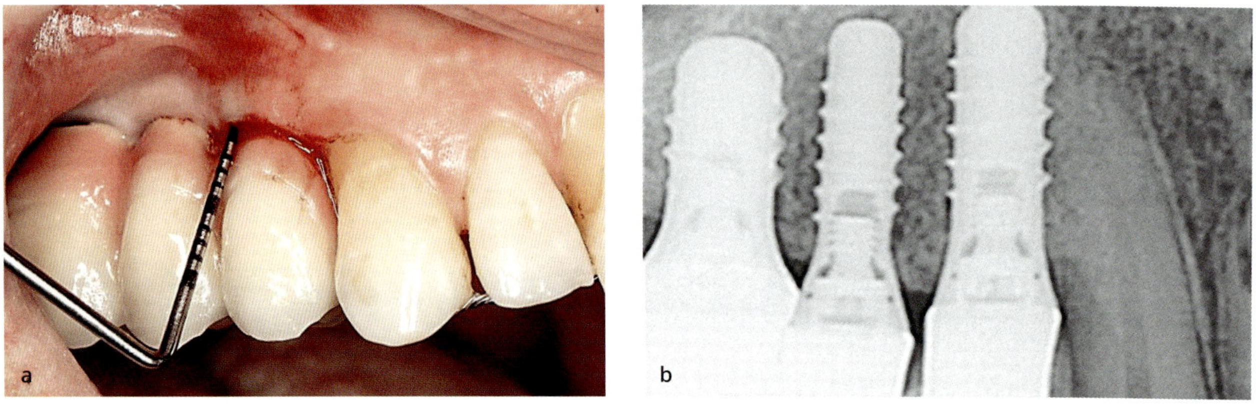

Figs 3-8a, b Clinical and radiographic images of peri-implant mucositis. BOP can be observed from the peri-implant sulci, while no bone loss is detected radiographically.

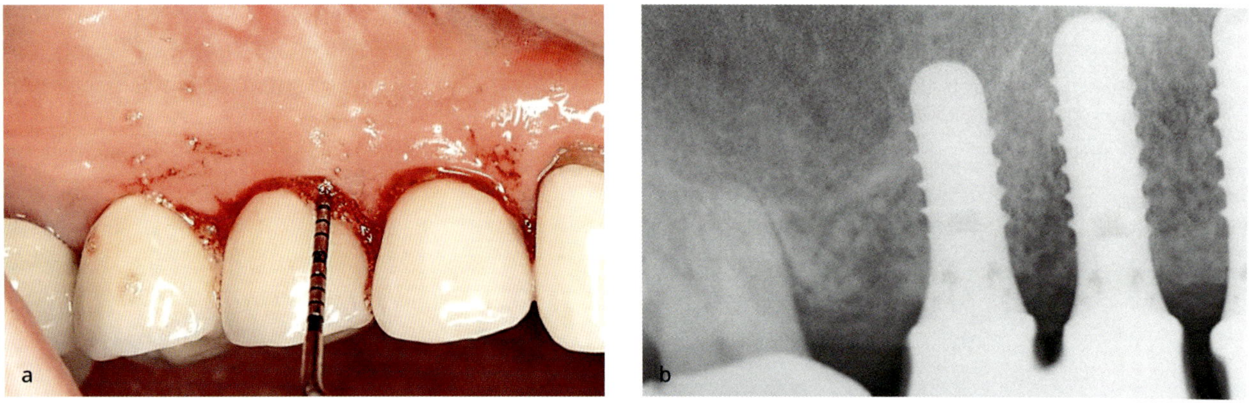

Figs 3-9a, b Clinical and radiographic images of peri-implant mucositis. Probing of peri-implant sulci leads to bleeding, while no bone loss is detected radiographically.

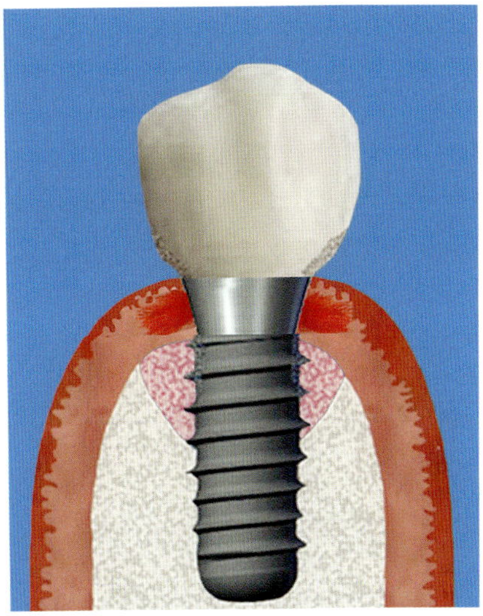

Fig 3-10 Schematic representation of peri-implantitis. Bone loss and exposure of the implant threads to the pocket environment can be observed. The microbial biofilm extends to the surface of the implant, over the exposed threads.

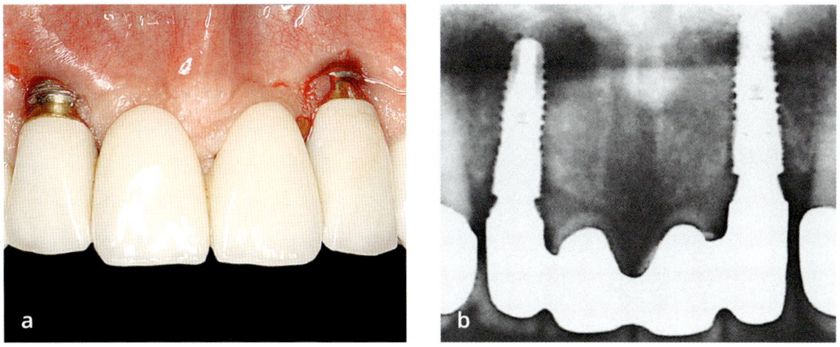

Figs 3-11a, b Clinical and radiographic images of peri-implantitis. There is a loss of soft peri-implant tissue attachment and BOP, while the radiograph reveals bone loss.

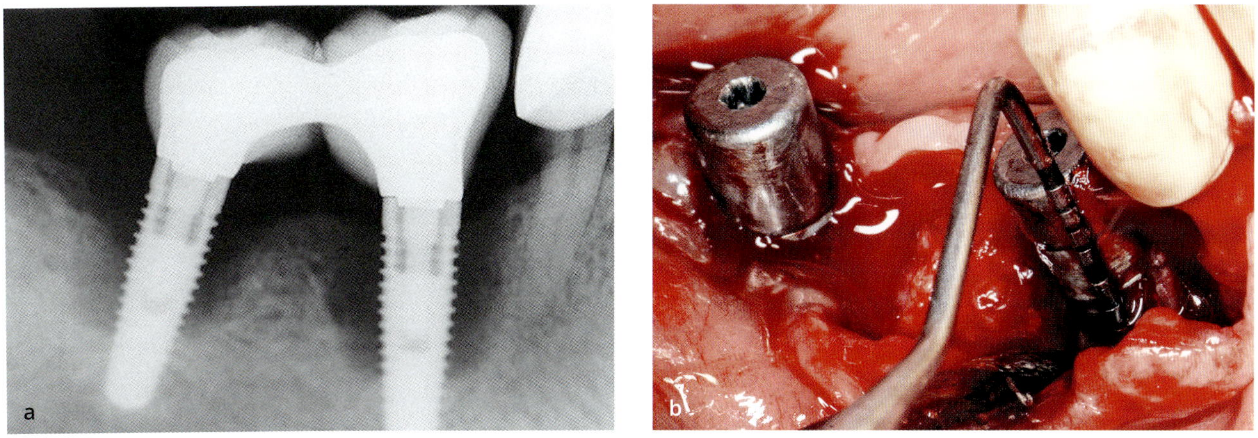

Figs 3-12a, b Radiographic and clinical images of peri-implantitis. Peri-implant bone loss in the fourth quadrant is evident in this patient who, for 10 years, remained without maintenance care. This is peri-implantitis due to biofilm accumulation.

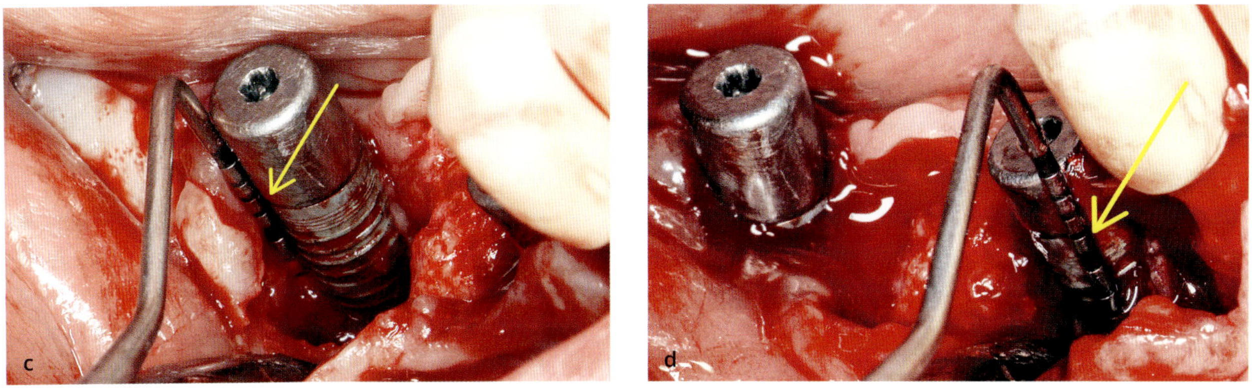

Figs 3-12c, d In addition to the extensive destruction of the peri-implant bone, the periodontal probe (yellow arrow) indicates 11 mm bone loss (for both implants) from the point of contact with the bone to the point of contact with the implant healing screw. The implants are 13 mm long. Therefore, the remaining bone support is only 2 mm.

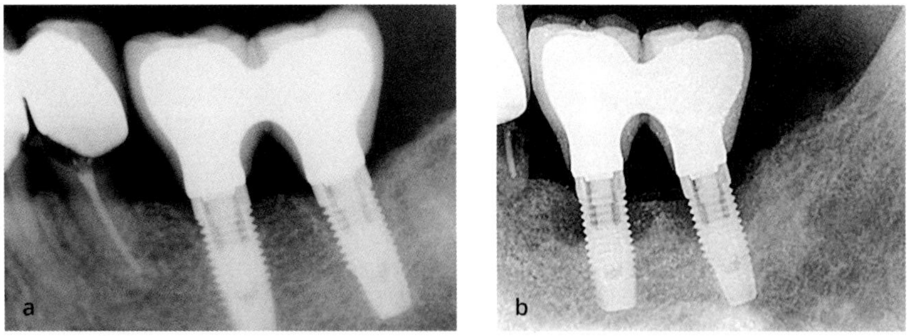

Figs 3-13a, b Radiographic image of implants **(a)** 7 and **(b)** 10 years after placement. Bone loss increased significantly, while caries destroyed tooth 35.

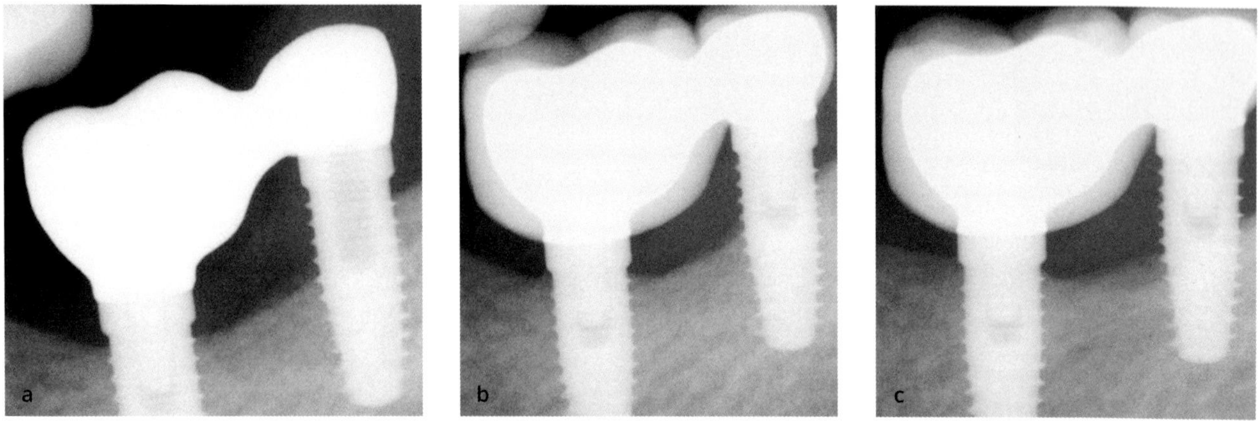

Figs 3-14a–c **(a)** Images of a patient's implants 6 years after placement. The implant in site 37 was placed incorrectly from the beginning and did not fully enter the alveolar bone. **(b)** The same area 1 year later, without having undergone any maintenance care. **(c)** Three years after implant placement, further bone loss is evident as peri-implantitis remained untreated. The case review continues in Chapter 10.

Peri-implantitis affects implants that have a prosthetic restoration and have undergone functional loading (Figs 3-15a–d and 3-16). It should not be confused with cases of early implant failure, where osseointegration is not achieved. In addition, during the first year after placement, a small amount of bone loss may be expected as part of the normal bone remodeling process. This is a radiographic finding but may not be accompanied by inflammation of the peri-implant mucosa.[8,9]

In this book, the term "iatrogenic peri-implantitis" is introduced to describe diseases caused by poorly designed or executed treatment. The most common case of iatrogenic peri-implantitis is that resulting from the presence of cement residue in the peri-implant sulcus. Because this is not a separate disease with different manifestations, signs, and symptoms, this topic is developed further in Chapter 5.

Some publications speak of "apical retrograde peri-implantitis". The term refers to the description of bone loss at the apical part of the implant due to the extension of peri-apical lesions from an adjacent tooth or from an incorrectly placed implant in an area with residual bone pathology of dental origin. These cases are rare, are managed with treatment of the primary lesion, and do not constitute a special category of peri-implantitis because they do not have a corresponding etiopathogenesis (Fig 3-17).[10–12]

Another category of peri-implant lesions includes cases of peri-implant bone loss and pocket formation due to periodontal pathology of an adjacent tooth. Periodontal pathology refers to cases of exacerbation of preexisting periodontitis or tooth fractures. In these cases, the term "secondary peri-implantitis" or "peri-implantitis due to an extension of inflammation from an adjacent tooth" may be used because the cause of peri-implant bone loss is inflammation and has a microbial etiology but the primary lesion is in an adjacent tooth and not on the implant surface (Figs 3-18a–n and 3-19).

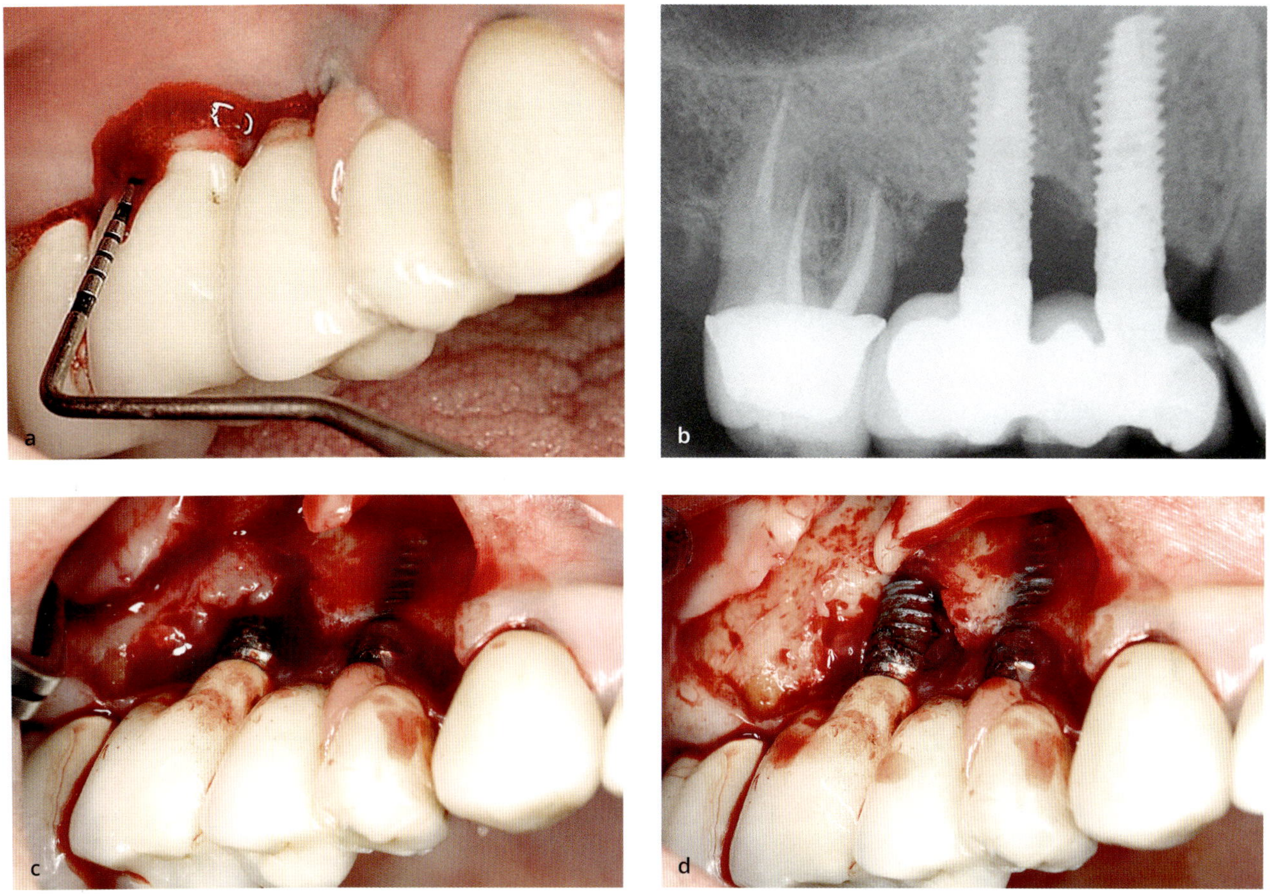

Figs 3-15a–d **(a and b)** Clinical and radiographic images of peri-implantitis. The deep expansion of the inflammation leads to bone loss and pocket formation while bleeding on probing is also detected. Radiographs give information about the size of the bone defect. **(c and d)** After the flap is elevated, the clinical inspection shows that the size of the defect was underestimated.

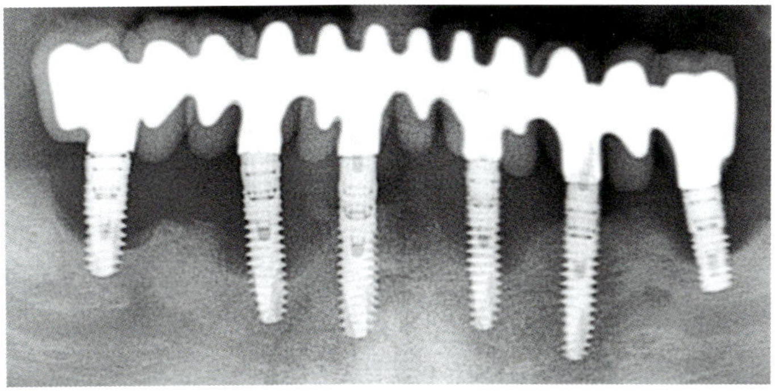

Fig 3-16 Radiograph showing peri-implantitis. Bone loss is extensive with characteristic saucer-shaped defects. Most implants now have little residual bone support.

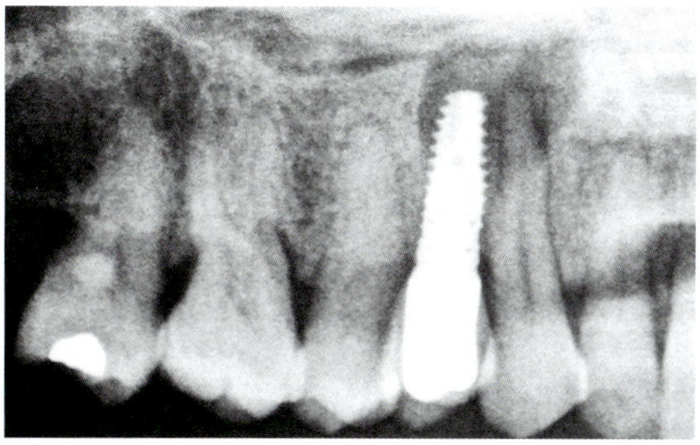

Fig 3-17 Radiograph of a patient with a lesion surrounding the apical part of implant 14 and tooth 13. This condition has also been described as "periapical peri-implantitis".

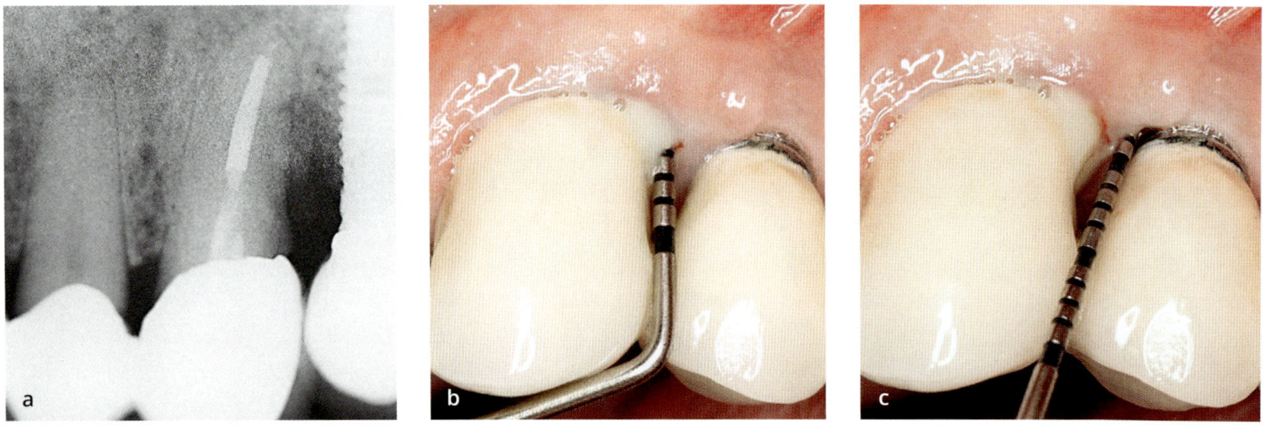

Figs 3-18a–c **(a)** Bone loss can be observed between tooth 23 and implant 24. **(b and c)** An 11-mm periodontal pocket is detected with suppuration from tooth 23 and the peri-implant sulcus at implant 24. Pus formation distal of tooth 23 is evident.

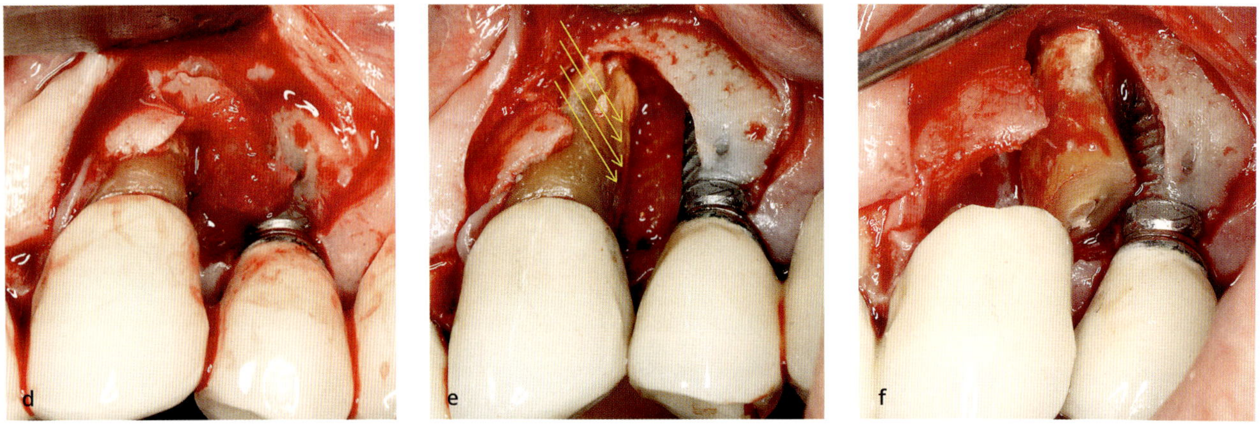

Figs 3-18d–f **(d)** After elevation of a diagnostic flap, a large amount of granulation tissue is found in the area where bone loss was shown radiographically. **(e)** After removal of the granulation tissue, a vertical fracture on the root of tooth 23 (yellow arrows) becomes visible, as well as extensive bone loss extending to the implant, leading to exposure of many threads. The palatal bone plate and the part of the buccal plate that is intact are visible. **(f)** The root of the tooth was amputated and carefully extracted so that the partial denture remained in situ.

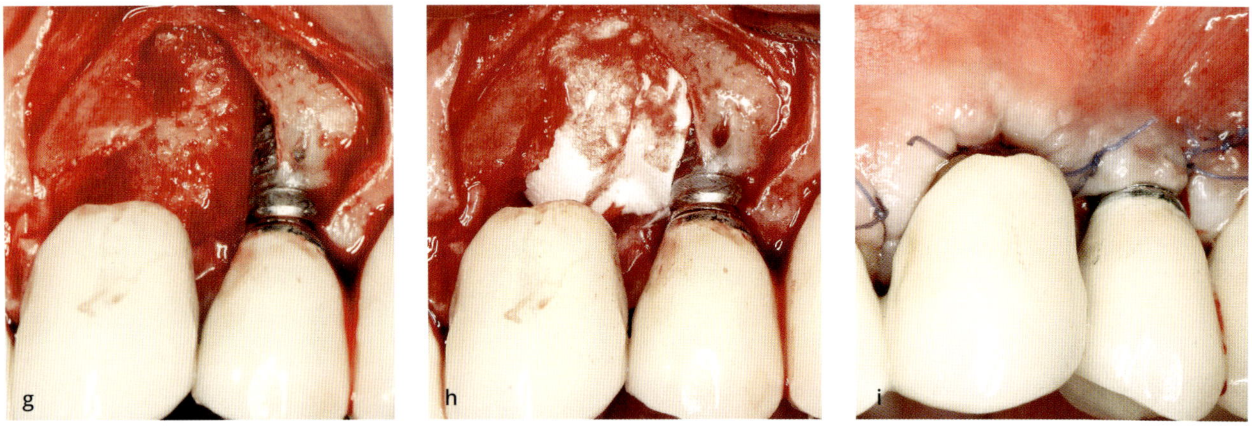

Figs 3-18 g–I **(g)** The root extraction area is visible. **(h)** Collagen graft placement. **(i)** Coronally repositioned flap and suturing.

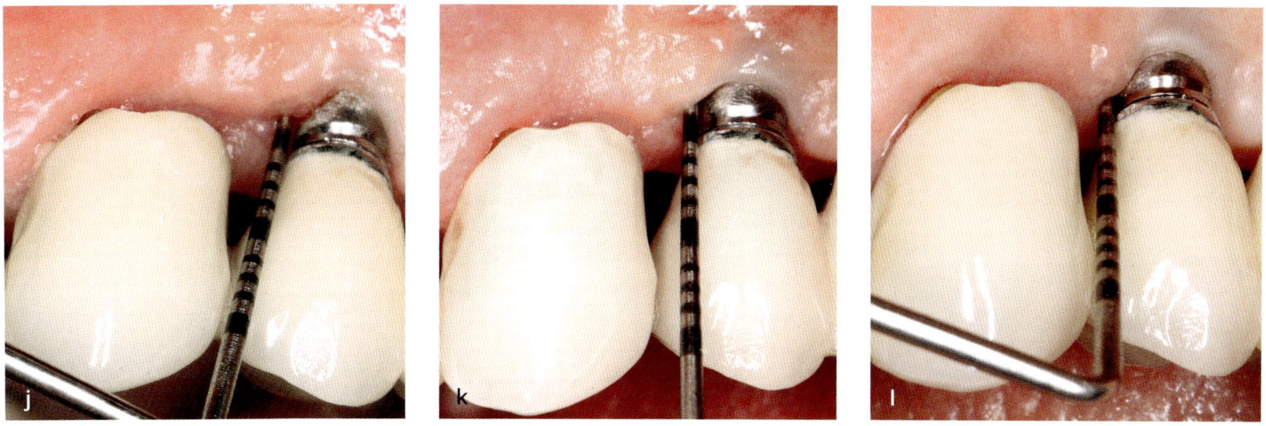

Figs 3-18j–l Peri-implant sulcus probing after **(j)** 3, **(k)** 6, and **(l)** 12 months shows peri-implant tissue stability.

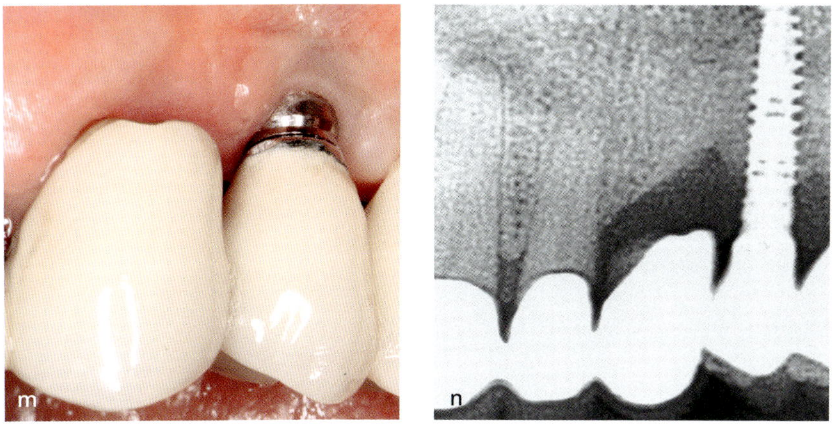

Figs 3-18m, n Clinical and radiographic images taken 2 years after surgery confirm that the peri-implant tissues are healthy and the bone–implant contact has been restored.

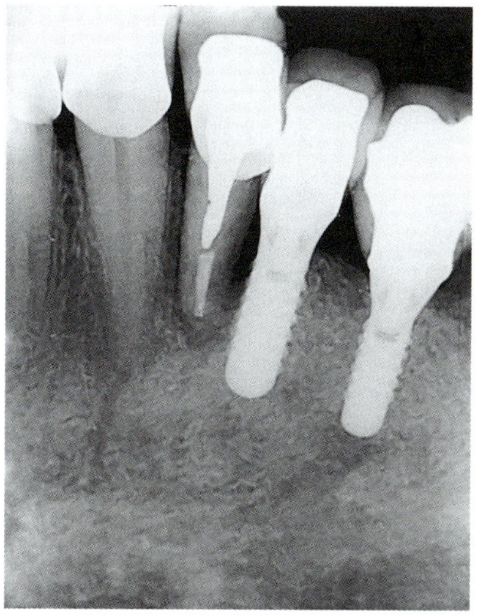

Fig 3-19 Radiographic image of secondary peri-implantitis. Bone loss is observed near the implant due to the pathology of tooth 34.

References

1. Heitz-Mayfield LJA, Salvi GE. Peri-implant mucositis. J Clin Periodontol 2018;45(suppl 20):S237–S245.
2. Pontoriero R, Tonelli MP, Carnevale G, Mombelli A, Nyman SR, Lang NP. Experimentally induced peri-implant mucositis. A clinical study in humans. Clin Oral Implants Res 1994;5:254–259.
3. Meyer S, Giannopoulou C, Cancela J, Courvoisier D, Müller F, Mombelli A. Experimental mucositis/gingivitis in persons aged 70 or over: microbiological findings and prediction of clinical outcome. Clin Oral Investig 2019;23:3855–3863.
4. Caton JG, Armitage G, Berglundh T, et al. A new classification scheme for periodontal and peri-implant diseases and conditions—Introduction and key changes from the 1999 classification. J Clin Periodontol 2018;45(suppl 20):S1–S8.
5. Renvert S, Persson GR, Pirih FQ, Camargo PM. Peri-implant health, peri-implant mucositis and peri-implantitis: case definitions and diagnostic considerations. J Clin Periodontol 2018;45(suppl 20):S278–S285.
6. Lindhe J, Meyle J. Peri-implant diseases: consensus report of the Sixth European Workshop on Periodontology. J Clin Periodontol 2008;35:282–285.
7. Lang NP, Bosshardt DD, Lulic M. Do mucositis lesions around implants differ from gingivitis lesions around teeth? J Clin Periodontol 2011;38:182–187.
8. Ericsson I, Lindhe J. Probing depth at implants and teeth. An experimental study in the dog. J Clin Periodontol 1993;20:623–627.
9. Berglundh T, Lindhe J, Ericsson L, Marinello CP, Liljenberg B, Thomsen P. The soft tissue barrier at implants and teeth. Clin Oral Implants Res 1991;2:81–90.
10. Singh R, Pandey V, Kumar V, Mishra AK. Retrograde peri-implantitis—A review of literature and an update. J Adv Med Dent Scie Res 2016;4:47–49.
11. Mohamed JB, Shivakumar B, Sudarsan S, Arun KV, Kumar TSS. Retrograde peri-implantitis. J Indian Soc Periodontol 2010;14:57–65.
12. Marshall G, Canullo L, Logan RM, Rossi-Fedele G. Histopathological and microbiological findings associated with retrograde peri-implantitis of extra-radicular endodontic origin: a systematic and critical review. Int J Oral Maxillofac Surg 2019;48:1475–1484.

4 Etiologic and Risk Factors for Peri-Implant Diseases

Understanding the biologic mechanism of osseointegration made a decisive contribution to expanding the use of implants to rehabilitate partially and completely edentulous patients. Implant placement is now common practice, and this has led to the implementation of protocols such as immediate implant placement, immediate loading, and regenerative techniques. Implant-supported prosthetic restorations are becoming increasingly popular as the high success rates of dental implants are confirmed by research data from long-term clinical trials. Clearly, biologic, technical, and esthetic complications are still a reality. Their incidence varies depending on the category of complications. Nevertheless, the ever-increasing and often excessive selection and use of implants has led to a significant increase in their number worldwide; consequently, this has resulted in a considerable rise in the number of complications and, at the same time, the need for dental care.

Epidemiologic data on biologic complications are discussed in Chapter 5. Complications affect many implants and patients. The recording and evaluation of all possible factors that may jeopardize the success of implant treatment is crucial when developing a treatment plan, and during the maintenance care phase.

The most severe biologic complication affecting implants is peri-implantitis. Peri-implantitis is a disease with a multifactorial etiology, with the main etiologic factor being oral biofilms. In addition to oral biofilms, other factors have been studied as risk factors regarding the establishment and development of peri-implant pathology, which can ultimately result in implant loss if the required treatment is not implemented in a timely and effective manner. Risk factors for the development of peri-implantitis are as follows:

- history of periodontitis;
- factors related to systemic health;
- genetic factors;
- factors related to patient behavior;
- presence of keratinized tissue around implants;
- factors related to implant geometry;
- factors related to the prosthetic design and performing an optimal reconstruction.[1]

The disease occurs more often in specific subsets of the general population, in which one or more risk factors can be identified. Their effect not only increases the incidence of the disease, but also complicates its treatment. Identification and successful control of all factors that lead synergistically to the manifestation and progression of the disease are essential (Figs 4-1a–g).

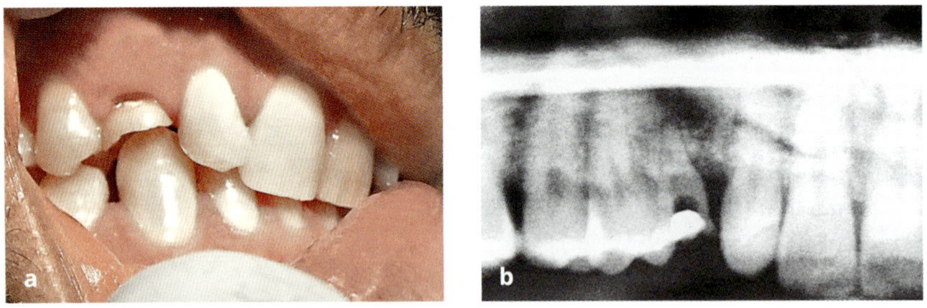

Figs 4-1a, b Initial **(a)** clinical and **(b)** radiographic images of a patient who did not want orthodontic treatment. The primary no. 53 and the impacted no. 13 can be seen.

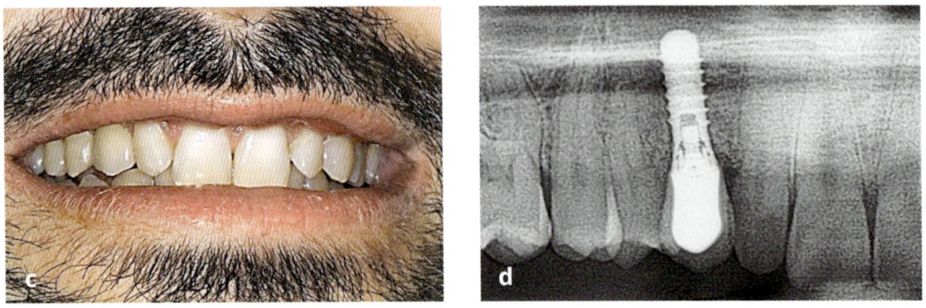

Figs 4-1c, d **(c)** Clinical and **(d)** radiographic images after completion of implant rehabilitation. Assessment of the risk factors foretells a good outcome of the implant treatment: nonsmoker status; consistency in oral hygiene; compliance with the maintenance program; thick soft tissue phenotype; and no history of periodontitis.

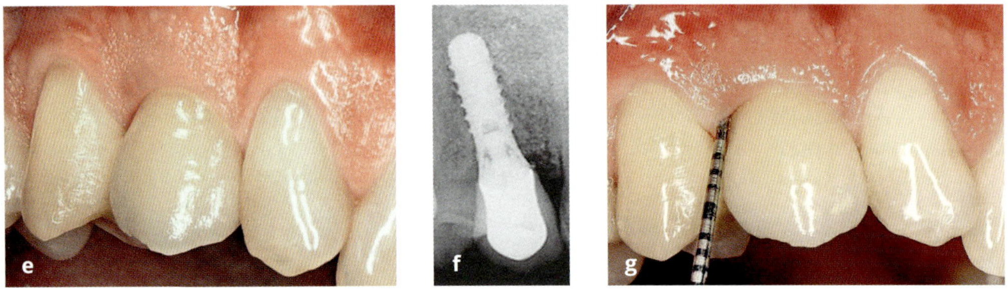

Figs 4-1e–g Maintenance of the results 3 years after implant placement. Note the absence of inflammation, alveolar margin stability, presence of a peri-implant sulcus, and absence of bleeding on probing.

4.1 Oral biofilms: the main etiologic factor for peri-implant diseases

Oral biofilms are the main etiologic factor for peri-implant diseases, as shown by many experimental and clinical studies. Dental plaque is a biofilm of organized microbial colonies that adhere to any hard, non-shedding surface in the fluid system of the oral cavity. Accordingly, calcification of biofilm occurs on these surfaces and gives rise to more abundant biofilm formation (Figs 4-2a, b).[2]

Immediately after implant placement, glycoproteins in saliva adhere to the titanium surfaces exposed to the oral cavity. These are high-molecular-weight mucins, α-amylases, and glycoproteins rich in proline; saliva albumin also plays an important role in the organization of the biofilm structure, mainly in the presence of free calcium ions. On these glycoproteins, microorganisms that will eventually form a biofilm adhere and multiply, like biofilm formation on teeth or restorations. Once microorganisms are organized in a biofilm, they behave like a multicellular organism that has defense mechanisms and regulated metabolic behavior to cope with a periodic lack of substrates and heterogeneous subpopulations, with a different functional purpose.

The composition of the microbiome colonizing the peri-implant sulcus in partially edentulous patients may qualitatively and quantitatively differ from the peri-implant microbiome of completely edentulous patients. Microbiologic studies have shown that the microbiota detected around osseointegrated implants shortly after being placed in totally edentulous patients is the same as that found in edentulous areas of patients without implants. The first microorganisms to adhere to the surface of implants are facultative organisms: Gram-positive cocci, mainly streptococci (ie, *Streptococcus sanguis* and *Streptococcus mitis*) and actinomycetes. Within a short time, implants are colonized by motile rod-shaped bacteria and spirochetes. In completely edentulous patients,

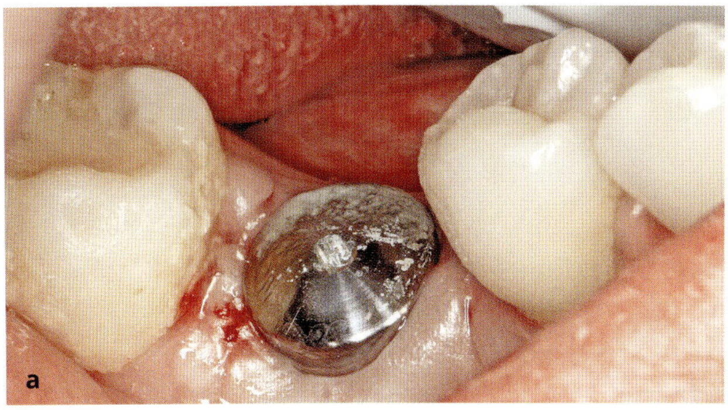

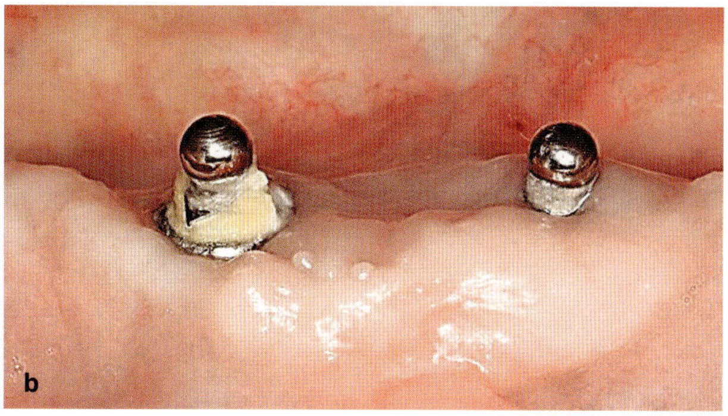

Figs 4-2a, b The biofilm is deposited on any surface in the oral cavity. Calculus can form around implants or their various components, such as healing screws or the transmucosal abutments of the removable prosthetic restorations.

periodontal pathogens such as *Aggregatibacter actinomycetemcomitans* and *Porphyromonas gingivalis* are detected less frequently than around implants in partially edentulous patients.

Gradually, the thickness of the dental biofilm increases, with proliferation of the already attached microbes and the addition of new microorganisms. The various species of streptococci and fusobacteria, mainly *Fusobacterium nucleatum*, play an important role in the growth of biofilm because they can attach and hold on to all other microorganisms, although they also co-aggregate. As the volume of dental biofilm increases, oxygen-deficient areas appear, thereby favoring the quantitative increase of strictly anaerobic microorganisms, such as *Veillonella* and actinomycetes. In most dentate patients, a higher percentage of black-pigmented bacteria and strains of the genus *Capnocytophaga* have been detected using anaerobic culturing techniques.

The dental biofilm on the surface of implants is gradually organized, especially in the absence of effective oral hygiene, resulting in the predominance of strictly anaerobic microbes, such as *Prevotella intermedia*, *F. nucleatum*, *Peptostreptococcus micros*, *P. gingivalis*, and *A. actinomycetemcomitans*.

Depending on the surface characteristics of implants (coating material, treatment method, degree of roughness, shape), the composition of the microbiome may be modified in completely and partially edentulous patients.[3] However, no specific correlation has been established between the type of implant or the roughness of its surface and the composition of the microbiome of the implant sulcus. If the rough part of the implant is placed inside the alveolar bone, roughness does not play a role in the colonization pattern of the biofilm. In experimental models where rough surfaces were placed supracrestally, there was an increase in the rate of biofilm accumulation but no qualitative change in its composition. As for the effect of implant surface roughness on the composition of the submucosal microbiome, it is clear that bone loss precedes exposure of the implant surface to the environment of the pocket.

Fitting of the implant-supported prosthetic restoration and the smoothness of the prosthetic accessories and restorations play an important role in the composition of the microbiome. Poor fitting or retention of cement around implant-supported prosthetic restorations favor the growth and proliferation of anaerobic periodontal pathogens (Figs 4-3a–d).

The factor that plays the most decisive role in the formation of the peri-implant microbiome is the composition of preexisting periodontal lesions serving as a reservoir for pathogens. In partially edentulous patients treated for chronic periodontitis, a similarity has been confirmed between the percentages of periodontal pathogens detected in the peri-implant sulci and those found in the residual periodontal pockets of teeth. In these patients, the biofilm follows the same pattern of maturation in teeth and at implants.[4]

The microbiome in peri-implantitis is similar to that associated with periodontitis. Gram-negative anaerobic microorganisms, such as *A. actinomycetemcomitans*, *P. gingivalis*, and *P. intermedia*, predominate. Several studies support the existence of *F. nucleatum*, *Staphylococcus aureus*, enterococci, and actinomycetes in peri-implant sulci. Regardless of the condition of the peri-implant tissues, in partially edentulous patients higher percentages of *P. gingivalis* and *Leptotrichia buccalis* were detected.[5,6]

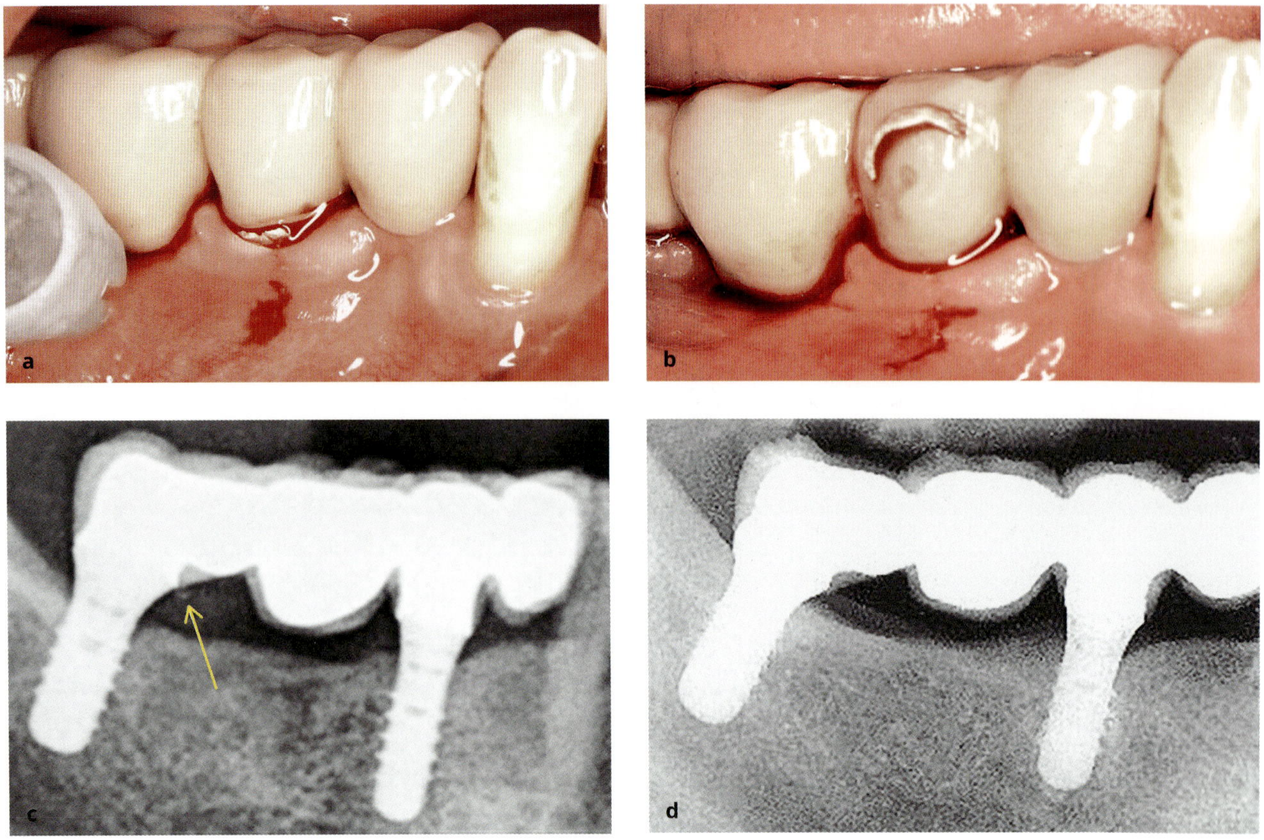

Figs 4-3a–d (a) In the first scheduled maintenance appointment after placement of the fixed dental prosthesis, intense inflammation and bleeding on probing were detected, which were caused by microbial challenge due to the presence of cement residue. (b) Cement can be seen around the neck of the implant. (c) Radiograph taken immediately after placement of the prosthesis. Detection of even a minimal radiopaque deposit in the contact area of the implant/prosthesis should raise suspicion of the presence of cement (yellow arrow). (d) Radiograph taken 6 years later showing preservation of the integrity of the alveolar bone.

In addition, higher percentages of *A. actinomycetemcomitans*, *P. gingivalis*, and *P. intermedia* were isolated from implants with deeper pockets and clinical signs of inflammation. Therefore, restoration of periodontal health must precede implant placement.[7] Implant placement in untreated periodontal patients constitutes a breach of the accepted standards of care.[8,9]

4.2 Risk factors for the development of peri-implant diseases

4.2.1 Patient history of periodontitis

Many patients in need of implant-supported restorations have lost some or all of their teeth from chronic or aggressive periodontitis. The predictability of long-term effectiveness of implant therapy in patients with a history of periodontitis has aroused considerable research interest. The main questions are whether or not a history of periodontitis is a risk factor for a higher rate of implant loss and for the incidence of peri-implantitis.

Many studies have confirmed that periodontal pathogens may be transferred from a patient's teeth to their implants. The previous section described the striking resemblance between the microbiome detected in residual periodontal pockets and that isolated from implants affected by peri-implantitis. In fact, significantly higher rates of motile rod-shaped microorganisms and spirochetes have been reported in the peri-implant areas of patients with a history of advanced chronic periodontitis.

The first studies examining the possibility of a history of chronic periodontitis affecting the prognosis of implants found high survival rates; this was

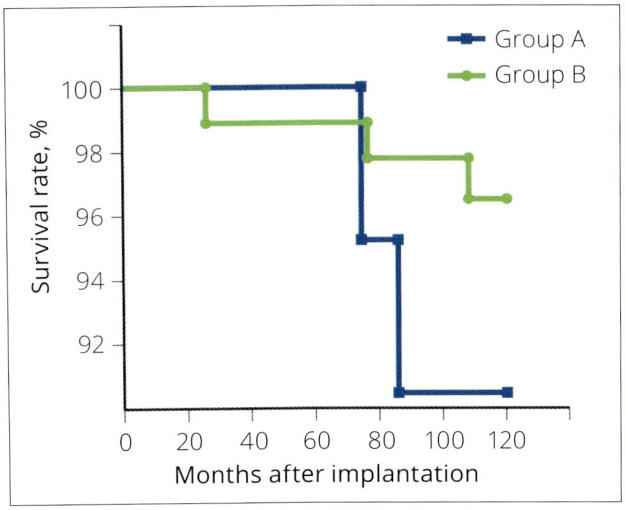

Fig 4-4 Difference in the survival rate of implants in patients with a history of periodontitis (group A, blue line) and in periodontally healthy patients (group B, green line). This difference supports the finding that a history of periodontitis is a risk factor for implant survival and is indirectly connected to the development of peri-implantitis (adapted from Karoussis et al[10]).

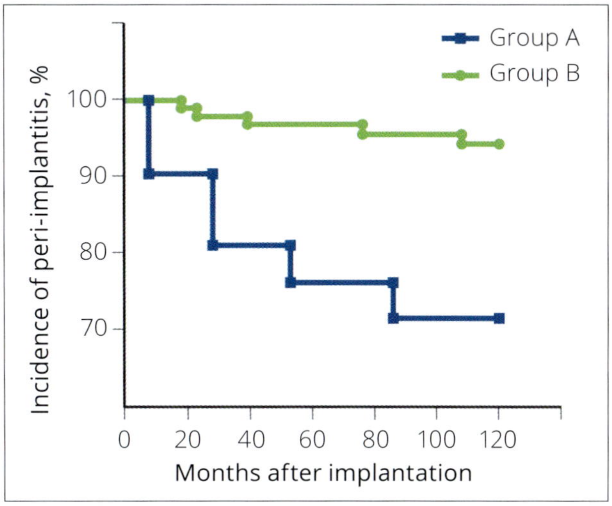

Fig 4-5 Difference in the incidence rate of peri-implantitis in patients with a history of periodontitis (group A, blue line) and implants in periodontally healthy patients (group B, green line). This difference is statistically significant and confirms that a history of periodontitis is a risk factor for implant placement (adapted from Karoussis et al[10]).

mistakenly described as "success" (details on survival and success are described in Chapter 6). The literature clearly concludes that implant placement is not contraindicated in patients who have previously developed and undergone treatment for chronic periodontitis.

In the early 2000s, the effect of a history of chronic periodontitis on the outcome of implant therapy was documented.[10] In the first prospective study published on this subject, a failure rate (implant loss) of 3.5% was reported after 10 years of observation for implants placed in patients without a history of periodontitis; the corresponding rate for implants placed in patients with a history of chronic periodontitis was close to 9.5% (Fig 4-4).

Implant success was examined according to several different criteria. Depending on the rigor of the criteria, success rates ranged from 52.4% to 81.0% for implants in patients with a history of chronic periodontitis and from 79.0% to 96.7% in patients without such a history. For each set of criteria selected, there was a significant difference in success rates between the two groups of patients. In patients with a history of chronic periodontitis, deterioration of clinical parameters was observed, such as peri-implant pocket depth, bleeding on probing, and progressive, radiographically established bone loss. In this study, a history of chronic periodontitis was shown to be a risk factor for peri-implantitis. The incidence of peri-implantitis was 5.8% and 28.6% in implants placed in individuals without and with a history of chronic periodontitis, respectively (Fig 4-5).[10]

Further analysis of the data led to evidence of a synergistic, negative impact of smoking on implant prognosis because smokers with a history of periodontitis had lower survival rates than non-smokers. In addition, smokers with a history of periodontitis had higher rates of peri-implantitis than smokers without a history of periodontitis.[10]

Several clinicians argued that implants were not affected by patients' preexisting periodontal status, even going so far as to express opinions in favor of a prognosis of implants than that of the existing teeth. This discrepancy may be explained by the fact that the views of these clinicians were based on sporadic observations and not on well-designed retrospective or even prospective cohort studies. After all, the influence of the history of chronic periodontitis on implant prognosis was confirmed in studies a few years later. Some of these studies were performed on patients with smooth-surface implants. In one study with a follow-up period of up to 14 years, a significant difference in implant survival was confirmed; in addition, the crucial role of patient inclusion in an individualized maintenance program was emphasized.

As shown, the risk of developing peri-implantitis does not differ depending on the roughness of the implant surface. The host's susceptibility to the disease is the leading cause of peri-implantitis.[11,12]

Although the presence of microorganisms is necessary for the initiation of peri-implant diseases, it is not sufficient in itself to affect the incidence of peri-implantitis. The presence of periodontal pathogens in residual periodontal pockets does not necessarily imply future bone loss or implant failure. It determines the composition of the peri-implant microbiome. The risk of implant loss or peri-implantitis is related more to patient characteristics than to implant-related factors.

An interesting study conducted in patients with implants affected by peri-implantitis compared to implants surrounded by healthy peri-implant tissues confirmed this. Microbiological analysis of the submucosal microbiome showed that the periodontal pathogens *Prevotella nigrescens*, *P. micros*, and *F. nucleatum*, and some mediators of inflammation (prostaglandin E_2, interleukin-1β, and tumor necrosis factor-α) were detected in the gingival fluid of implants affected by peri-implantitis and at implants with healthy peri-implant tissues. In implants with peri-implantitis, a higher number of periodontal pathogens and higher concentrations of mediators of inflammation were observed. That is, in the mouth of each patient, the same microorganisms were isolated regardless of the degree of peri-implant health, but at increased levels in diseased peri-implant tissues. Systematic reviews provided conclusive evidence that the history of chronic periodontitis is a risk factor for the incidence of peri-implantitis. In one of these systematic reviews, even though implant survival rates in patients with a history of aggressive periodontitis were acceptable for a follow-up period of up to 5 years, the deterioration of peri-implant tissue health did not follow the same pattern as in patients with a history of chronic periodontitis. This was the first study to report on a more cautious long-term implant prognosis for patients with aggressive periodontitis, something that was further researched in the years that followed.[13]

To date, there is no evidence to prove that the prognosis for implants may be better than that of periodontally treated teeth. Teeth and implants that coexist in the mouth of the same patient follow a common model in the deterioration of periodontal health. This, in turn, means that when a maintenance program is followed, any condition observed in the teeth may be reflected at implants also. If there is a deterioration in clinical and radiographic parameters in a patient's dentition, a similar deterioration may be observed at their implant sites. Therefore, the paradigm to extract teeth "while there is still adequate bone" is on weak grounds. Successful periodontal treatment may predictably maintain teeth that were previously periodontally affected for a long time.

Clinicians should exhaust the range of therapeutic approaches offered by modern periodontology and general dentistry to save and maintain the natural dentition. They should not consider tooth extraction and implant placement as a primary objective (Figs 4-6a–g).

4.2.2 Specifics of implant treatment of patients with aggressive periodontitis (stage III or IV, grade C)

According to the available data, regarding the outcome of implant placement in patients with aggressive periodontitis, research has concluded that after implant placement, the survival rate in the short term and up to 3 years is acceptable (95% to 100%), whereas for 5 years it is reduced (88%).[52]

Consequently, the implant bone loss observed in patients with a history of aggressive periodontitis is at levels similar to those observed in healthy controls or patients treated for chronic periodontitis for up to 3 years. However, 3 years after implant placement, there is a significant change in pocket depth and attachment loss. According to data from a long-term prospective study,[52] patients with a history of aggressive periodontitis were five times more likely to lose an implant over a follow-up period of 3 to 16 years, despite involvement in a quarterly maintenance care program. In addition, they were three times more likely to develop peri-implant mucositis and 14 times more likely to develop peri-implantitis than healthy controls.

In contrast to patients with a history of chronic periodontitis, teeth and implants that coexist in the mouth of a patient with a history of aggressive periodontitis do not follow a common pattern for the

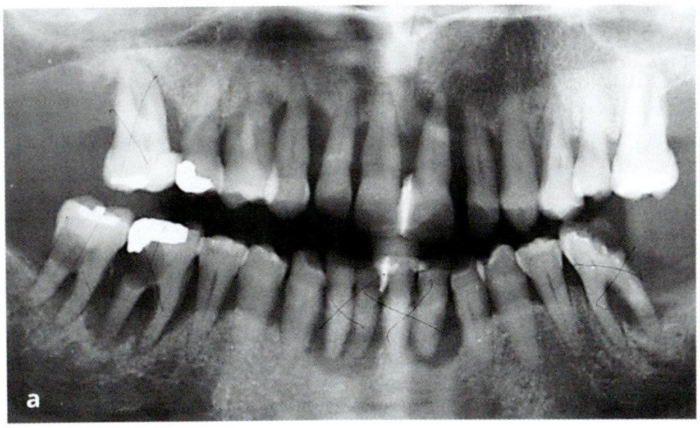

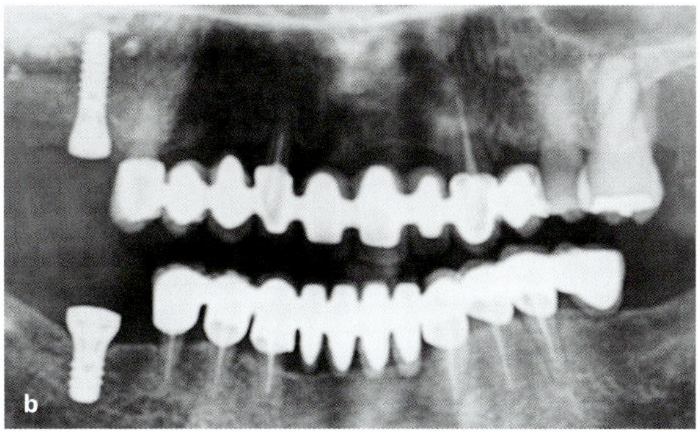

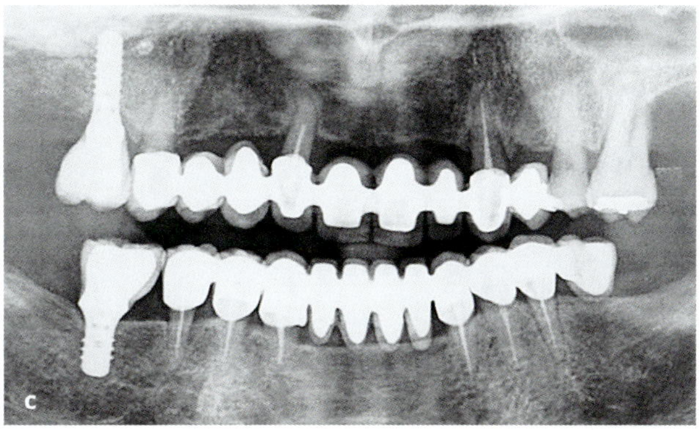

Figs 4-6a–c **(a)** Radiographic image of a patient with advanced chronic periodontitis (according to the 2017 classification: stage IV, grade C). The condition is a risk factor for the outcome of implant treatment. **(b)** One year after completion of perio-prosthetic treatment, implants are placed. Periodontal treatment must be completed and any risk factors must be addressed. **(c)** Radiographic image of the patient 6 years after implant placement.

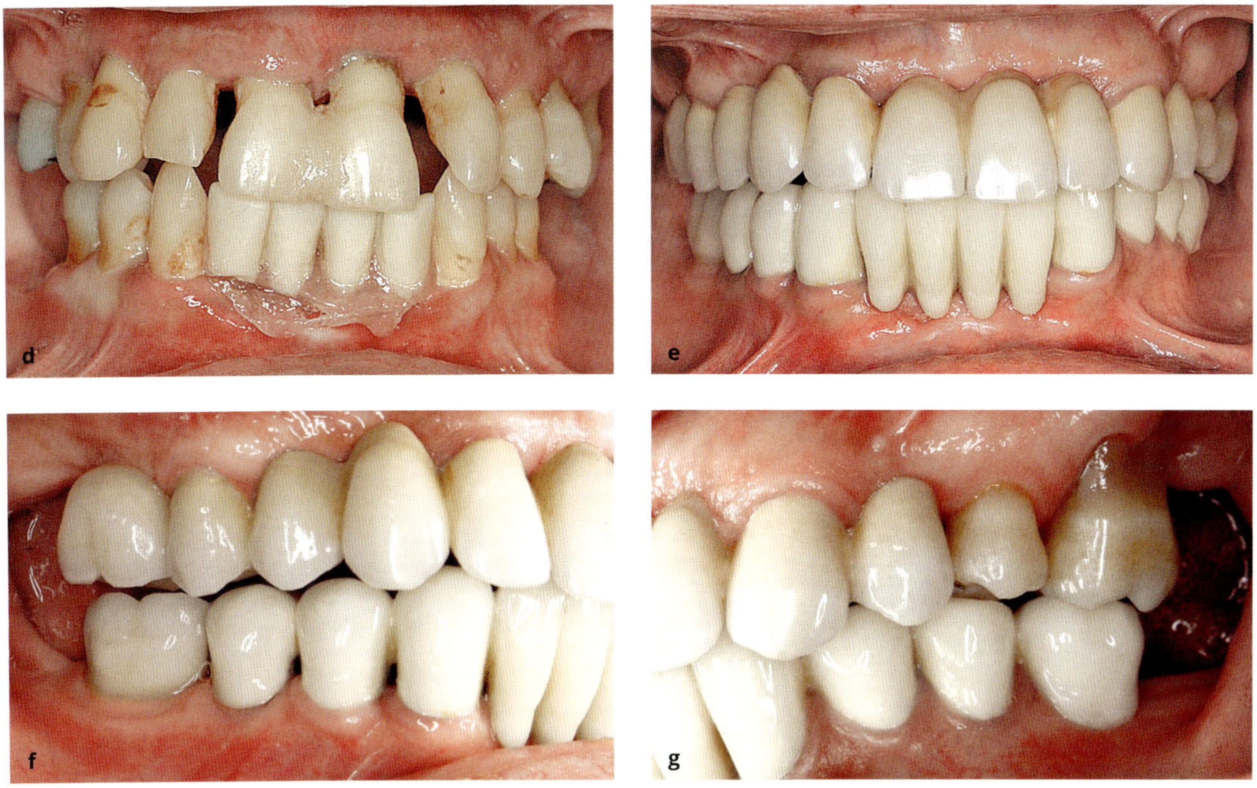

Figs 4-6d–g **(d)** Clinical picture of the patient before perio-prosthetic treatment, after placement of a temporary prosthetic restoration in the mandibular anterior teeth and temporary immobilization of nos. 11 and 21 to avoid spontaneous extraction. **(e)** Clinical picture 7 years after completion of perio-prosthetic treatment. **(f and g)** Images showing the healthy periodontal and peri-implant tissues due to careful compliance with the rules during the design and development of the treatment plan and the patient's consistency in performing oral hygiene on a daily basis and attending maintenance appointments every 3 months for 7 years.

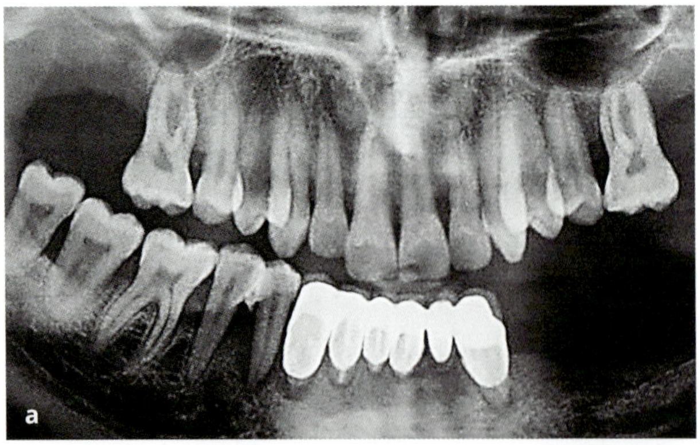
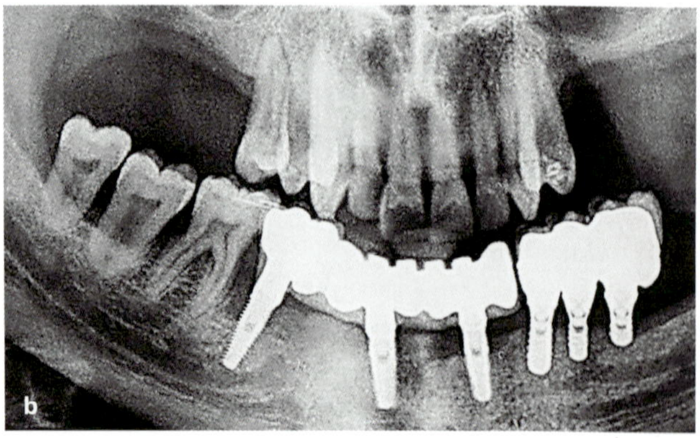
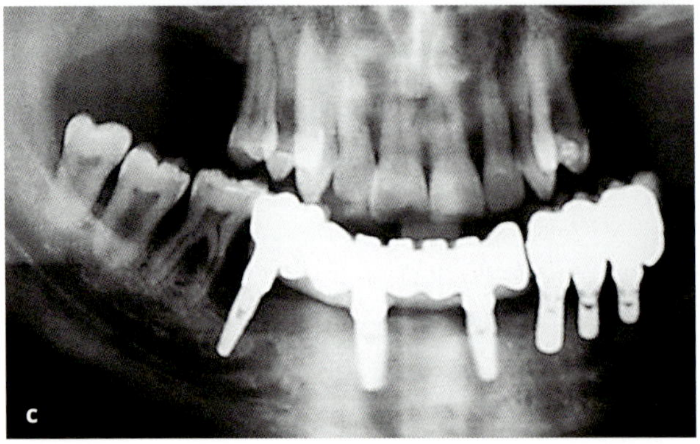

Figs 4-7a–c **(a)** Radiographic image of a 25-year-old patient with generalized aggressive periodontitis (according to the 2017 classification: stage IV, grade C). **(b)** Radiographic image taken just 3 years after implant placement. Bone loss is evident and the long-term survival of the implants is not assured. **(c)** Four years after placement of the prosthetic restoration, the radiographic image shows further deterioration of the implant bone support. In patients with aggressive periodontitis, implant prognosis is worse than in periodontally healthy patients or patients with a history of chronic periodontitis.

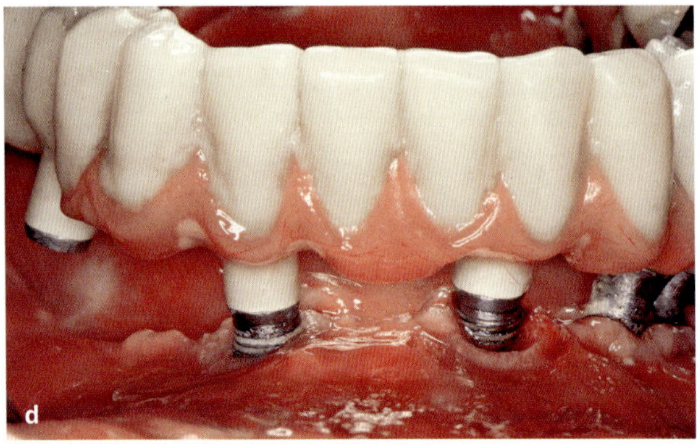
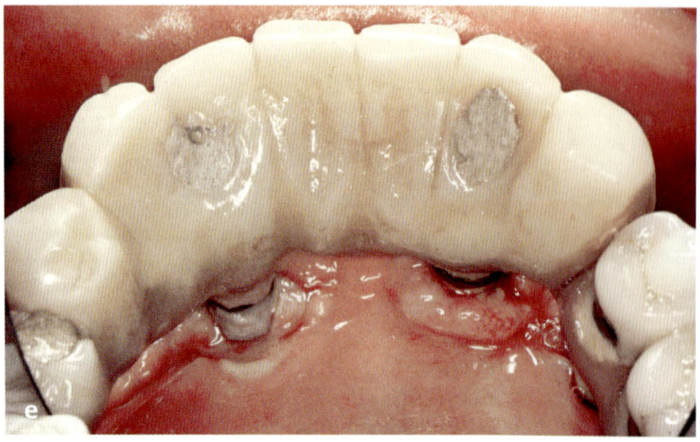

Figs 4-7d, e Clinical images 5 years after implant placement. The case is the same as shown in Fig 9-14 of Chapter 9. The condition is now very serious; implant removal and planning of a new treatment must be considered.

development of periodontal and peri-implant tissue pathology. The deterioration of the clinical and radiographic parameters observed in implants is likely greater than that observed in the teeth of the same patient.[14]

The choice of a treatment plan that includes implants for a patient with aggressive periodontitis should be made with particular caution because the implant survival rate is lower in the long term and the expected incidence rates of peri-implantitis are higher (Figs 4-7a–e).

4.2.3 Systemic health

The influence of specific systemic factors on the initiation and development of peri-implant diseases is a point of particular interest. However, the available evidence on the subject is limited because of the very small number of prospective studies. In contrast, many studies have provided clear answers about the effect of various diseases and conditions on the success of osseointegration, that is, whether or not these diseases contribute to early failure of implants.

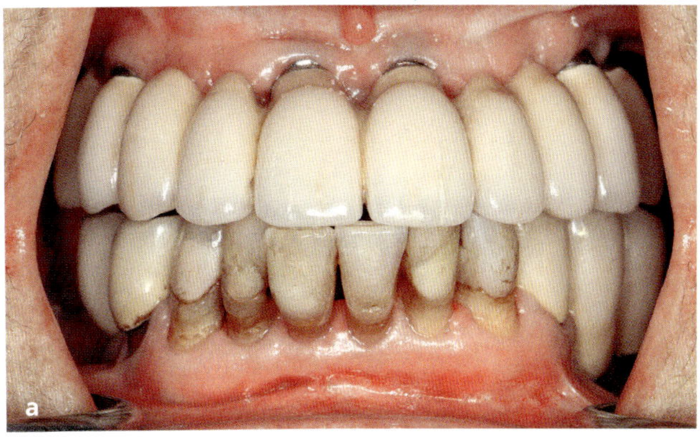

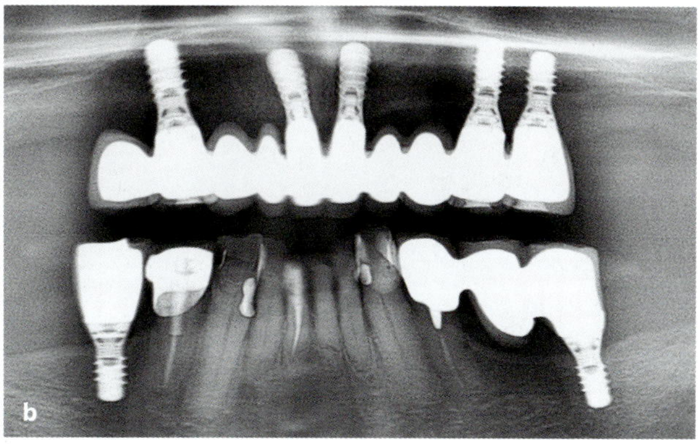

Figs 4-8a, b Clinical and radiographic images of a patient with scleroderma. The implants were placed gradually over a period of 4 to 10 years. Despite the difficulty in opening the mouth and the stiffness of the fingers, the consistency in the application of effective oral hygiene on a daily basis and the continuous participation in the maintenance program led to an excellent therapeutic result.

Uncontrolled diabetes has been blamed for the increased incidence of peri-implantitis. Therefore, special care should be taken to maintain acceptable blood sugar levels, with regular monitoring of glycosylated hemoglobin and inclusion of patients with diabetes in a strictly individualized maintenance care program. The effect of osteoporosis, radiotherapy, and several autoimmune diseases on the development of peri-implantitis is contradictory. Many more studies are needed to characterize these or other systemic diseases or conditions as risk factors for the incidence of peri-implantitis (Figs 4-8a, b).[15]

4.2.4 Genetic factors

Biofilms being the main etiologic factor for peri-implantitis is certainly a necessity but not a sufficient condition (on its own) to cause bone loss. The latter, in fact, is due to the host's immune response. This suggests a possible correlation of each patient's sensitivity to peri-implantitis with their genetic background, emphasizing the possible involvement of genetic factors in the establishment and development of peri-implantitis. Despite conflicting results, this view is further substantiated by the highly unequal distribution of the disease in the general population. According to existing research, polymorphisms in the interleukin-1 (IL1) gene complex play an important role in smokers. Research has supported the association of IL1 genetic polymorphisms with the occurrence of peri-implantitis and with a reduced response to treatment. In addition, the presence of elevated levels of proinflammatory cytokines, such as IL-1, in the peri-implant sulcus, indicated inflammatory activity and predicted the onset of peri-implant disease.[16,17] However, these results are not universally accepted, as other studies focusing on assessing the possible involvement of genetic factors did not reveal any association between peri-implantitis and IL1 polymorphisms or other gene polymorphisms such as tumor necrosis factor alpha.[18]

Finally, special attention should be paid to the ethnic origin of patients in different studies because certain alleles occur with different frequencies between ethnic groups.[19–22]

4.2.5 Behavioral factors

As the main etiologic factor for peri-implantitis is dental biofilm, its successful removal contributes significantly to maintaining peri-implant tissue health. Practicing effective oral hygiene will prevent the establishment and organization of microorganisms that contribute to peri-implant mucositis and its progression to peri-implantitis. A very strong association between ineffective oral hygiene and the onset and severity of peri-implantitis has been documented, as the Plaque Index is associated not only with soft tissue inflammation but also with peri-implant bone loss. In addition, there is a synergistic effect of poor oral hygiene with smoking. In particular, smokers who do not perform effective oral hygiene experience three times more implant bone loss. Implant placement in patients who either cannot or do not want to perform effective oral hygiene on a daily basis should be avoided (Figs 4-9a–c).

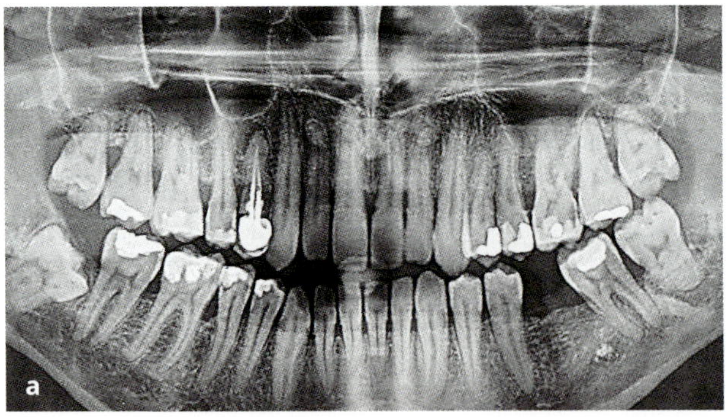

Figs 4-9a–c (a) Radiographic image showing that placement of an implant in the position of the missing no. 36 is possible. However, the patient's attitude precluded such a treatment plan. **(b)** Clinical image showing the condition in which the patient came for treatment. Soft tissue inflammation and the accumulation of large amounts of biofilm causing it are evident. **(c)** Clinical image showing the completely ineffective oral hygiene applied by the patient despite having received multiple sessions dedicated to this exercise for this purpose.

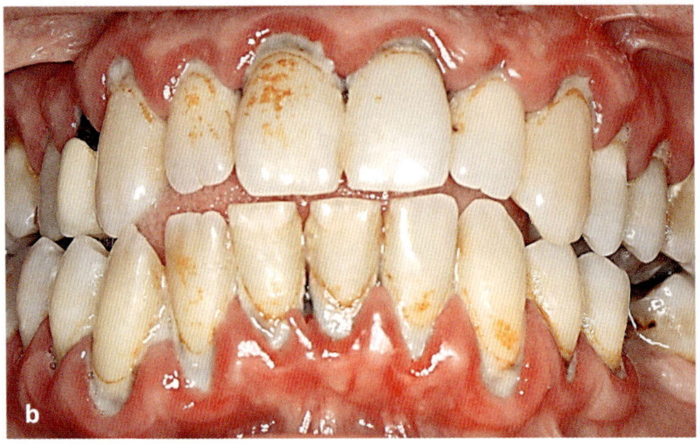

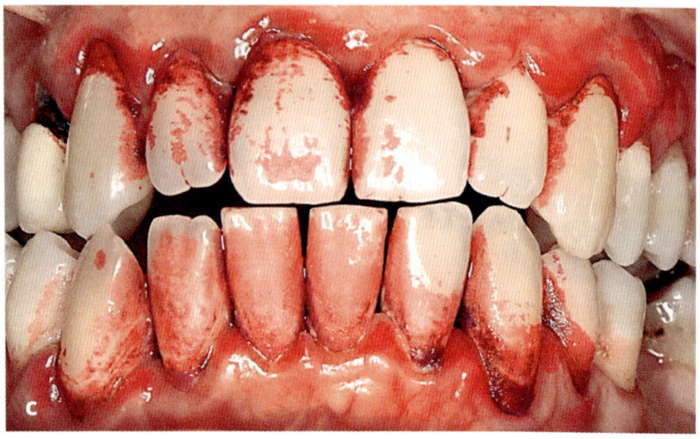

A particularly important factor related to human behavior is smoking. The extremely aggravating effect of smoking on both periodontal and peri-implant tissues has been demonstrated in several relevant prospective and retrospective studies, the results of which showed a dramatic increase in the risk of implant loss, especially in heavy smokers (20 cigarettes or more per day). The risk of implant loss due to peri-implantitis in smokers, after implant loading, has been estimated to be from 2.5 to 4.6 times higher than in non-smokers. In other words, smokers have a 250% to 460% higher risk of developing peri-implantitis.[11,23–25] Some studies reported that heavy smokers have a 31% chance of implant loss, whereas light and moderate smokers have a 10% chance of losing implants. Regardless of the percentages reported in different studies, they all point to a particularly high risk of complications in smokers having implants placed, regardless of the number of cigarettes they smoke per day. The risk is greater for implants placed in the maxilla (Figs 4-10a, b).[11,23–25]

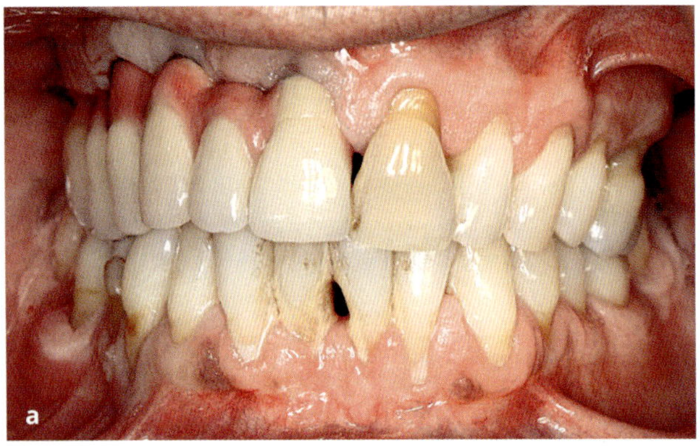

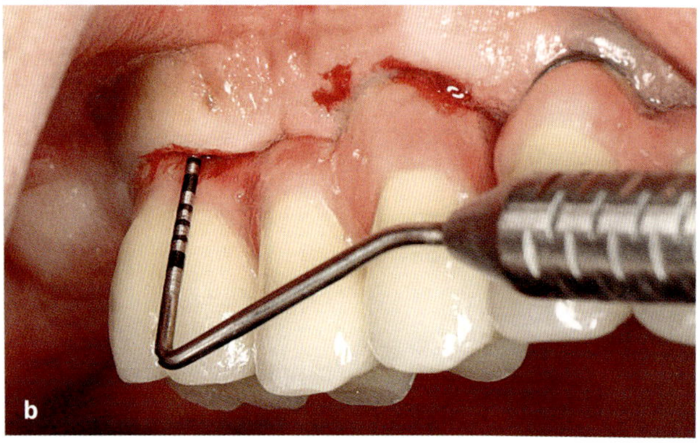

Figs 4-10a, b (a) A heavy smoker, who was inconsistent in performing daily oral hygiene and presented with a history of periodontitis. Implant prognosis was doubtful. **(b)** Despite the fibrous consistency of the soft peri-implant tissues, deep pockets and bleeding on probing were detected.

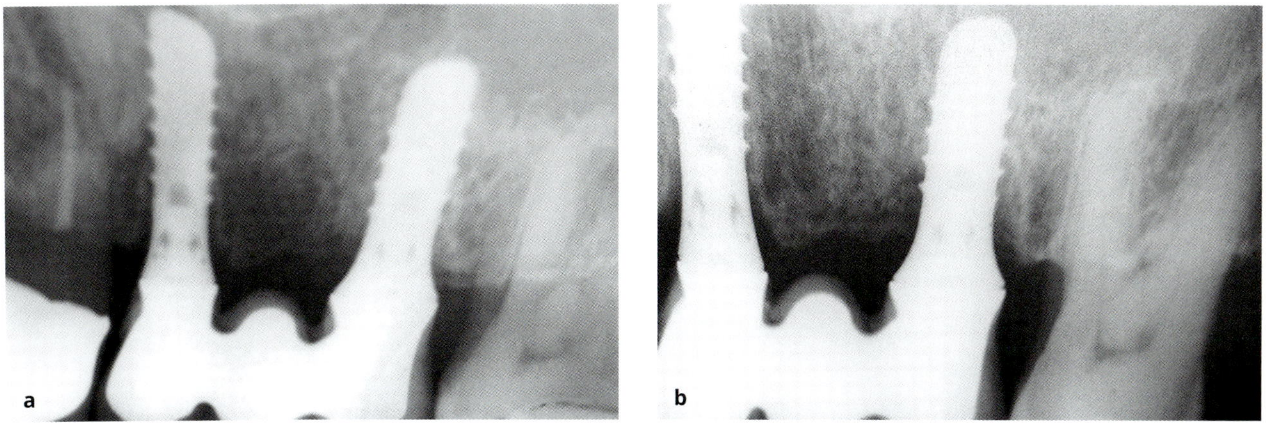

Figs 4-11a, b Implants **(a)** 5 and **(b)** 7 years after placement in a heavy smoker. The patient came for treatment (cumulative interceptive supportive therapy protocol, A and B) but did not agree to surgery or smoking cessation. The establishment and development of peri-implantitis is obvious.

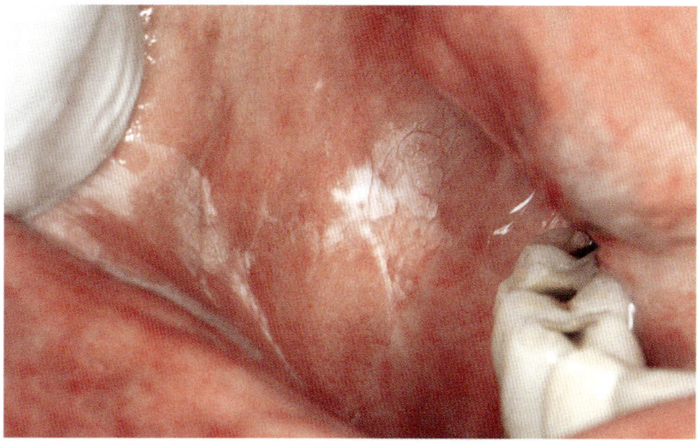

Fig 4-11c Image showing leukoplakia lesions attributed to smoking. However, the patient did not intend to quit.

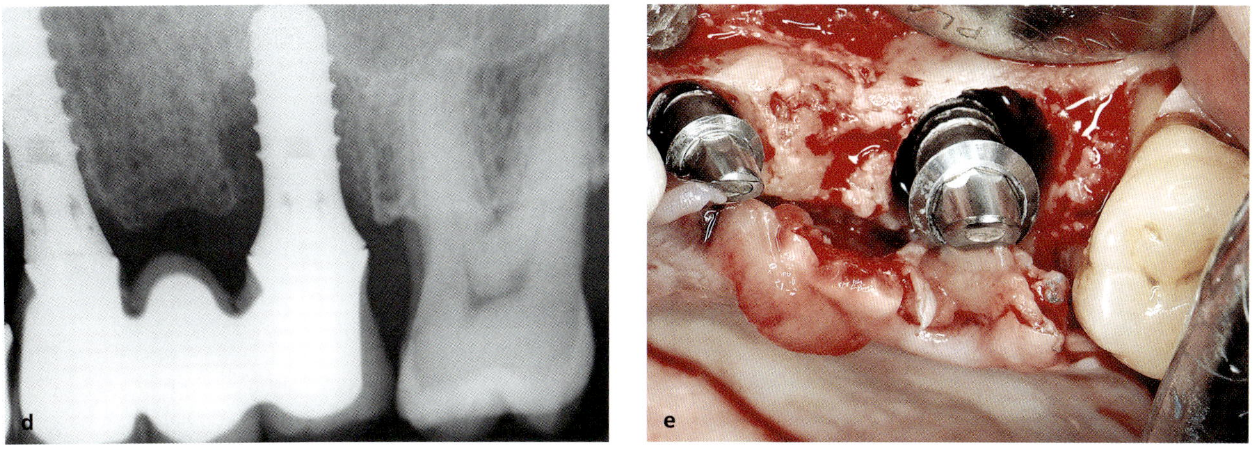

Figs 4-11d, e Eight years after implant placement and after the patient agreed to surgery but not smoking cessation. Increased bone loss within a year is evident.

In addition, the effectiveness of peri-implantitis therapy is limited in smokers. Consequently, implant survival rates are expected to be lower in smokers (Figs 4-11a–i).[26]

The negative effect of tobacco consumption on peri-implant tissues is exacerbated by the simultaneous use of alcohol. There is a statistically significant association between smoking, alcohol

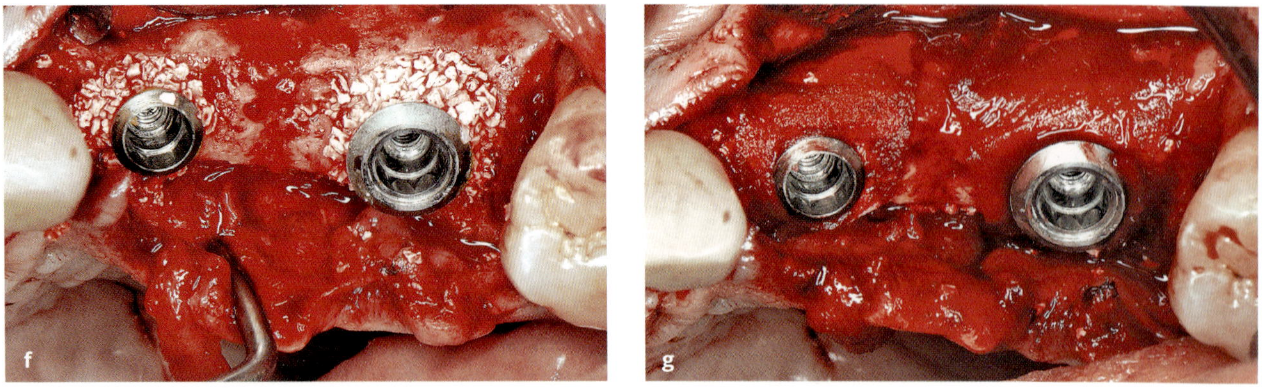

Figs 4-11f, g An attempt was made to regenerate the lost bone with guided bone regeneration.

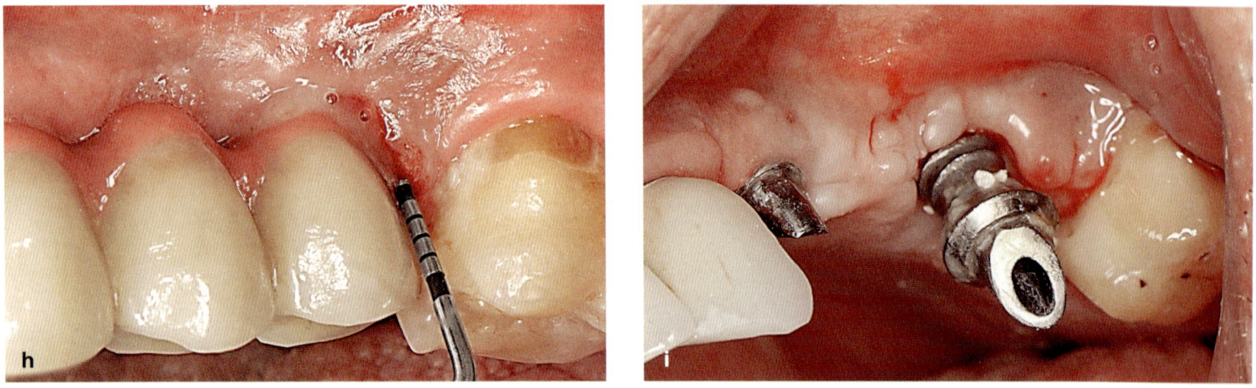

Figs 4-11h, I Three months after surgery, the implant was removed due to failure as it had become mobile.

consumption, and poor oral hygiene with the occurrence of peri-implantitis. According to some studies, daily consumption of alcohol (> 10 grams) can cause more extensive implant bone loss than smoking. However, as a single parameter, the effect of alcohol consumption on the occurrence of peri-implantitis is difficult to investigate because most patients who consume alcohol daily are also smokers.[27]

Another factor that reflects patient behavior is compliance with an individualized maintenance program. Studies involving periodontal patients in either university clinics or private clinics recorded particularly low patient response rates to the recall system, especially after the first 5 years of treatment. Only one-third of patients were fully responsive, whereas almost 45% of patients never returned for follow-up appointments. This parameter is very important because implants placed in patients who do not participate in such programs show signs of peri-implantitis in the 5-year radiographic images, at a rate that reaches 70%.[53] Well-designed prospective studies that record particularly high survival or success rates of various implant systems have been performed in large university research centers, with well-organized and structured patient recall programs. Unfortunately, these rates are rarely confirmed in the daily clinical practice of private dental clinics. Clinical experience shows that many patients receive implants without ever coming back for reexamination as part of the maintenance phase, either because of personal negligence or because they were poorly informed of the importance of complying with the recall program or the negative consequences of not doing so. Sadly, patients' complete lack of compliance is due to negligence (Figs 4-12a–h).[28–30]

Dental practitioners lacking or avoiding information relating to the risk factors for peri-implantitis or, ultimately, implant failure, is unacceptable. Informing

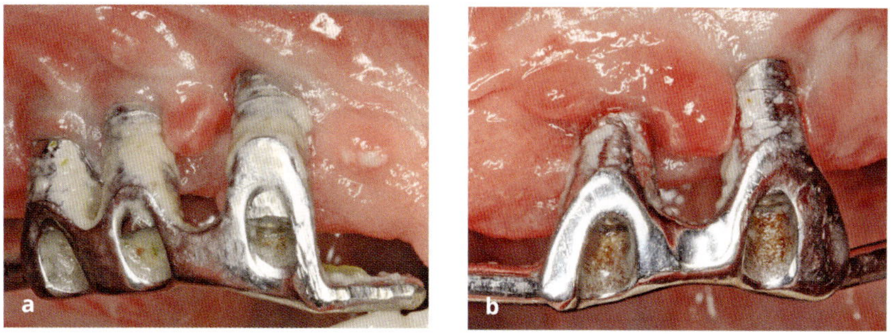

Figs 4-12a, b Clinical images of peri-implantitis in a patient who did not apply oral hygiene and did not undergo periodontal monitoring. The accumulation of biofilm for several years led to the development of peri-implantitis. Soft tissue inflammation and thread exposure are evident; these are covered by large amounts of biofilm.

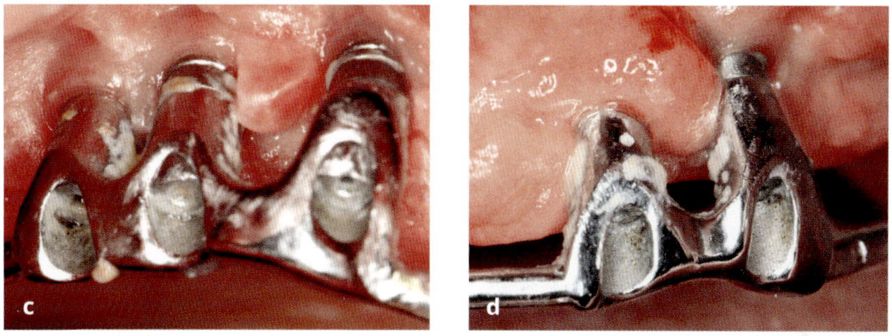

Figs 4-12c, d One year after repeated attempts, the patient was not successful in maintaining oral hygiene.

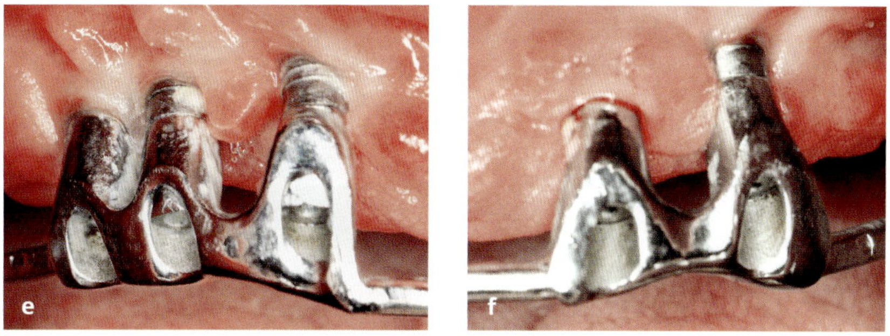

Figs 4-12e, f Eighteen months after the start of cause-related therapy, any improvement in the clinical appearance of the tissues was due to regular attendance at the dental office. Oral hygiene remained poor. Long-term implant prognosis was poor.

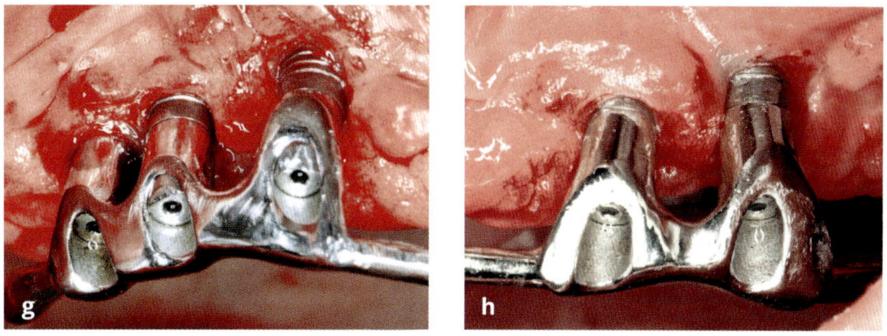

Figs 4-12 g, h Application of AIRFLOW (EMS Dental, Nyon, Switzerland) at regular intervals (every 1 to 2 months) is an essential solution however, it cannot replace optimal oral hygiene.

the patient about the importance of effective oral hygiene, and compliance with the individual recall program during the maintenance phase, should be an integral part of the initial treatment plan; non-compliance contributes significantly to the development of peri-implant tissue inflammation. Awareness of the need to attend recall appointments, highlighted during the first session with the new patient, doubles the percentage of patients who consistently attend maintenance sessions. In addition, the clinician should discourage the prospective patient from undergoing any treatment if they do not intend to practice effective oral hygiene on a daily basis and attend the recall sessions consistently. The patient is highly appreciative of this frank approach on the part of the clinician and is then prompted to a significant degree to collaborate with them.

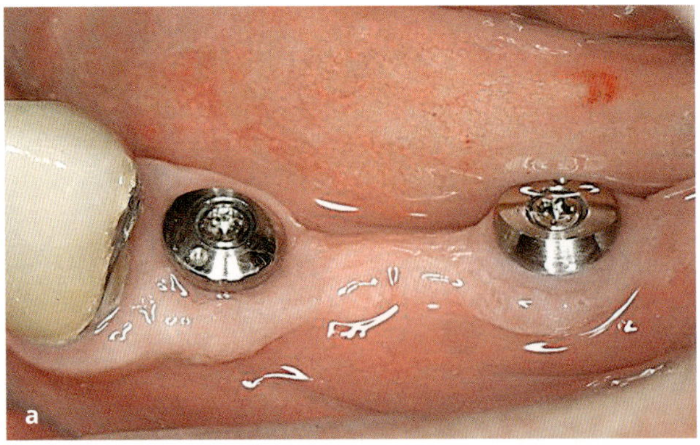

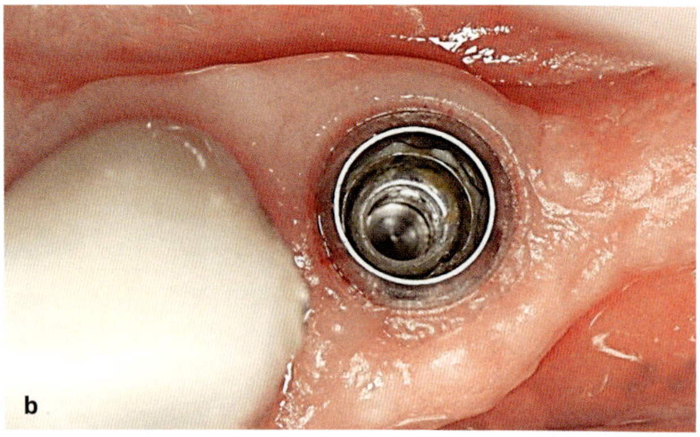

Figs 4-13a, b Adequate keratinized mucosa width around implants.

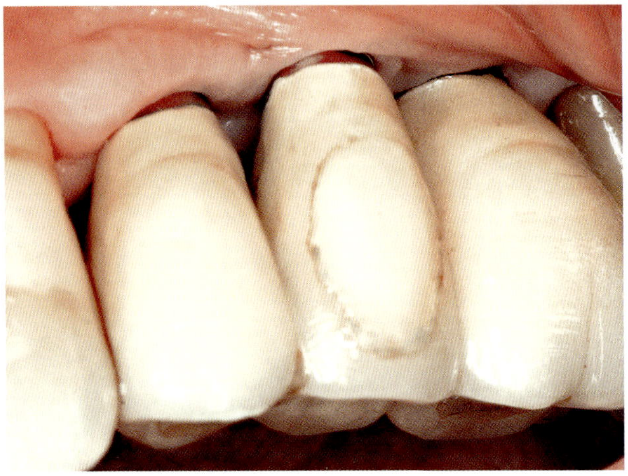

Fig 4-14 Implant health in the absence of keratinized mucosa when oral hygiene was administered effectively on a daily basis and the patient complied with an individualized maintenance program. Clinical picture taken 10 years after implant placement. The image also shows poor esthetics buccally of site no. 25 because a screwed restoration was chosen, while there was buccal deviation during implant placement.

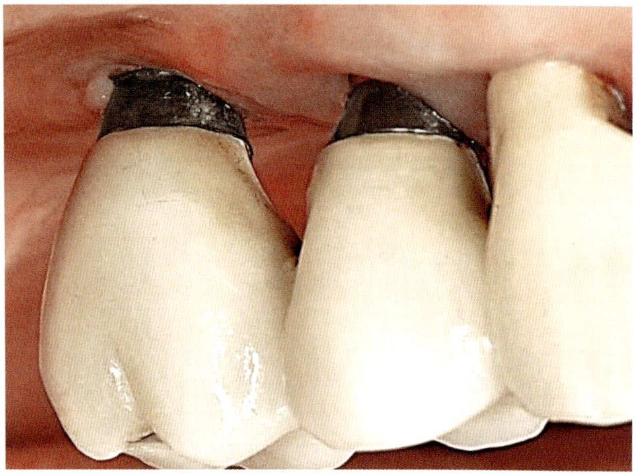

Fig 4-15 Image of a patient treated for peri-implantitis in implants in sites 14, 15, and 16. In addition, a free gingival graft was placed, which did not cover implant no. 16. Peri-implantitis recurred in this implant. Purulent exudate can be seen. (This is an image from the case described in Fig 4-17.)

4.2.6 Presence of keratinized mucosa around implants

The importance of having an adequate zone of keratinized mucosa around implants to maintain the health of peri-implant tissues has been the subject of intense research (Figs 4-13a, b).

Many studies have suggested that the presence of an adequate zone of keratinized tissue is not necessary to maintain the health of peri-implant tissues, provided that successful removal of dental biofilm is ensured daily and that the patient complies with an individualized maintenance care program (Fig 4-14).

In contrast, studies where experimental peri-implantitis was created using submucosal ligatures around the necks of implants in test animals found that peri-implant bone loss was greater in areas with a lack of keratinized mucosa.[31] Nevertheless, a significant number of clinical observations and studies support the view that the presence of even the slightest thickness of keratinized mucosa (1 to 2 mm) is desirable to avoid the occurrence of recession or attachment loss; if it is completely absent, performing oral hygiene is particularly difficult (Fig 4-15).[32]

For this reason, a preventive increase in the dimensions of keratinized tissues is advised before implant placement or during the second stage of implants placed using a two-stage protocol, along with the placement of free grafts and gingival or connective tissue (Figs 4-16a–f).

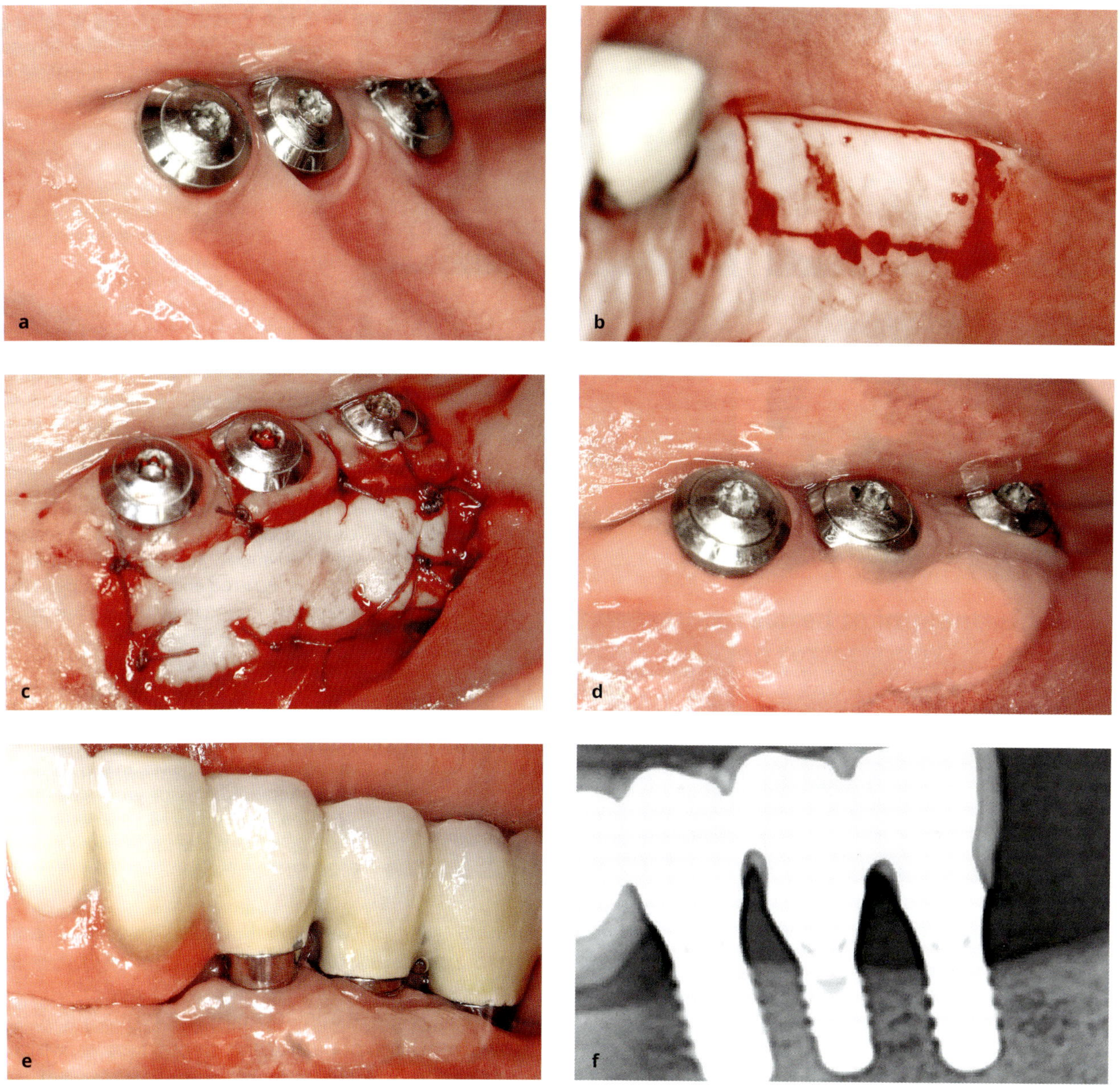

Figs 4-16a–f (a and b) The traction of the cheek causes tension to the nonattached peri-implant mucosa and favors food entrapment and makes it difficult to administer oral hygiene. To prevent peri-implantitis, a free gingival graft was obtained from an edentulous area of the maxillary alveolar ridge, after a partial thickness flap was prepared at the recipient site. **(c)** Graft suturing. **(d)** Clinical image of the area 1 month later. **(e and f)** Four years after graft placement, peri-implant health was maintained.

Even though there are differing views on the importance of the presence of adequate keratinized tissue width around implants, any changes in the morphology of the area should be taken into account, for example due resorption of the alveolar ridge, but also the possible complexity of implant-supported prosthetic rehabilitation, all conditions that may compromise the implementation of effective oral hygiene. The consequence, in the absence of keratinized mucosa, is usually injury of the peri-implant mucosa and a high concentration of biofilm, making the presence of keratinized tissues desirable. Daily clinical experience confirms this; the presence of keratinized tissues facilitates implant care. Finally, in cases of implants with peri-implantitis that are surrounded by a zone with inadequate width or thickness of keratinized mucosa, increasing the keratinized tissue zone is beneficial for inhibiting the progression or recurrence of disease (Fig 4-17a-f).

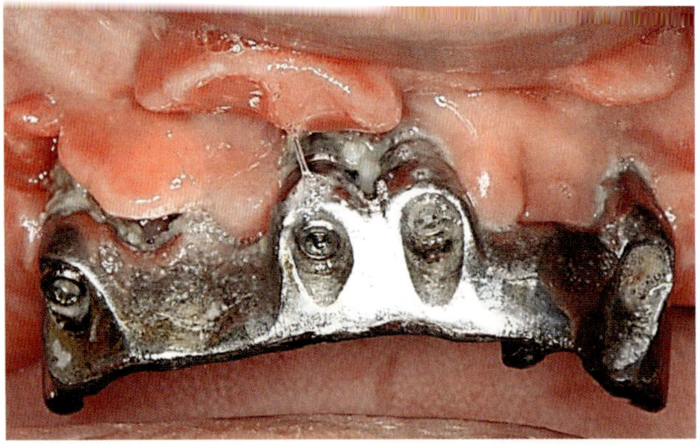

Fig 4-19 Poor construction of a bar for an implant-supported overdenture, which does not allow the administration of oral hygiene. In addition, the design of the denture is shorter, resulting in hyperplasia.

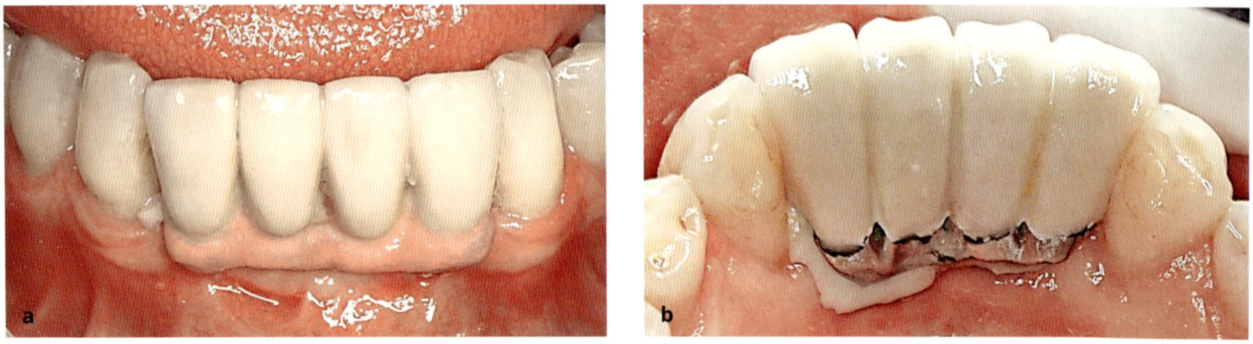

Figs 4-20a, b Poorly constructed fixed prosthetic restoration without any provision for maintaining the space for an interdental brush to maintain good oral hygiene.

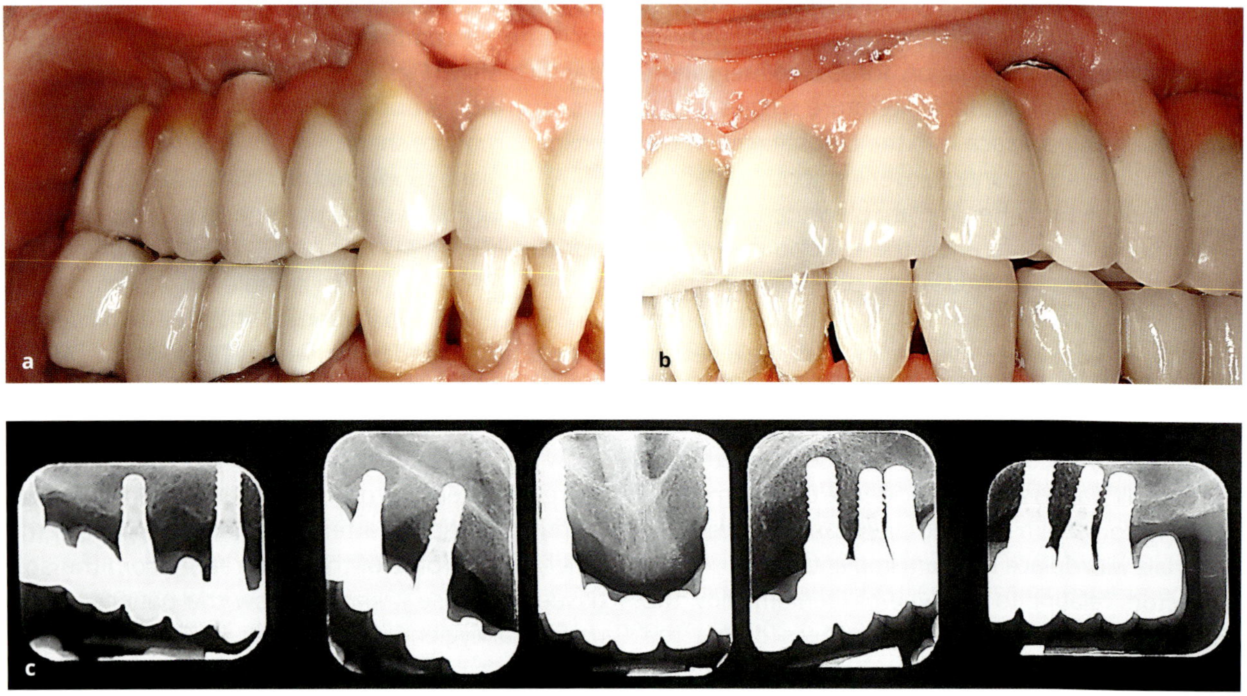

Figs 4-21a–c Clinical and radiographic images of a patient in whom all the rules of proper placement and implant rehabilitation were observed. The design of the prosthesis serves the esthetic and functional needs of the patient, while at the same time allowing the application of effective oral hygiene with an anatomic contour that enables interdental cleaning.

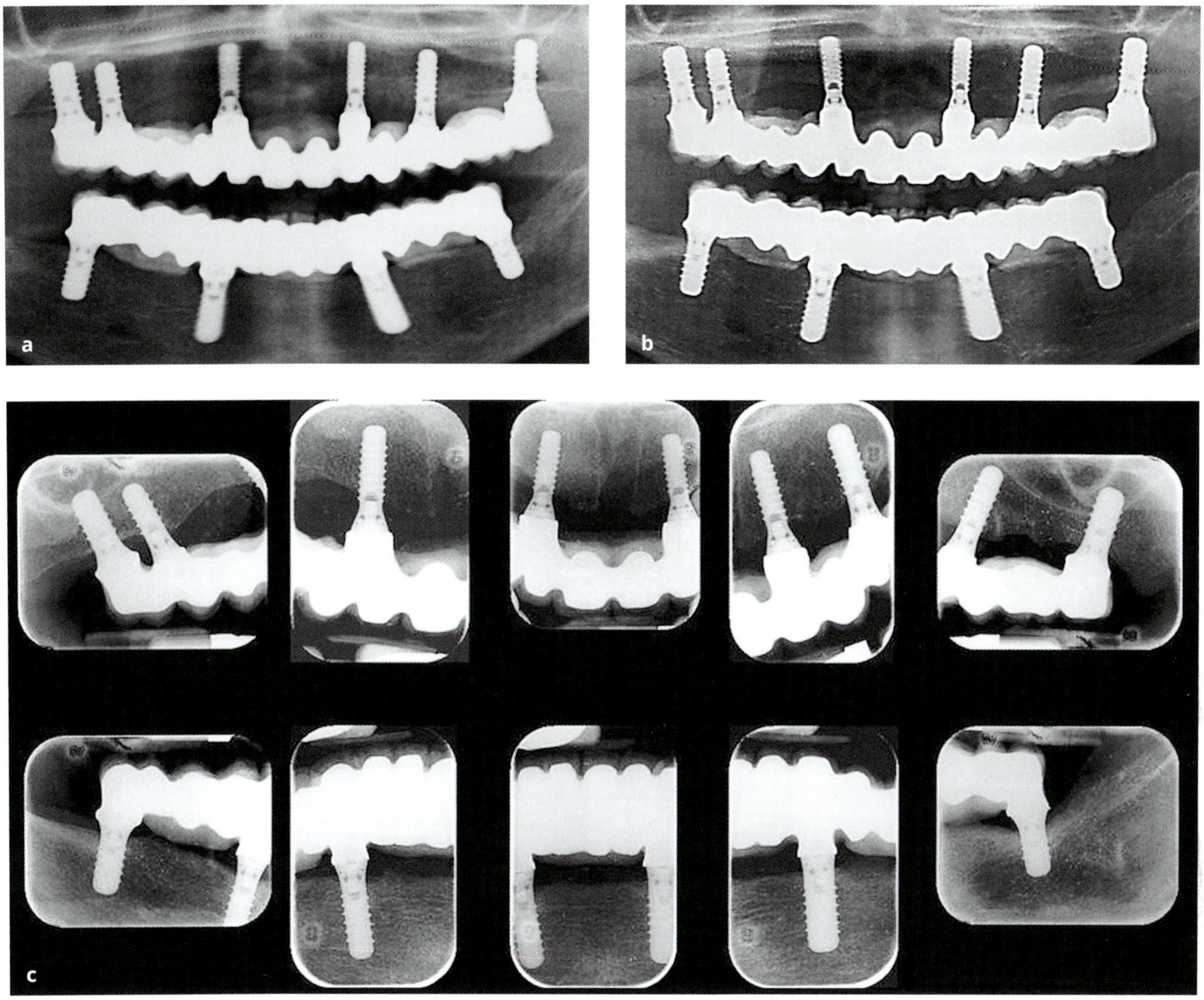

Fig 4-22a–c (a) Radiographic image of a patient taken immediately after implant placement. **(b)** Radiographic image taken 5 years after implant placement. **(c)** Radiographic image captured 12 years after implant placement. Stability of osseointegration had been achieved due to the correct choice of case, effective application of treatment, effective oral hygiene, consistency in attending the recall appointments, and effective removal of the microbial load every 3 months. The design and implementation of the prosthetic restoration played a crucial role in the successful outcome of this implant treatment.

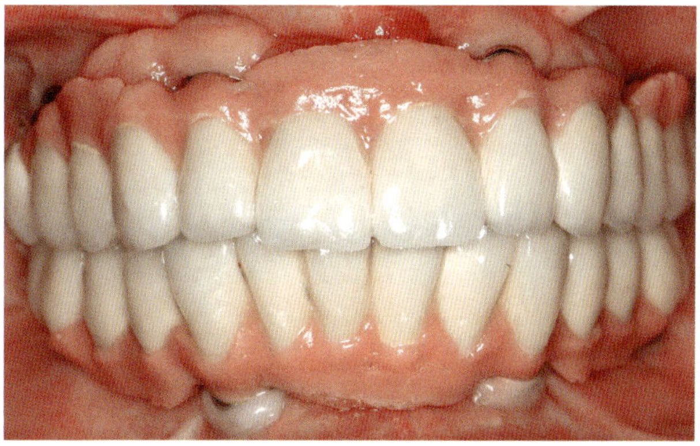

Fig 4-22d Clinical image of the patient taken 12 years after implant placement. Implant maintenance and prosthetic restoration were carried out under biologically, functionally, and esthetically acceptable conditions.

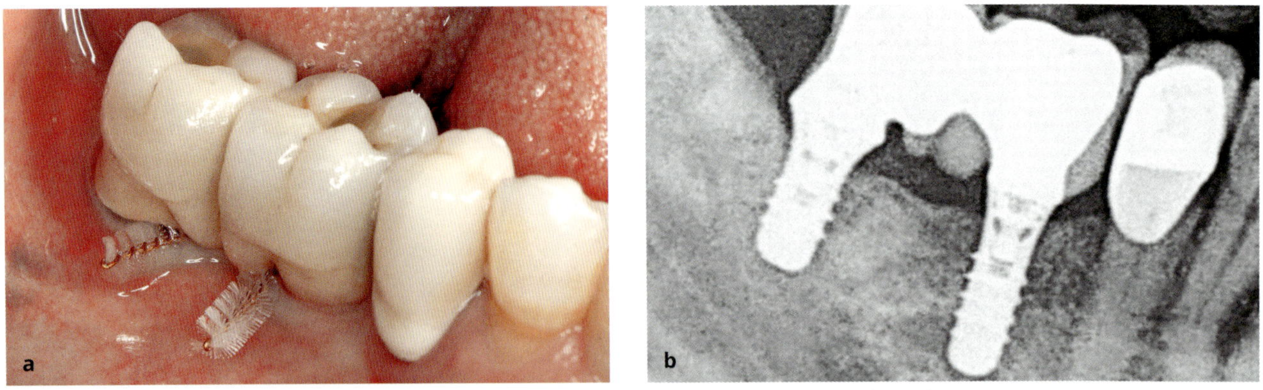

Figs 4-23a, b (a) Clinical image of a properly designed implant-supported fixed dental prosthesis that allows the application of effective oral hygiene. (b) Radiographic image showing the stability of osseointegration 10 years after functional loading.

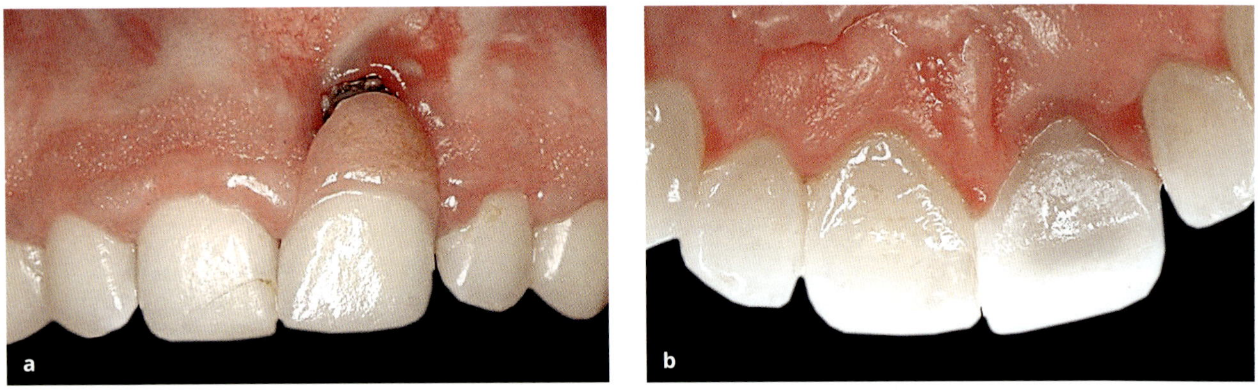

Figs 4-24a, b Clinical images of the anterior maxilla of a young patient in whom incorrect, buccal, and deep implant placement was performed. Recession, implant thread exposure, an absence of keratinized mucosa, and a poorly designed prosthetic restoration can be observed. The wrong treatment plan led to an increased chance of developing peri-implantitis.

For implant-supported fixed dental prostheses, the implant should be placed in an area corresponding to the location of the tooth and not in the interdental space (Figs 4-25a, b). For this purpose, the following steps should be followed: a thorough preoperative examination; preparation of a diagnostic wax-up; creation of a radiographic image; and finally, the manufacture of a surgical stent, always based on the additional guidance provided by the diagnostic wax-up (Figs 4-26a, b).

Related to this is the avoidance of regenerative techniques when these are needed, through selection of obliquely placed implants. The implant sites, in these cases, and the position of the implant neck, make access for oral hygiene devices extremely difficult, with subsequent inflammation and increased risk of peri-implantitis (Figs 4-27a, b and 4-28a–d).[40,41]

The choice of the retention type for implant-supported restorations (cemented or screw-retained) is often determined by the direction of the implants. Buccal deviation of the implants due to the anatomic limitations of the placement area, as it is typical for the anterior maxilla, or due to surgical inexperience, significantly limits the options for implant-supported prostheses (Fig 4-14). To avoid this, placement of cemented implant-supported restorations should be chosen, making it possible to achieve a harmonious esthetic result. The main disadvantage of cemented implant-supported restorations is the possible retention of cement residue in the peri-implant sulcus. The cement acts as a retaining agent for dental biofilm and will contribute to the development of inflammation in the area. If the cement is not promptly removed, peri-implant mucositis may be observed. If not treated in a timely fashion, this will develop into peri-implantitis (Figs 4-29a–d).[42–44]

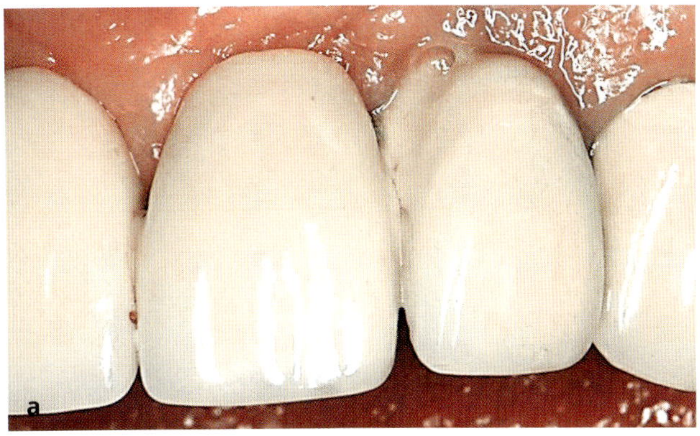

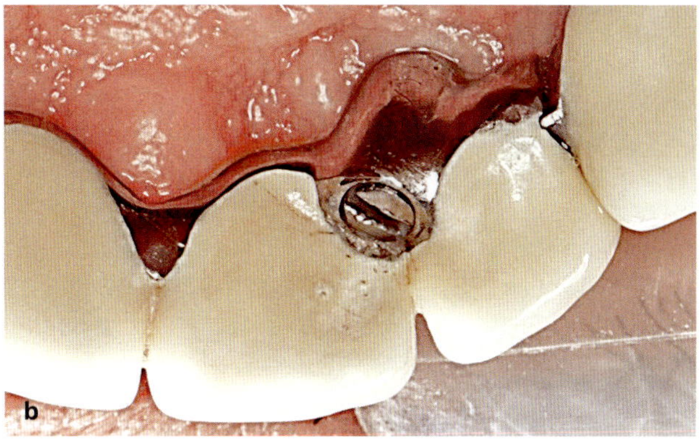

Figs 4-25a, b Buccal and palatal clinical image of an implant-supported prosthetic restoration. The position of the implant, when its placement was not prosthetically guided, created significant difficulties in the implementation of effective oral hygiene and was a risk factor for the development of inflammation.

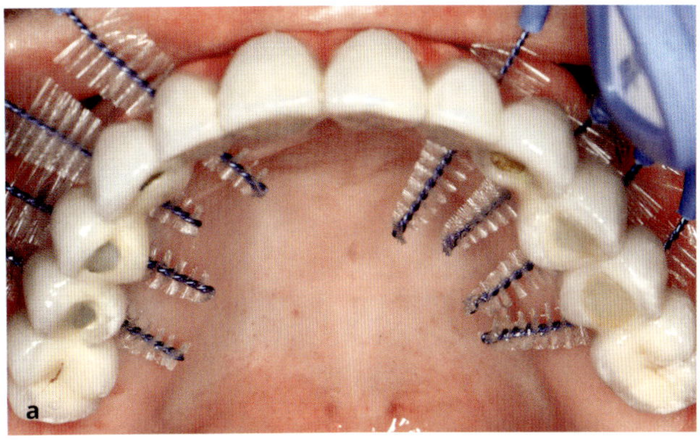

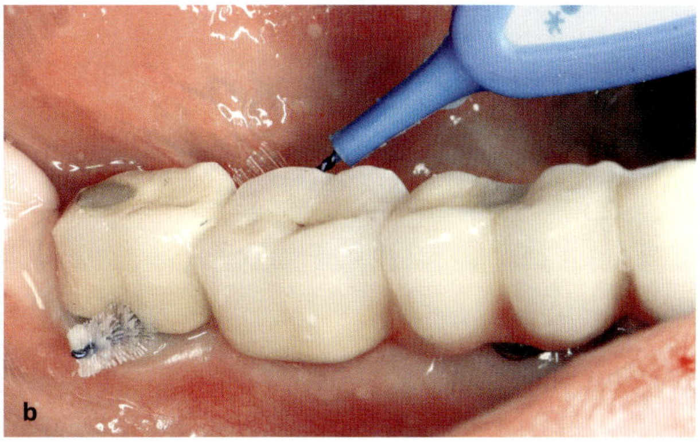

Figs 4-26a, b The use of a surgical splint and the correct design of the restoration are extremely important for cleaning efficiency, a cornerstone of long-term success.

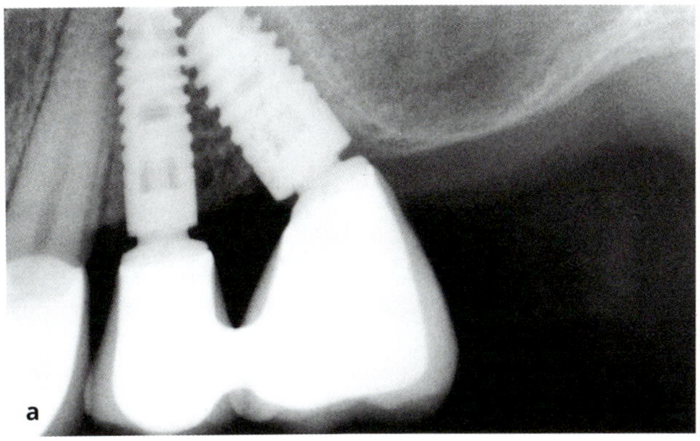

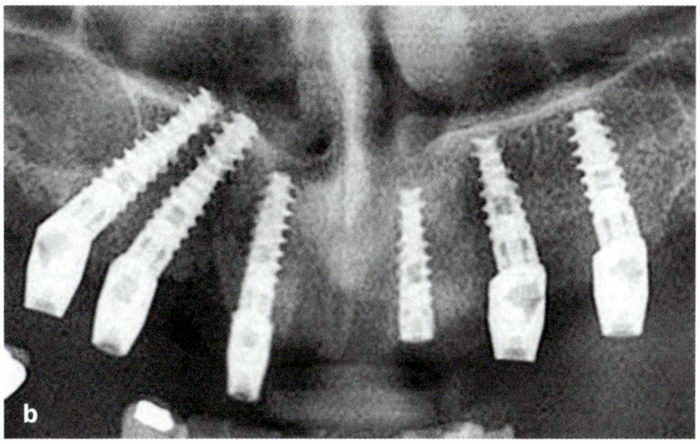

Figs 4-27a, b The direction of implant placement can cause difficulties with oral hygiene.

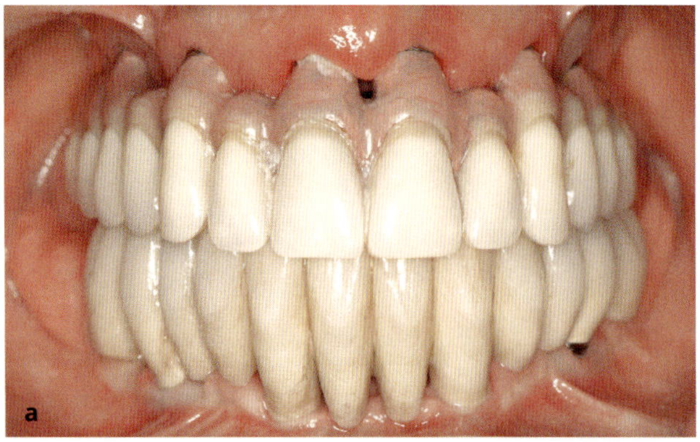

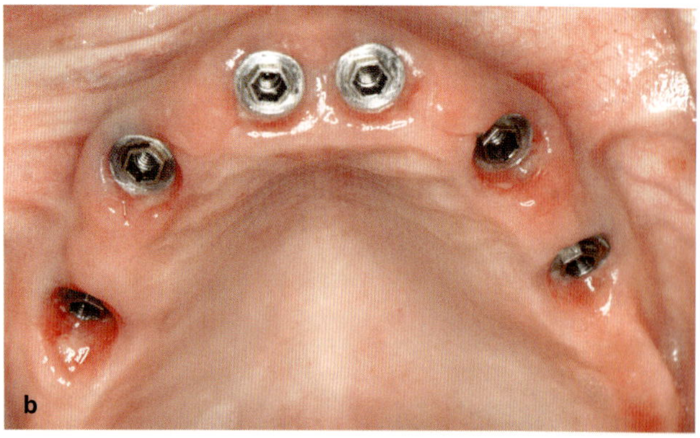

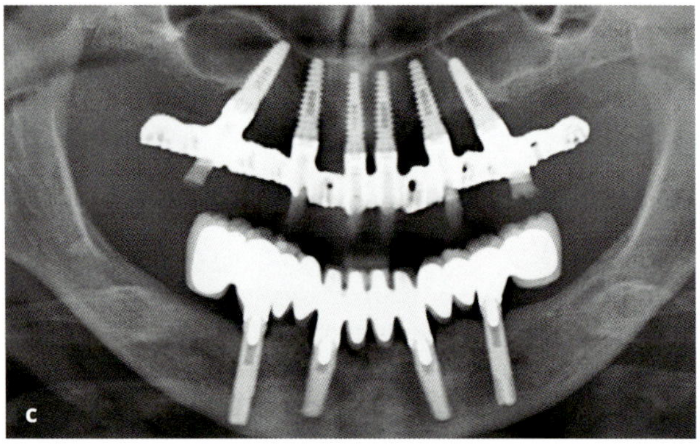

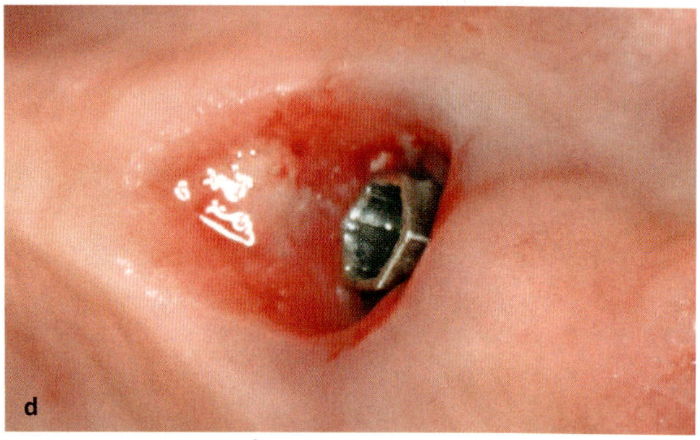

Figs 4-28a–d The choice of a fixed implant-supported dental prosthesis in the case of a wide cross-arch distance due to bone loss, as well as the angular placement of implants, are risk factors for soft tissue inflammation and subsequent peri-implantitis because oral hygiene is difficult to perform. Bone loss and intense soft tissue inflammation occurred over a few years in the areas of the implants placed with severe inclination.

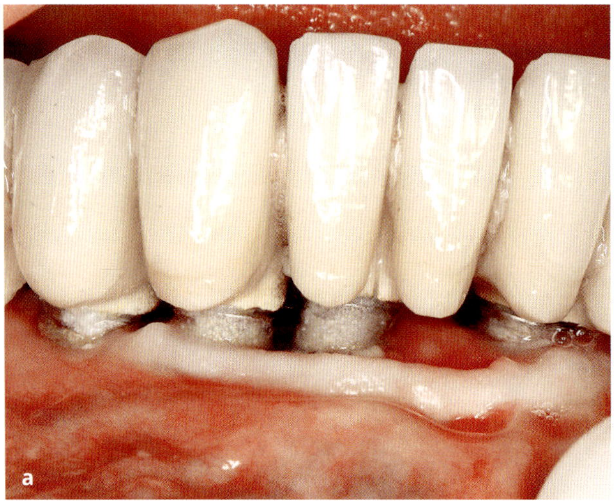

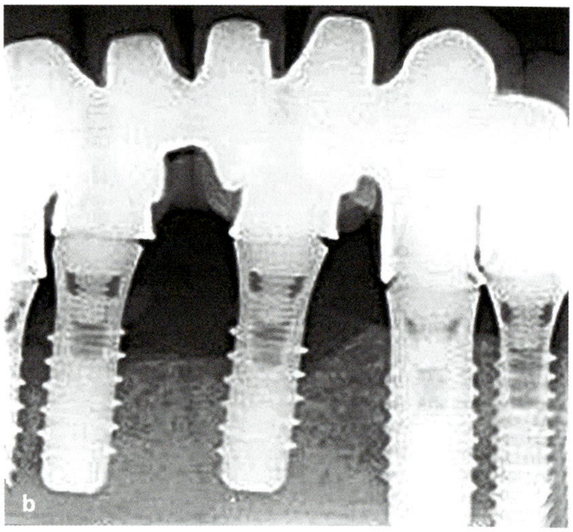

Figs 4-29a, b Clinical and radiographic images of a patient referred by her endocrinologist for periodontal examination before starting treatment for osteoporosis. An absence of oral hygiene was ascertained. On the radiograph, a radiopaque mass can be observed around the implant in site no. 42, which likely depicts cement that entered the peri-implant sulcus and contributed to the establishment and development of peri-implantitis.

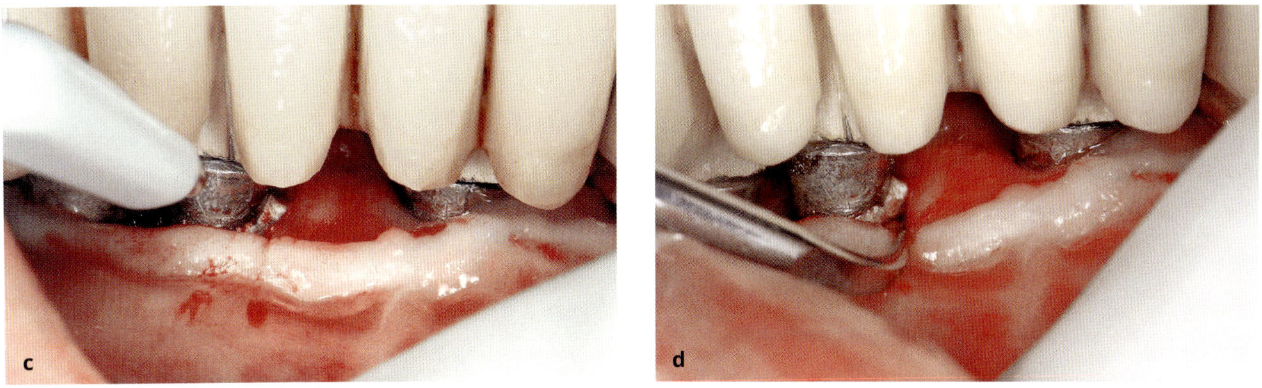

Figs 4-29c, d After the removal of the biofilm and with the help of an air syringe, the soft tissues were removed and the cement in the peri-implant pocket was revealed. The image on the right shows the removal of the cement.

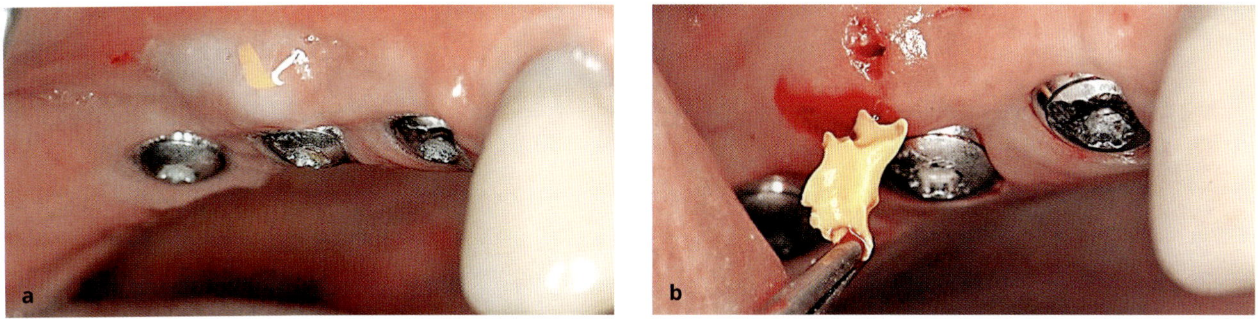

Figs 4-30a, b Remnant of the impression material that penetrated the peri-implant pocket by excess pressure, leading to inflammation and abscess formation, and ultimately, to bone loss ('iatrogenic peri-implantitis').

The risk of peri-implantitis from cement retention in the peri-implant sulcus is higher in patients with a history of periodontitis. A similar situation may arise from the presence of impression material left within the peri-implant sulcus. As for cement residue, these remnants act as biofilm retaining factors (Figs 4-30a, b).

A common mistake is choosing a fixed prosthetic restoration in cases of increased edentulous inter-arch space or severe skeletal Class II or III, but also in cases of extensive resorption of the alveolar ridge, leading to skeletal Class III (Figs 4-31a–f).

Regardless of the patient's desire for "fixed teeth", the choice of removable restorations in these cases will be beneficial for both function and esthetics; at the same time, it will allow effective oral hygiene. A common mistake is forgetting to inform patients to remove their dentures at nighttime to avoid chronic irritation of the oral mucosa. This omission, or a lack of compliance on the part of the patient, can lead to fungal infections and stomatitis and indirectly limit the effectiveness of oral hygiene because of the discomfort caused by the toothbrush to already irritated mucosa (Figs 4-32a–d).[45–47]

An issue that has been of particular concern in clinical implant dentistry is the potential effect of trauma from occlusion on functional implants. Although evidence is minimal and findings from experimental studies are mostly negative, clinical experience has occasionally suggested an effect of excessive occlusal forces on the integrity of peri-implant tissues. This condition usually presents as a sudden sensation of implant mobility, which is accompanied by tenderness in the area, without detecting an increase of the peri-implant sulcus depth. Radiographic images reveal a radiopaque zone cir-

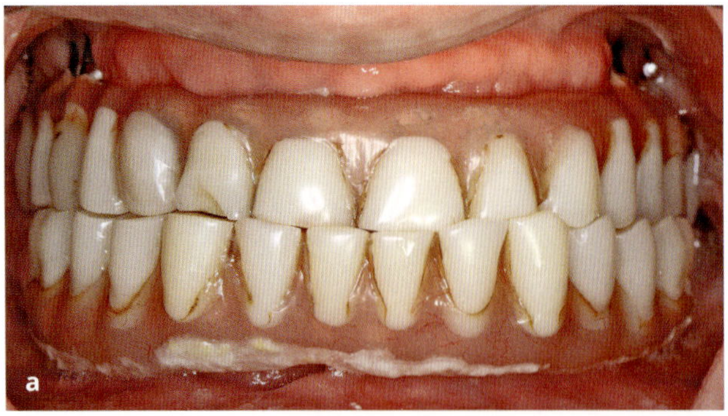

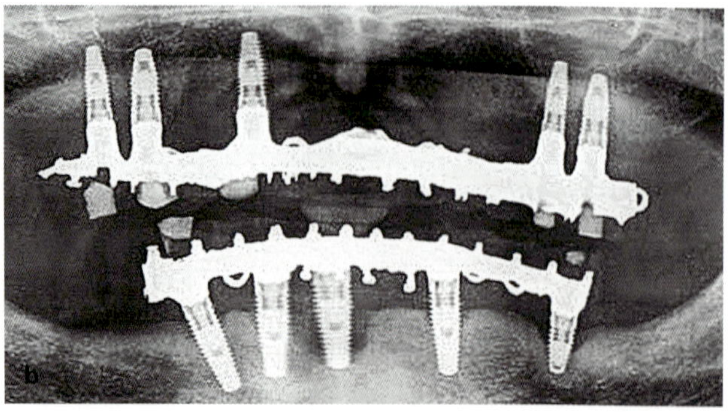

Figs 4-31a, b Clinical and radiographic images of fixed implant-supported prosthetic restorations that were manufactured without respect for the rules of biology, occlusion, and esthetics. The extent of peri-implantitis is obvious. In this case, the choice of a fixed implant-supported prosthetic restoration was inappropriate.

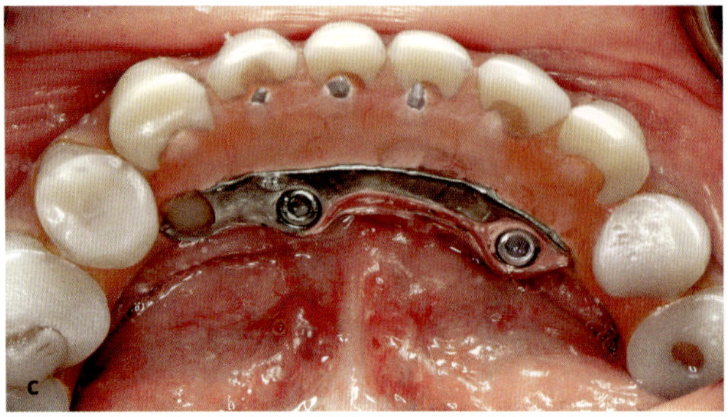

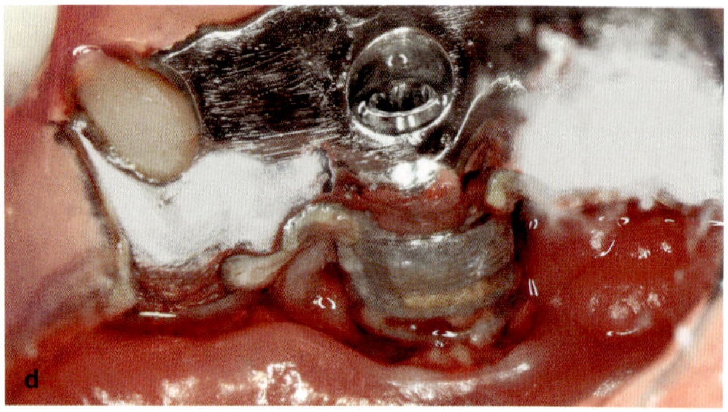

Figs 4-31c, d Application of any oral hygiene, especially in the mandibular anterior implants, is practically impossible.

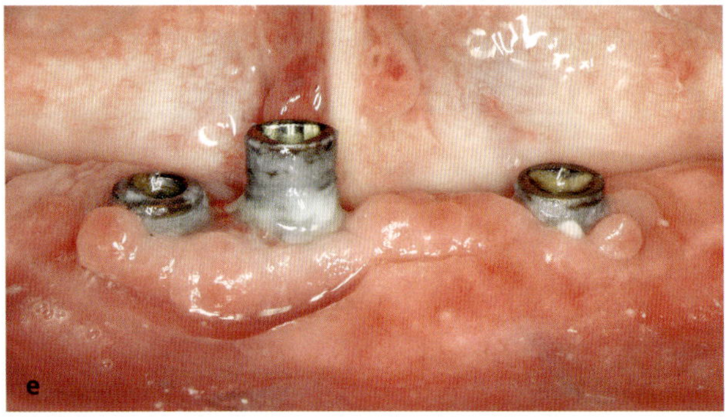

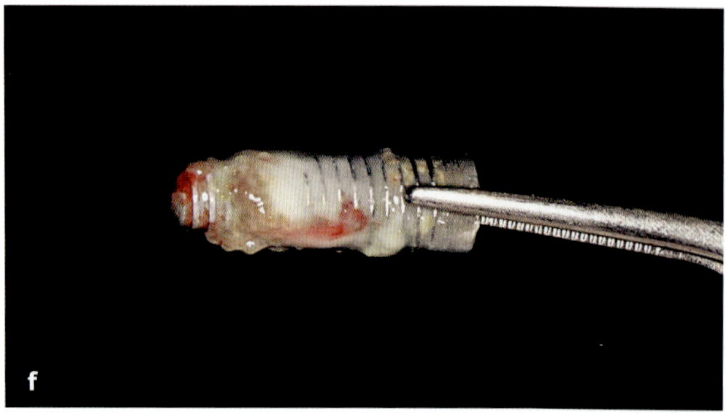

Figs 4-31e, f Poor construction and a lack of oral hygiene resulted in the progressive and ultimate destruction of osseointegration.

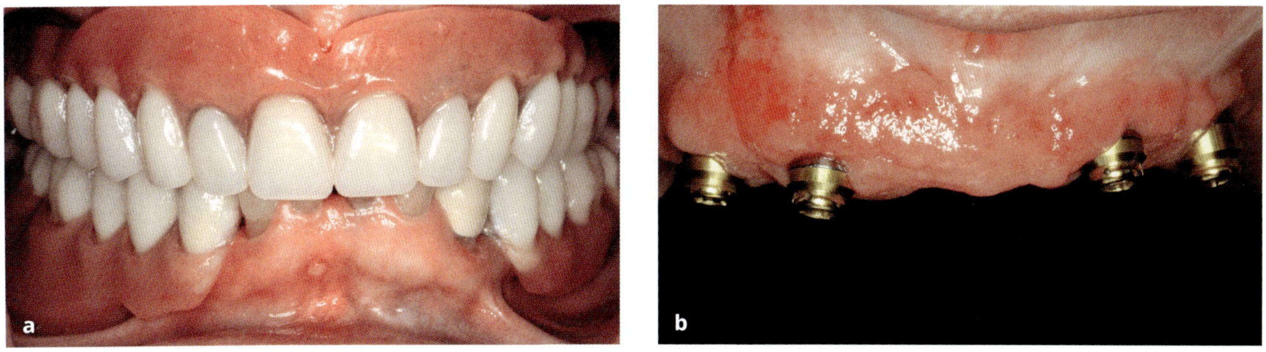

Figs 4-32a, b **(a)** Clinical image of a patient with a 5-year-old implant-supported overdenture in the maxilla **(b)**. Clinical image after removal of the denture where redness and swelling of the mucosa are evident (denture stomatitis) because of chronic irritation caused by the patient being unable to remove the restoration, except to apply oral hygiene **(b)**.

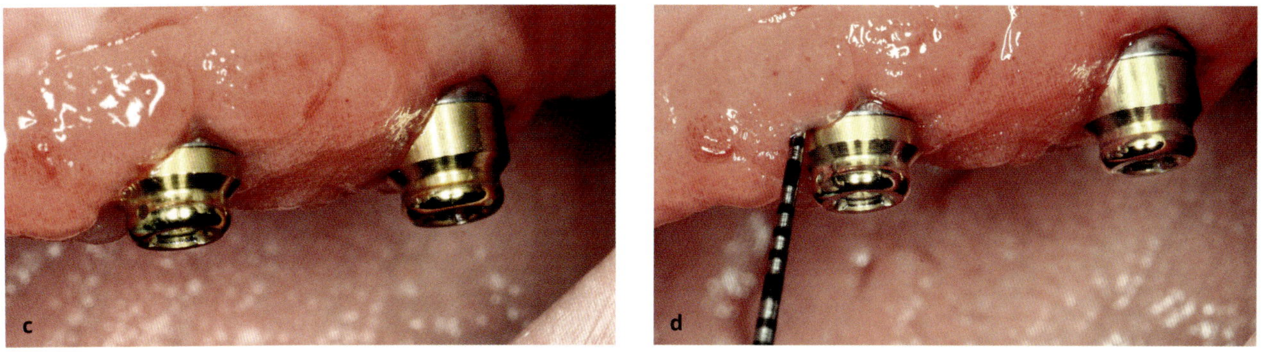

Figs 4-32c, d **(c)** An image characteristic of inflammation. **(d)** Effective oral hygiene can be proved by the absence of pockets and bleeding on probing. However, instructions were given to remove the denture at nighttime to reduce the possibility of chronic irritation.

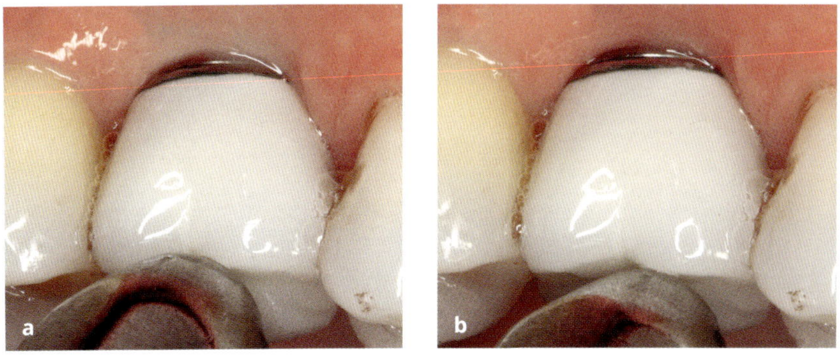

Figs 4-33a, b **(a)** In the implant, which had been in situ for 6 years, mobility and pain appeared. Application of excessive force buccally caused ischemia in the free peri-implant mucosa. **(b)** Application of force toward the palate led to the return of the pink gingiva.

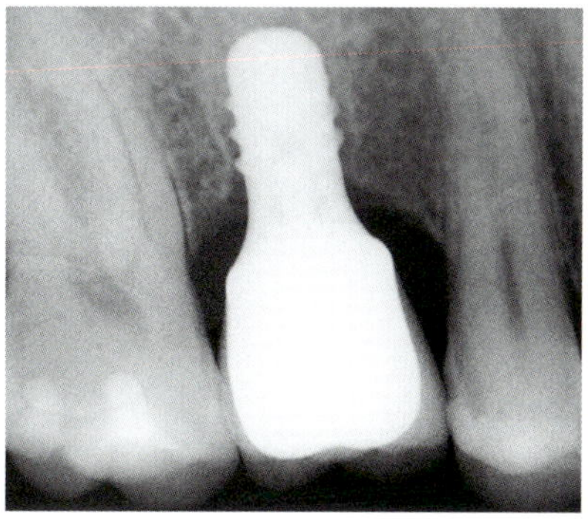

Fig 4-33c A radiograph did not reveal bone loss, but a thin radiopaque space can be seen between the implant and the surrounding bone, a condition diagnosed as a rare case of excessive loading.

cumferential to the implant. This phenomenon is a very rare condition and has been referred to as "overloading" (Figs 4-33a–i and 4-34a–d).[48]

In the only experimental study in monkeys that has documented this phenomenon, histologic images of a connective tissue capsule surrounding the implant resulting in sudden mobility were described.[49–51] Three similar experimental studies in dogs did not confirm an effect of excessive forces leading to implant loss.[48]

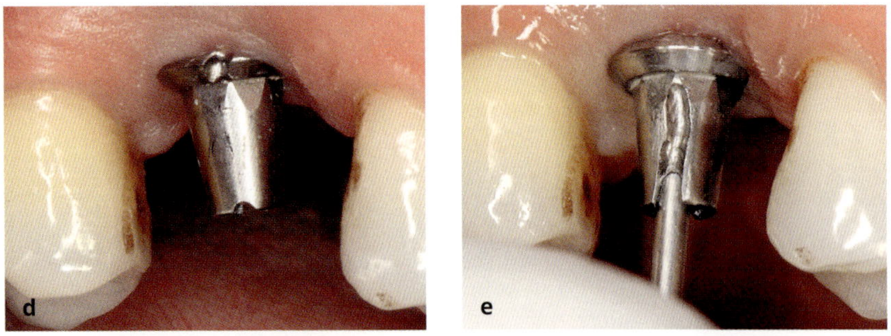

Figs 4-33d, e Corresponding modification of the color of the mucosa, achieved with the application of pressure and after removal of the crown. To be removed, the crown was cut through, leaving behind a slot (right) on the abutment surface. In the first rotation the patient reported pain, which then subsided.

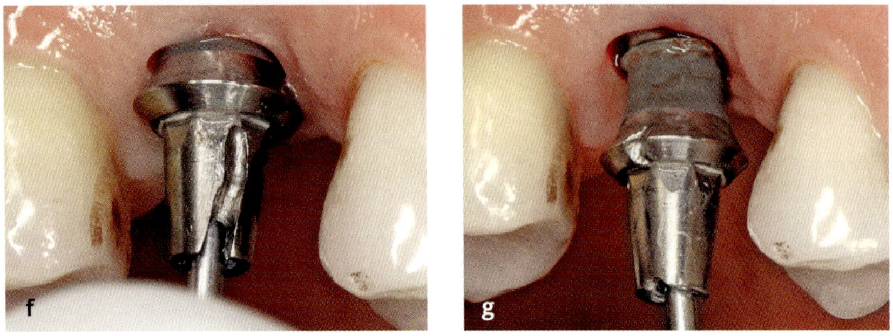

Figs 4-33f, g Next, the implant was loosened by applying a low torque.

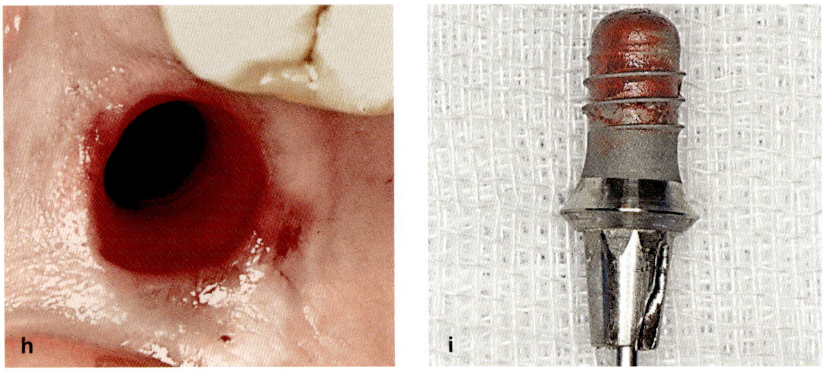

Figs 4-33h, i (h) Imprint of the implant thread on the alveolar socket and soft tissues without the characteristic inflammation can be observed, even after implant removal. **(i)** The implant immediately after its removal. The clean implant surface can be seen, without biofilm deposits and calculus but with blood residues from the removal process.

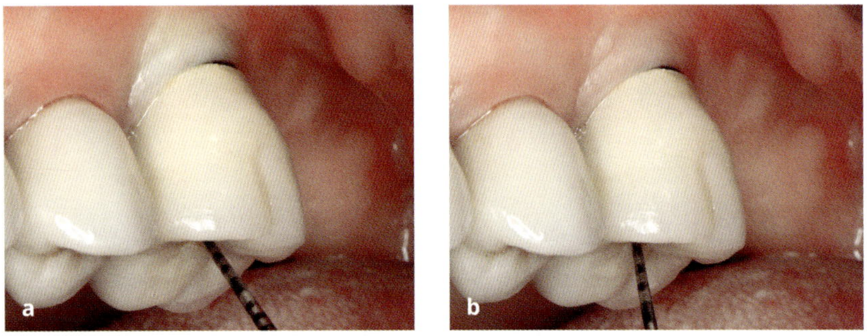

Figs 4-34a, b (a) Mobility and pain occurred in implant no. 26 of a patient with bruxism, in situ for 10 years. Application of force buccally caused ischemia in the free peri-implant mucosa. **(b)** Application of force toward the palate led to the return of the pink gingiva.

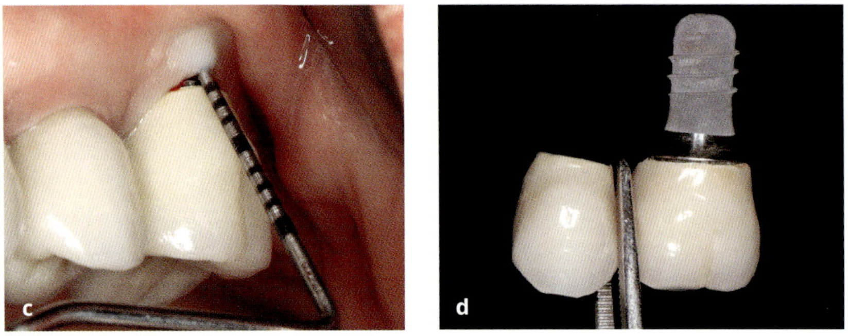

Figs 4-34c, d (c) No inflammation (redness, swelling, bleeding on probing) could be observed, while the peri-implant pocket was 5 mm deep. The crown on implant no. 25 came loose. **(d)** By pulling with the fingers, the two joined crowns together with implant no. 26 were removed. No accumulation of biofilm can be seen. The implant was simply rinsed with water.

References

1. French D, Grandin HM, Ofec R. Retrospective cohort study of 4,591 dental implants: analysis of risk indicators for bone loss and prevalence of peri-implant mucositis and peri-implantitis. J Periodontol 2019;90:691–700.
2. Carcuac O, Abrahamsson I, Albouy J-P, Linder E, Larsson L, Berglundh T. Experimental periodontitis and peri-implantitis in dogs. Clin Oral Implants Res 2012;24:363–371.
3. Quirynen M, Bollen CM. The influence of surface roughness and surface free energy on supra- and subgingival plaque formation in man. A review of the literature. J Clin Periodontol 1995;22:1–14.
4. Papaioannou W, Quirynen M, Nys M, Van Steenberghe D. The effect of periodontal parameters on the subgingival microbiota around implants. Clin Oral Implants Res 1995;6:197–204.
5. Rakic M, Grusovin MG, Canullo L. The microbiologic profile associated with peri-implantitis in humans: a systematic review. Int J Oral Maxillofac Implants 2016;31:359–368.
6. Sanz M, Newman MG, Nachnani S, Holt R, Stewart R, Flemmig T. Characterization of the subgingival microbial flora around endosteal sapphire dental implants in partially edentulous patients. Int J Oral Maxillofac Implants 1990;5:247–253.
7. Hultin M, Gustafsson A, Hallström H, Johansson L-A, Ekfeldt A, Klinge B. Microbiological findings and host response in patients with peri–implantitis. Clin Oral Implants Res 2002;13:349–358.
8. Papaioannou W, Quirynen M, Van Steenberghe D. The influence of periodontitis on the subgingival flora around implants in partially edentulous patients. Clin Oral Implants Res 1996;7:405–409.
9. Tamrakar AK, Murali G, Singh S, Shakila R. Evaluation of subgingival microbiota around single tooth implants. J Oral Biol Craniofac Res 2020;10:180–183.
10. Karoussis IK, Salvi GE, Heitz-Mayfield LJ, Brägger U, Hämmerle CHF, Lang NP. Long-term implant prognosis in patients with and without a history of chronic periodontitis: a 10-year prospective cohort study of the ITI Dental Implant System. Clin Oral Implants Res 2003;14:329–339.
11. Karoussis IK, Müller S, Salvi GE, Heitz-Mayfield LJA, Brägger U, Lang NP. Association between periodontal and peri-implant conditions: a 10-year prospective study. Clin Oral Implants Res 2004;15:1–7.
12. Ferreira SD, Martins CC, Amaral SA, et al. Periodontitis as a risk factor for peri-implantitis: systematic review and meta-analysis of observational studies. J Dent 2018;79:1–10.
13. Renvert S, Polyzois I, Claffey N. How do implant surface characteristics influence peri-implant disease? J Clin Periodontol 2011;38:214–222.
14. Swierkot K, Lottholz P, Flores-de-Jacoby L, Mengel R. Mucositis, peri–implantitis, implant success, and survival of implants in patients with treated generalized aggressive periodontitis: 3- to 16-year results of a prospective long-term cohort study. J Periodontol 2012;83:1213–1225.
15. Dreyer H, Grischke J, Tiede C, et al. Epidemiology and risk factors of peri–implantitis: a systematic review. J Periodontal Res 2018;53:657–681.
16. Feloutzis A, Lang NP, Tonetti MS, et al. IL-1 gene polymorphism and smoking as risk factors for peri-implant bone loss in a well-maintained population. Clin Oral Implants Res 2003;14:10–17.
17. Jacobi-Gresser E, Huesker K, Schütt S. Genetic and immunological markers predict titanium implant failure: a retrospective study. Int J Oral Maxillofac Surg 2013;42:537–543.
18. Dereka X, Mardas N, Chin S, Petrie A, Donos N. A systematic review on the association between genetic predisposition and dental implant biological complications. Clin Oral Implants Res 2012;23:775–788.
19. Mo Y-Y, Zeng X-T, Weng H, Cen Y, Zhao Q, Wen X. Association between tumor necrosis factor-alpha G-308A polymorphism and dental peri-implant disease risk: a meta-analysis. Medicine 2016;95:e4425.
20. Petkovic-Curcin A, Zeljic K, Cikota-Aleksic B, Dakovic D, Tatic Z, Magic Z. Association of cytokine gene polymorphism with peri-implantitis risk. Int J Oral Maxillofac Implants 2017;32:e241–e248.
21. Fourmousis I, Vlachos M. Genetic risk factors for the development of periimplantitis. Implant Dent 2019;28:103–114.
22. Chang Z, Jiang D, Zhang S, et al. Genetic association of the epidermal growth factor gene polymorphisms with peri-implantitis risk in Chinese population. Bioengineered 2021;12:8468–8475.
23. Lindquist LW, Carlsson GE, Jemt T. Association between marginal bone loss around osseointegrated implants and smoking habits: a 10-year follow-up study. J Dent Res 1997;76:1667–1674.
24. Klinge B, Meyle J, Working Group 2. Peri-implant tissue destruction. The Third EAO Consensus Conference 2012. Clin Oral Implants Res 2012;23(suppl 6):108–110.
25. Schwarz F, Derks J, Monje A, Wang H-L. Peri-implantitis. J Periodontol 2018;89:S267–S290.
26. Strietzel FP, Reichart PA, Kale A, Kulkarni M, Wegner B, Küchler I. Smoking interferes with the prognosis of dental implant treatment: a systematic review and meta-analysis. J Clin Periodontol 2007;34:523–544.
27. Galindo-Moreno P, Fauri M, Avila-Ortiz G, Fernández-Barbero JE, Cabrera-León A, Sánchez-Fernández E. Influence of alcohol and tobacco habits on peri-implant marginal bone loss: a prospective study. Clin Oral Implants Res 2005;16:579–586.
28. Costa FO, Takenaka-Martinez S, Cota LOM, Ferreira SD, Silva GLM, Costa JE. Peri-implant disease in subjects with and without preventive maintenance: a 5-year follow-up. J Clin Periodontol 2012;39:173–181.
29. Monje A, Aranda L, Diaz KT, et al. Impact of maintenance therapy for the prevention of peri-implant diseases: a systematic review and meta-analysis. J Dent Res 2016;95:372–379.

30. Sheth N, Tabassum R, Mistry G, Shetty O. Dental-implant maintenance: a critical factor in long-term treatment success. Int J Life Sci Scienti Res 2018;4:1585–1588.
31. Warrer K, Buser D, Lang NP, Karring T. Plaque-induced peri-implantitis in the presence or absence of keratinized mucosa. An experimental study in monkeys. Clin Oral Implants Res 1995;6:131–138.
32. Isler SC, Uraz A, Kaymaz O, Cetiner D. An evaluation of the relationship between peri-implant soft tissue biotype and the severity of peri-implantitis: a cross-sectional study. Int J Oral Maxillofac Implants 2019;34:187–196.
33. Albrektsson T, Wennerberg A. Oral implant surfaces: Part 1—review focusing on topographic and chemical properties of different surfaces and in vivo responses to them. Int J Prosthodont 2004;17:536–543.
34. De Bruyn H, Christiaens V, Doornewaard R, et al. Implant surface roughness and patient factors on long-term peri-implant bone loss. Periodontol 2000 2017;73:218–227.
35. Albouy J-P, Abrahamsson I, Berglundh T. Spontaneous progression of experimental peri-implantitis at implants with different surface characteristics: an experimental study in dogs. J Clin Periodontol 2012;39:182–187.
36. Albouy J-P, Abrahamsson I, Persson LG, Berglundh T. Spontaneous progression of ligatured induced peri-implantitis at implants with different surface characteristics. An experimental study in dogs II: histological observations. Clin Oral Implants Res 2009;20:366–371.
37. Schwarz F, Alcoforado G, Guerrero A, et al. Peri-implantitis: summary and consensus statements of group 3. The 6th EAO Consensus Conference 2021. Clin Oral Implants Res 2021;32(suppl 21):245–253.
38. Yi Y, Koo K-T, Schwarz F, Ben Amara H, Heo S-J. Association of prosthetic features and peri-implantitis: a cross-sectional study. J Clin Periodontol 2020;47:392–403.
39. de Tapia B, Mozas C, Valles C, Nart J, Sanz M, Herrera D. Adjunctive effect of modifying the implant-supported prosthesis in the treatment of peri-implant mucositis. J Clin Periodontol 2019;46:1050–1060.
40. Thoma DS, Naenni N, Figuero E, et al. Effects of soft tissue augmentation procedures on peri-implant health or disease: a systematic review and meta-analysis. Clin Oral Implants Res 2018;29(suppl 15):32–49.
41. Romanos GE, Delgado-Ruiz R, Sculean A. Concepts for prevention of complications in implant therapy. Periodontol 2000 2019;81:7–17.
42. Kordbacheh Changi K, Finkelstein J, Papapanou PN. Peri-implantitis prevalence, incidence rate, and risk factors: a study of electronic health records at a U.S. dental school. Clin Oral Implants Res 2019;30:306–314.
43. De Martinis Terra E, Berardini M, Trisi P. Nonsurgical management of peri-implant bone loss induced by residual cement: retrospective analysis of six cases. Int J Periodontics Restorative Dent 2019;39:89–94.
44. Wadhwani C, Rapoport D, La Rosa S, Hess T, Kretschmar S. Radiographic detection and characteristic patterns of residual excess cement associated with cement-retained implant restorations: a clinical report. J Prosthet Dent 2012;107:151–157.
45. Kern J-S, Kern T, Wolfart S, Heussen N. A systematic review and meta-analysis of removable and fixed implant-supported prostheses in edentulous jaws: post-loading implant loss. Clin Oral Implants Res 2016;27:174–195.
46. Tsigarida A, Chochlidakis K. A comparison between fixed and removable mandibular implant-supported full-arch prostheses: an overview of systematic reviews. Int J Prosthodont 2021;34:s85–s92.
47. Fu J-H, Wang H-L. Breaking the wave of peri-implantitis. Periodontol 2000 2020;84:145–160.
48. Heitz-Mayfield LJA, Schmid B, Weigel C, et al. Does excessive occlusal load affect osseointegration? An experimental study in the dog. Clin Oral Implants Res 2004;15:259–268.
49. Isidor F. Loss of osseointegration caused by occlusal load of oral implants. A clinical and radiographic study in monkeys. Clin Oral Implants Res 1996;7:143–152.
50. Isidor F. Histological evaluation of peri-implant bone at implant subjected to occlusal overload or plaque accumulation. Clin Oral Implants Res 1997;8:1–9.
51. Isidor F. Influences of forces on peri-implant bone. Clin Oral Implants Res 2006;17:8–18.
52. Swierkot K, Lottholz P, Flores-de-Jacoby L, Mengel R. Mucositis, peri-implantitis, implant success, and survival of implants in patients with treated generalized aggressive periodontitis: 3- to 16-year results of a prospective long-term cohort study. J Periodontol 2012;83:1213–1225.
53. Roos-Jansåker AM, Lindahl C, Renvert H, Renvert S. Nine- to fourteen-year follow-up of implant treatment. Part II: presence of peri-implant lesions. J Clin Periodontol 2006;33:290–295.

5 Epidemiology of Peri-Implant Diseases

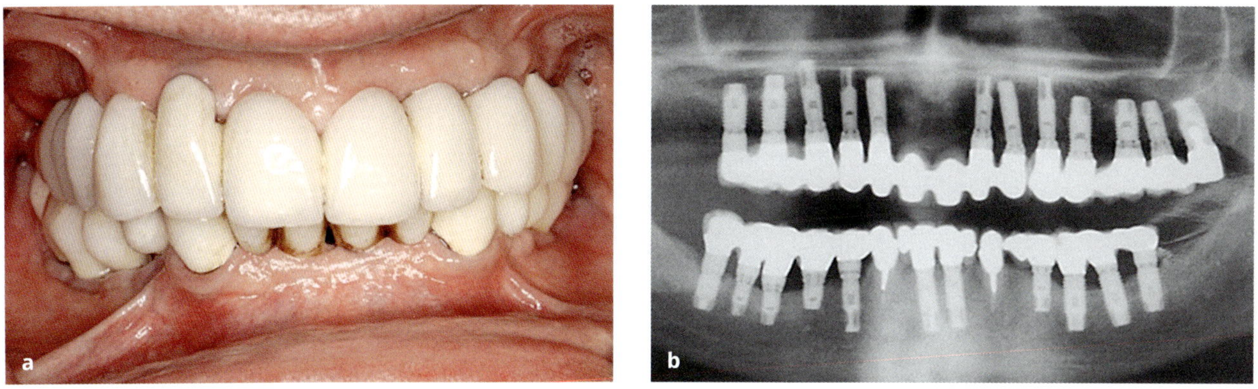

Figs 5-1a, b Clinical and radiographic images of a patient with an excessive number of implants placed in a treatment plan that clearly involved gross overtreatment.

According to current marketing statistics, the number of dental implants placed annually in the United States has reached five million; in the European Union, the figure has reached two million. Given the continuously rising world population, the increased marketing of the dental implant industry, the ease with which osseointegration is achieved, and the fact that implant placement has become a common treatment, these high numbers are expected to increase even further. This significant growth in popularity is demonstrated in the ease with which many patients opt for tooth extraction and implant placement, and the adoption of approaches that prevent malpractice in the dental profession (Figs 5-1a, b).[1]

The survival and success rates of dental implants are very high; however, the occurrence of inflammatory diseases, such as peri-implant mucositis and peri-implantitis, is a daily reality. In fact, the incidence of peri-implantitis increases for implants in situ for more than 5 years. Bleeding on probing (BOP), one of the clinical criteria for the presence of inflammation in the peri-implant area, is recorded—even sporadically—in very high percentages, affecting 90% of implants. In addition, at the patient level, the incidence of peri-implant mucositis has reached 77%.

The initial enthusiasm for achieving osseointegration was significant; indeed, for many years, researchers considered the mere fact that implants remained in the mouth and continued to provide support for prosthetic restorations a great success. Only the loss of implants was considered a failure, for example, as a result of complete loss of osseointegration. It took time for the scientific community to focus on individual studies on the stability of hard and soft tissues, and esthetics. Extensive reporting of implant survival and success is provided in Chapter 6.

For osseointegrated implants that have served the patient for some time, while the peri-implant tissues are in a healthy state, it is difficult to imagine that they might be suddenly "lost" as a result of an accident without ever showing signs or symptoms of disease. In fact, the exact opposite is true. The questions that arise are whether or not the clinician correctly evaluates the peri-implant site and whether or not the reexamination and reevaluation are carried out at regular intervals, and especially when the presence of the early signs of peri-implant pathology is detected. The answer is negative in most cases; otherwise, rates of peri-implantitis and implant loss would be much lower. Although the need for a regular follow-up by a clinician has been emphasized for several years, this is unfortunately not mandatory for most patients who already have implants.

Prevalence is defined as the number of diseased cases that exist in a population at a given period of time, whereas incidence is the rate at which a particular event or disease occurs, for example the number of new cases of a particular disease that occur during a specified period of time. Therefore, analysis of the prevalence of peri-implant diseases requires the collection of data from contemporary or descriptive studies, whereas longitudinal studies provide information on the incidence of the disease. Undoubtedly, the prevalence of peri-implant diseases is determined at a patient level and not at an implant level. The number of implants affected by peri-implantitis per patient describes the extent of the disease, whereas the degree of supporting bone loss expresses its severity.

However, the exact prevalence of peri-implantitis is difficult to determine accurately when evaluating data from existing studies. In other words, the results of these studies show significant variation in the numerical expression of the prevalence of peri-implant diseases. This discrepancy between studies is primarily attributed to the lack of standardized and universally accepted criteria for the diagnosis of peri-implant mucositis and peri-implantitis and, secondarily, to the different implant systems evaluated in different studies and at different time points.[2]

Regardless of the criteria that each research team has used to diagnose peri-implantitis, it is interesting to conclude that, as time passes, systematic reviews focusing on the individual have resulted in gradually increasing prevalence rates. For example, one of the first systematic reviews in 2002 identified a prevalence of peri-implantitis of 6.47%.[3] As revealed by a thorough evaluation of the literature, prevalence was often evaluated at an implant level, whereas it is good practice to evaluate it at a patient level, at which point it assumes a higher value. In the same year, in the first prospective study[4] published on the effect of a history of chronic periodontitis on the outcome of implant treatment, it was emphasized that depending on the criteria chosen more or less rigorously, different evaluations and therefore different conclusions may emerge for the same group of patients or implants. This conclusion underscored the need to establish universally accepted criteria for the diagnosis of peri-implantitis. Just 2 years later, a systematic review including a large number of studies found a higher prevalence of peri-implantitis, reaching 8.6% on the total of implants in function after 10 years.[4] A few years later, it was recognized around the world that the prevalence of peri-implantitis was close to or more than 10% after 10 years of function.[4–6]

Today, most clinicians and researchers agree that, despite the rigor of diagnostic criteria (see Chapter 6), peri-implantitis constitutes a serious problem for health systems globally. This problem arises 5 to 10 years after implant placement. The percentage of patients with the disease ranges from 28% to 56%, whereas in already placed implants, the percentage of those who exhibit bone loss due to peri-implantitis ranges from 12% to 43%.

Like periodontitis and gingivitis, peri-implantitis starts as peri-implant mucositis.[7] The prevalence of peri-implant mucositis is 80% at the patient level and 50% at the implant level. In addition, of implants that receive peri-implant mucositis treatment (even if patients are included in a maintenance care program), 18% will eventually develop peri-implantitis. In the event of poor compliance with the maintenance care program, this percentage increases dramatically and rises to 44% within 5 years.[8]

As concluded in a recent study, 33% of all patients who have implants and 20% of all implants placed will develop peri-implantitis.[9]

Two points of particular concern are the transition time from peri-implant mucositis to peri-implant-

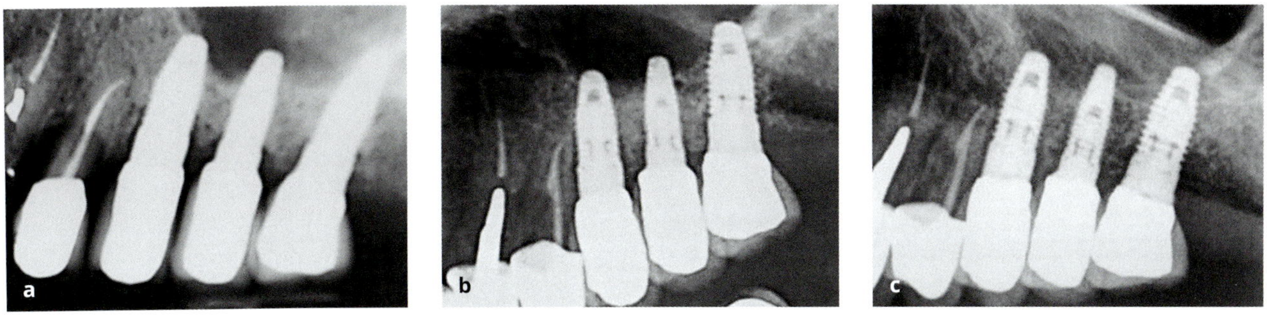

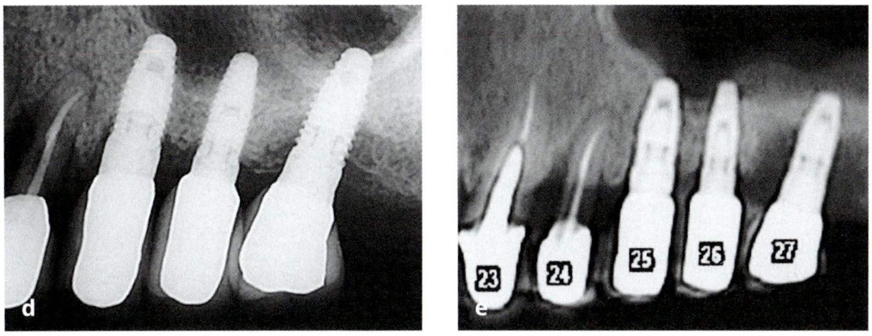

Figs 5-2a–e Development of peri-implantitis in a patient who did not consent to surgical treatment. Despite the application of stages A and B of the cumulative interceptive supportive therapy protocol every 3 to 4 months, the condition of implant no. 27 progressively deteriorated within a decade. Radiographs taken **(a)** 6, **(b)** 10, **(c)** 12, **(d)** 14, and **(e)** 16 years after implant placement.

itis and the rate of progression of peri-implantitis if left untreated. These factors remain unknown because it would be unethical to diagnose patients with peri-implantitis and leave them untreated to study the natural course of the disease. Regarding the time of onset of bone loss, as it remains unknown, the only countermeasure the clinician has is regular monitoring and recording of clinical and radiographic measurements and parameters and their comparison with the previous condition, in combination with the protocol to maintain care for peri-implant health (see Chapter 17). Regarding the rate of progression of peri-implantitis, all clinicians agree that it may be rapid (Figs 5-2a–e).[10] As treatment difficulty and the severity of bone loss increase, urgent diagnosis and immediate treatment are imperative.

These epidemiologic data should encourage those involved in implant dentistry to take all possible measures to prevent peri-implant mucositis, treat it in a timely fashion, and hence prevent the development of peri-implantitis. Combining these data with the information provided in Chapter 14 on the effectiveness of treatment, it is easy to understand how crucial it is to take the correct approach to implant treatment, which must be based on scientific evidence. The implementation of a proper treatment plan, including the identification and control of risk factors and pretherapeutic cause-related therapy, the selection of implant design and the type of prosthetic restoration, and proper implementation and maintenance care, play a crucial role in the effort to address the growing phenomenon of peri-implant pathology. Clinical experience indicates that a large percentage of peri-implantitis cases could be described as "iatrogenic"; in other words, these are cases that have been caused by a poor therapeutic approach due not only to ignoring the risk factors or failing to inform patients about the importance of oral hygiene and maintenance care, but also to poor placement of implants or poor prosthetic reconstructions. The number of cases of iatrogenic peri-implantitis cannot be calculated at the level of private practices (Figs 5-3 to 5-6a–d).

Further information on the subject of diagnosis of peri-implantitis at a research level is also worth mentioning. Current research is based on signs or combinations of signs to determine peri-implantitis. These signs are BOP from the peri-implant sulcus or pocket, pocket probing depth, and vertical bone loss as shown on a radiograph. BOP is characterized by many as a clinical sign of a particularly high presence of inflammation in implants as it has been

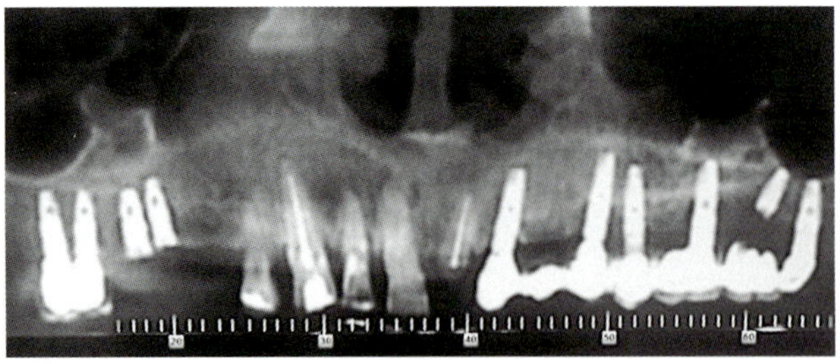

Fig 5-3 Placing two implants to restore no. 17 is not only unnecessary but also makes oral hygiene practices difficult to apply. The panoramic section also shows two implants placed to restore the missing no. 16. In the two-dimensional section, they are placed too close to each other.

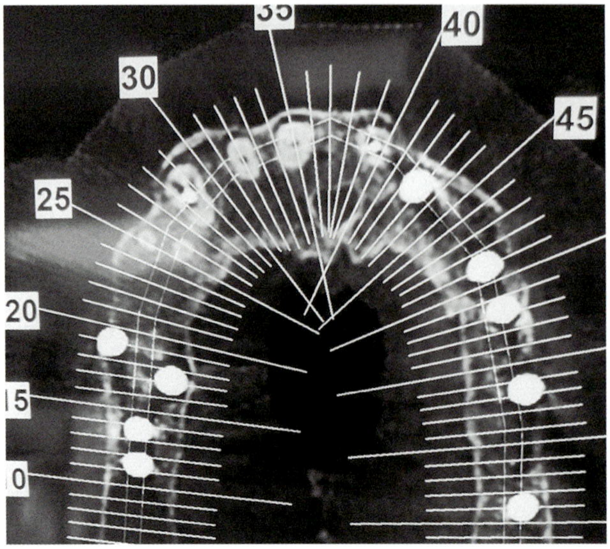

Fig 5-4 In the cross section, one of the implants that were used for the restoration of no. 16 was placed very palatally and the other was placed very buccally, to the point that the buccal surface of the implant was not covered by bone. The choice of placement sites made iatrogenic peri-implantitis highly likely.

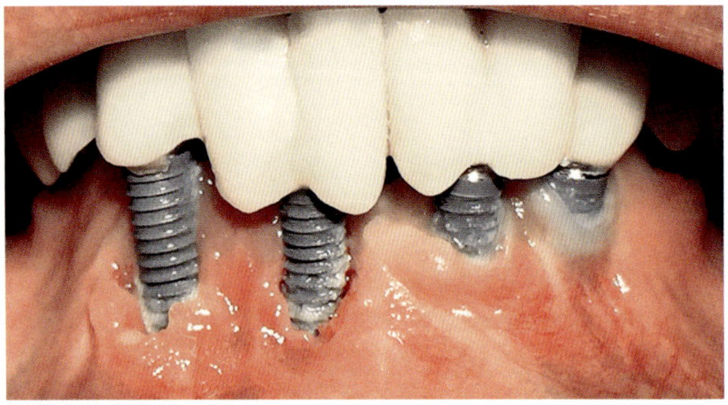

Fig 5-5 Case of a patient with terminal peri-implantitis. Several wrong choices were made with regard to patient selection, implant positioning, implant inclination, implant size, prosthesis type, and prosthesis design and placement. Hence, this condition may be described as iatrogenic peri-implantitis.

recorded in 80% of the implants studied. The notion that probing of a peri-implant sulcus leads more easily to a hemorrhagic reaction is of clinical significance. This, of course, does not underestimate the value of bleeding as a sign of inflammation. The most important element regarding BOP is its highly negative prognostic value; that is, its absence indicates not only healthy peri-implant tissues, as is the case with periodontal tissues, but also that peri-implant health may be stable for the future.

Studies differ in the criteria applied for diagnosis, so readers must carefully assess the definition criteria for peri-implant mucositis, peri-implantitis, and even peri-implant tissue health.[11,12]

As stated at the beginning of this chapter, the number of implants placed each year is now in the millions. As such, the number of implants and patients suffering from peri-implantitis globally is enormous, and the extent of therapeutic needs that already exist is likewise immense.

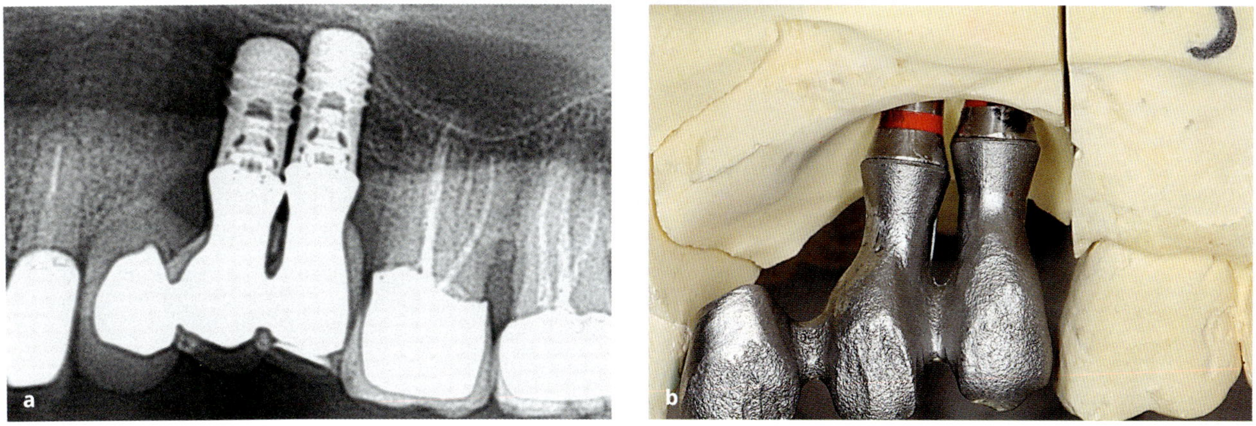

Figs 5-6a, b Incorrect implant proximity, which made placement of the partial denture and interdental cleaning very difficult.

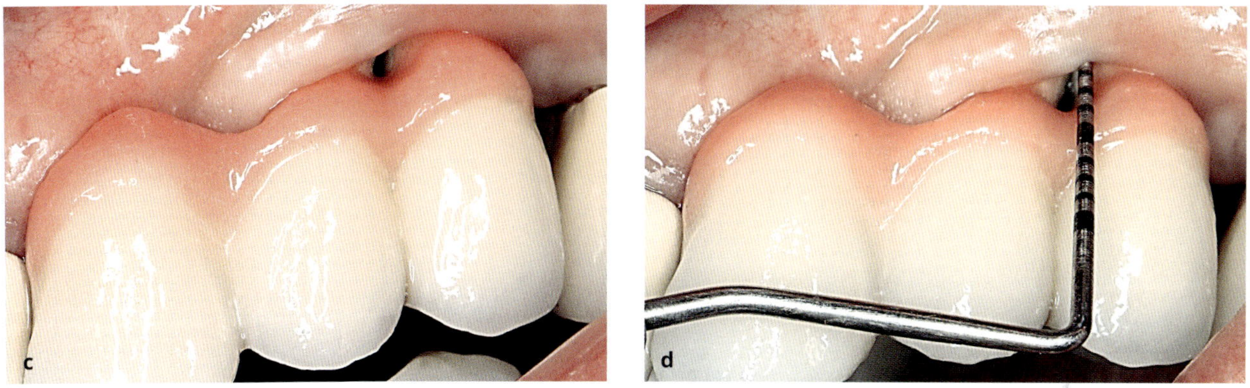

Figs 5-6c, d Even though the peri-implant tissues remain healthy 2 years after implant placement because the patient was consistent in their daily oral plaque removal and complied with the maintenance program, the possibility of developing peri-implantitis in the future is significant.

References

1. Pjetursson BE, Heimisdottir K. Dental implants—are they better than natural teeth? Eur J Oral Sci 2018;126(suppl 1):81–87.
2. Tomasi C, Derks J. Clinical research of peri-implant diseases—quality of reporting, case definitions and methods to study incidence, prevalence and risk factors of peri-implant diseases. J Clin Periodontol 2012;39(suppl 12):207–223.
3. Berglundh T, Persson L, Klinge B. A systematic review of the incidence of biological and technical complications in implant dentistry reported in prospective longitudinal studies of at least 5 years. J Clin Periodontol 2002;29:197–212.
4. Mombelli A, Cionca N. The prevalence of peri-implantitis: how big is the problem? Forum Implantol 2013;9:12–19.
5. Lee CT, Huang Y-W, Zhu L, Weltman R. Prevalences of peri-implantitis and peri-implant mucositis: systematic review and meta-analysis. J Dent 2017;62:1–12.
6. Mir-Mari J, Mir-Orfila P, Figueiredo R, Valmaseda-Castellón E, Gay-Escoda C. Prevalence of peri-implant diseases. A cross-sectional study based on a private practice environment. J Clin Periodontol 2012;39:490–494.
7. Vignoletti F, Di Domenico GL, Di Martino M, Montero E, de Sanctis M. Prevalence and risk indicators of peri-implantitis in a sample of university-based dental patients in Italy: a cross-sectional study. J Clin Periodontol 2019;46:597–605.
8. Zitzmann NU, Berglundh T. Definition and prevalence of peri-implant diseases. J Clin Periodontol 2008;35:286–291.
9. Kordbacheh Changi K, Finkelstein J, Papapanou PN. Peri-implantitis prevalence, incidence rate, and risk factors: a study of electronic health records at a U.S. dental school. Clin Oral Implants Res 2019;30:306–314.
10. Derks J, Schaller D, Håkansson J, Wennström JL, Tomasi C, Berglundh T. Peri-implantitis—onset and pattern of progression. J Clin Periodontol 2016;43:383–388.
11. Coli P, Sennerby L. Is peri-implant probing causing over-diagnosis and over-treatment of dental implants? J Clin Med 2019;8:11–23.
12. Heitz-Mayfield LJA. Peri-implant diseases: diagnosis and risk indicators. J Clin Periodontol 2008;35:292–304.

6 Success and Survival of Implants

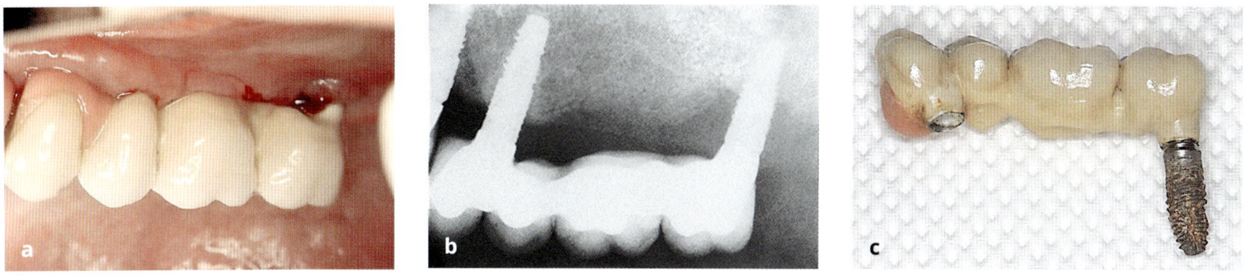

Figs 6-1a–c Clinical and radiographic image of implant no. 27. The implant remained in situ; therefore, it survived. **(c)** The unscrewing of the implant-supported partial denture from no. 24 shows that implant no. 27 has completely lost its osseointegration.

Tooth loss is the final consequence of untreated caries and periodontal disease. Several types of dental implants have been used to replace missing teeth. Implants in their current form appeared in the 1960s, beginning with the achievement of a direct structural and functional connection between a living bone and an implant surface as seen through the optical microscope, which was defined as osseointegration. Until the middle of the last century and before the introduction of osseointegrated implants, dental practitioners used mainly blade-type or subperiosteal implants that healed by fibrous encapsulation.

The outcome of implant placement is of interest to the dental profession because it is an invasive and concomitantly time-consuming procedure that incurs a significant cost. The definition of several terms used in implant dentistry to describe the outcome of implant therapy is relatively unclear. The terms "survival", "success", "failure", and "complication" have been used with different interpretations, resulting in confusion when reading scientific articles. For the same reason, it is difficult to compare the results of different studies. At the 3rd European Workshop on Periodontology, "survival rate" was defined as the proportion of implants that are still in situ at the time of the review, regardless of whether they met predetermined parameters of function, biology, or esthetics (Figs 6-1a–c and 6-2a–l).[1]

The achievement of specific biologic, functional, and esthetic criteria was defined as "success" (Figs 6-3a, b and 6-4a, b). However, what is defined as success of implant treatment is a matter of debate because no commonly accepted criteria have been established by the scientific community. Several

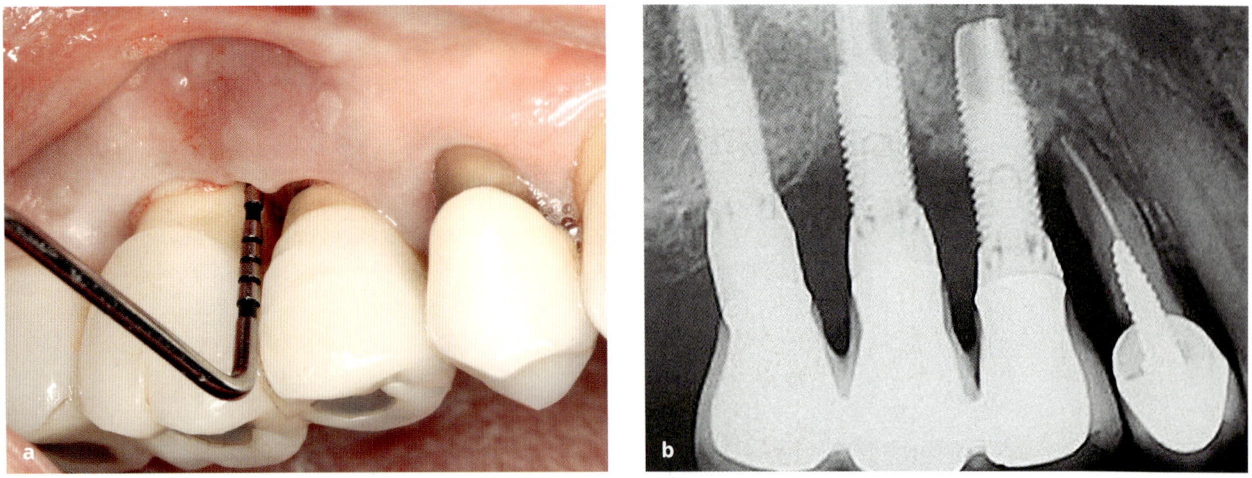

Figs 6-2a, b Clinical and radiographic images of peri-implantitis 10 years after implant placement. The incidence of peri-implantitis, even if it characterizes the implants as unsuccessful, does not change the fact that they survived.

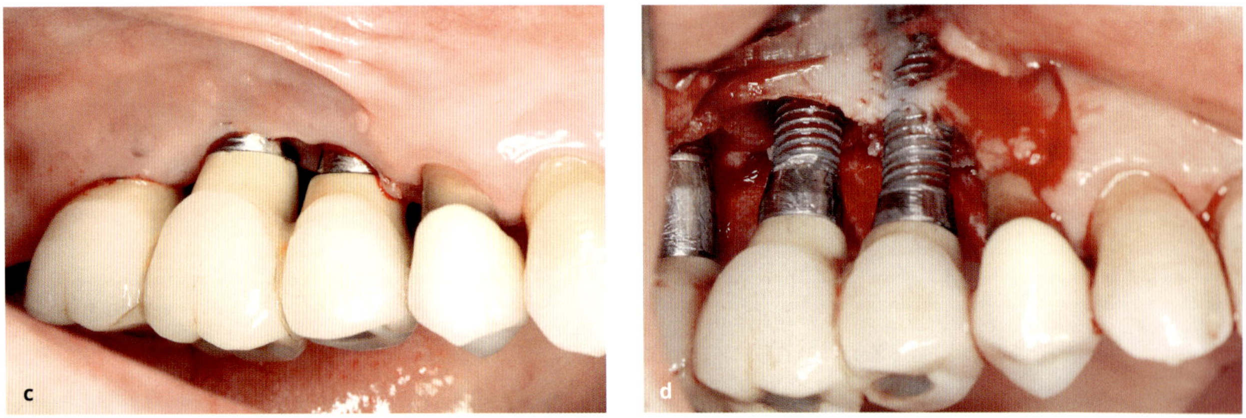

Figs 6-2c, d **(c)** After cause-related therapy and before surgery. **(d)** During surgery.

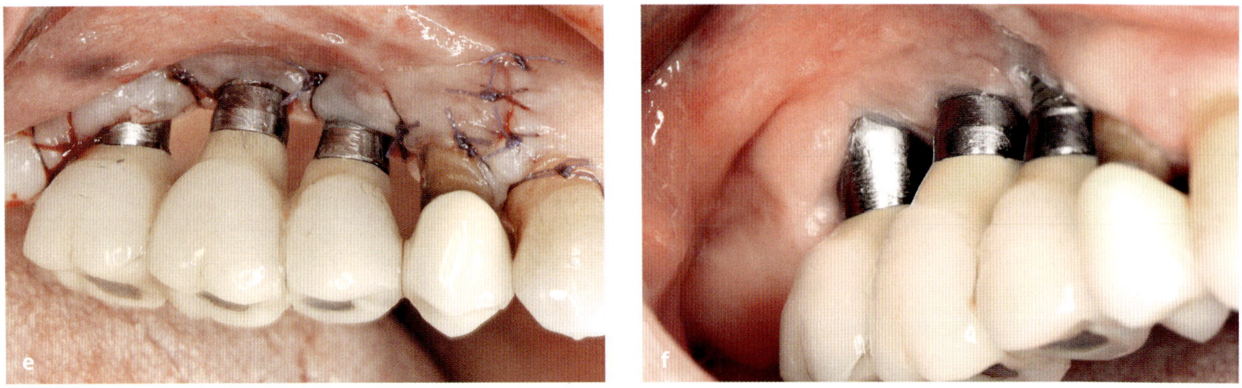

Figs 6-2e, f **(e)** Apically repositioned flap to eliminate pockets. **(f)** One year after surgery.

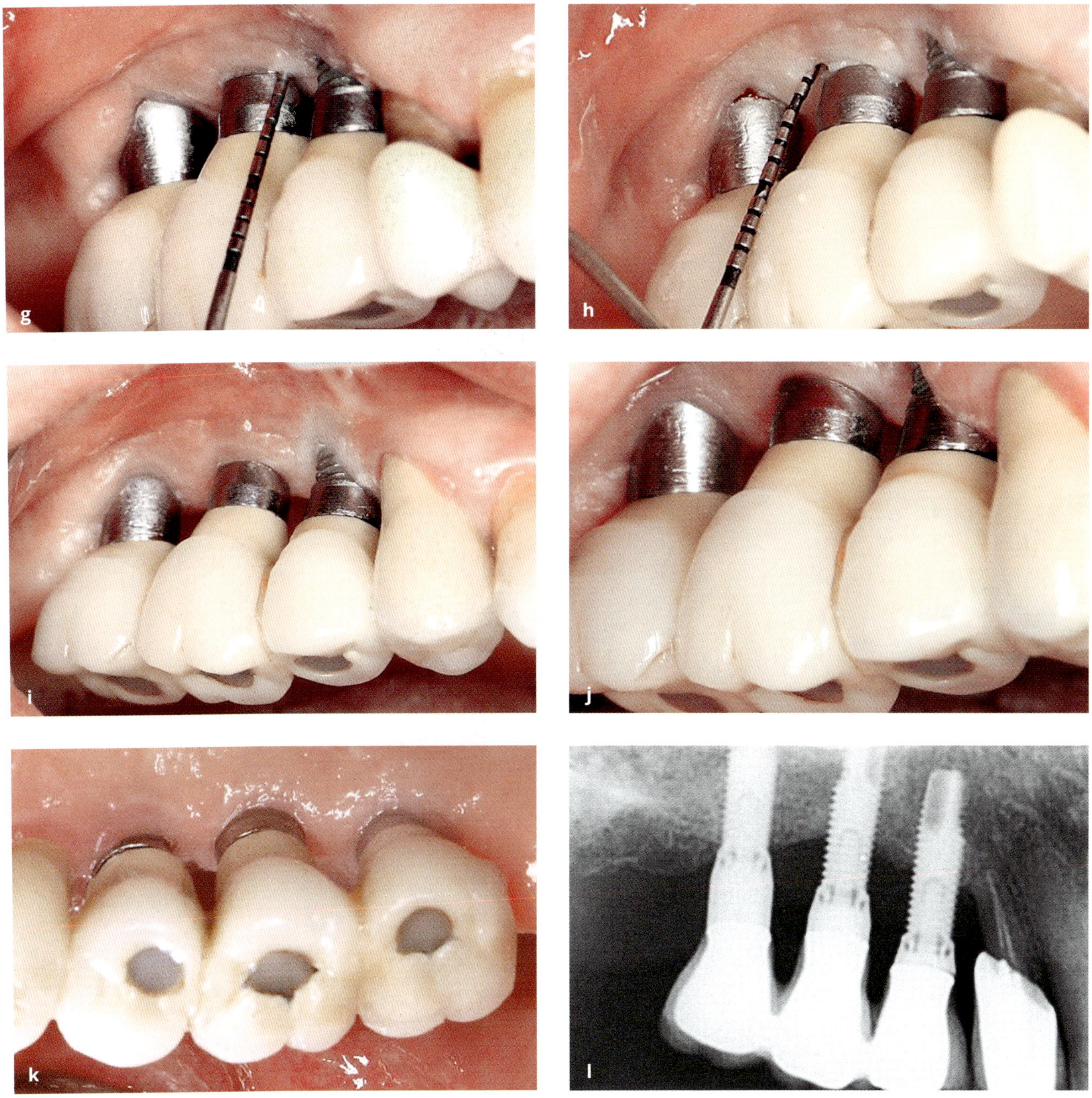

Figs 6-2g–l **(g)** Two years after surgery. **(h)** Three years after surgery. Inflammation was treated with the cumulative interceptive supportive therapy protocol, as described in this book. **(i)** Four years after surgery. The crown was replaced at no. 14. **(j to l)** Clinical images and radiograph taken 5 years after the therapeutic intervention and 15 years after implant placement. The implants maintained a remarkable survival rate. They survived but were no longer considered successful.

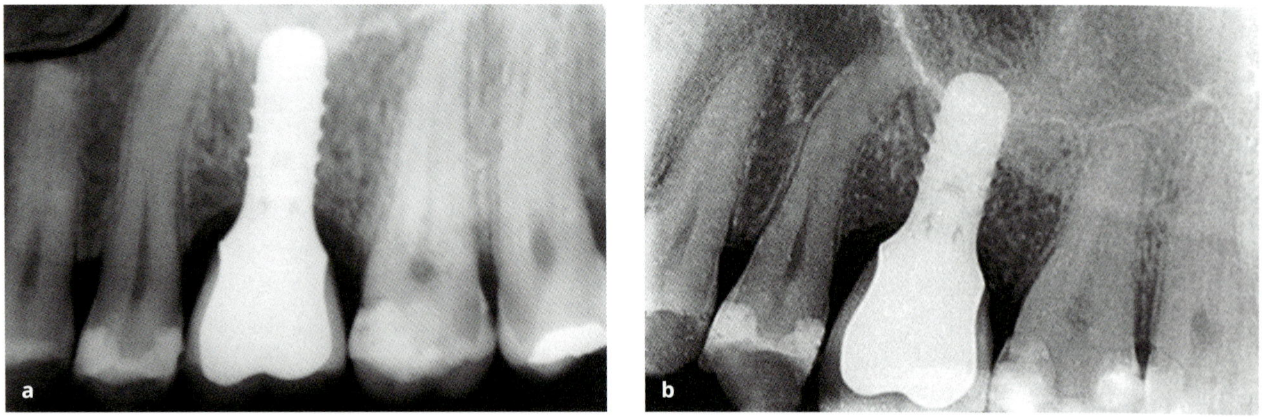

Figs 6-3a, b Radiographic images of a single implant **(a)** 5 years and **(b)** 10 years after placement. The fact that the patient's functional needs were met while the biologic parameters were fulfilled for 10 years meant that the implant is characterized as successful. The fillings of the adjacent teeth have been replaced.

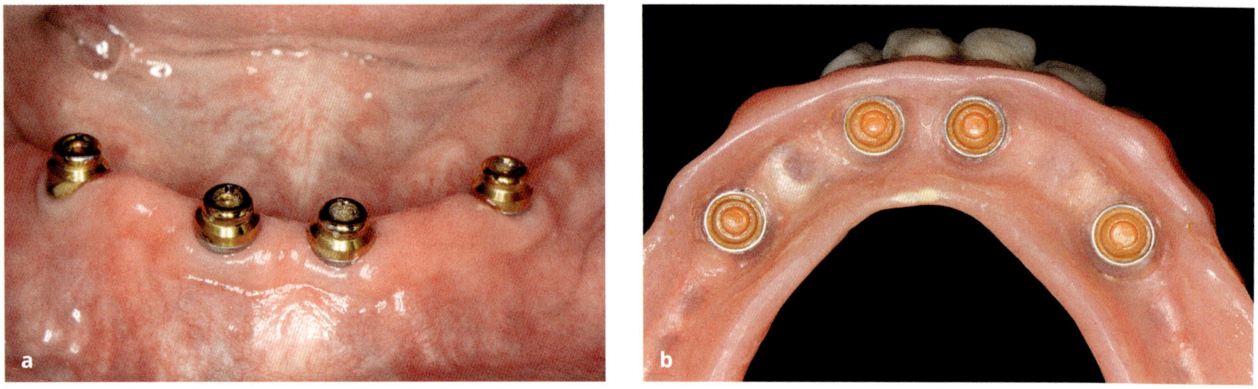

Figs 6-4a, b **(a)** Clinical image of a patient with an implant-supported overdenture, taken when they came for their scheduled maintenance care quarterly session. The health of the peri-implant tissues was maintained through daily administration of effective oral hygiene and compliance with the maintenance care program for 7 years. **(b)** The patient kept the denture free of soft or hard deposits.

Table 1 Implant success criteria as defined by Schnitman and Shulman[2]

Subjective	Objective
▪ Adequate function ▪ Absence of discomfort ▪ Satisfaction of the patient's subjective needs in terms of improving esthetics, and emotional and psychologic parameters	▪ Stable occlusion and proper vertical dimension ▪ Bone loss not greater than one-third of the implant's vertical height, absence of symptoms and functional stability after 5 years ▪ Mild soft tissue inflammation, mobility less than 1 mm ▪ Absence of symptoms, infection, injury of neighboring teeth, or paresthesia ▪ No violation of neighboring anatomic structures (inferior alveolar nerve, sinus cavity, and nasal floor)

criteria have been proposed, some objective and some more subjective.

It is interesting to see the historic development of stricter success criteria over time as knowledge on the subject has increased.

In one of the first attempts to establish success criteria, Schnitman and Shulman[2] (Table 1) defined objective and subjective criteria for evaluating implants, including subperiosteal and blade-type implants (Figs 6-5a–e).

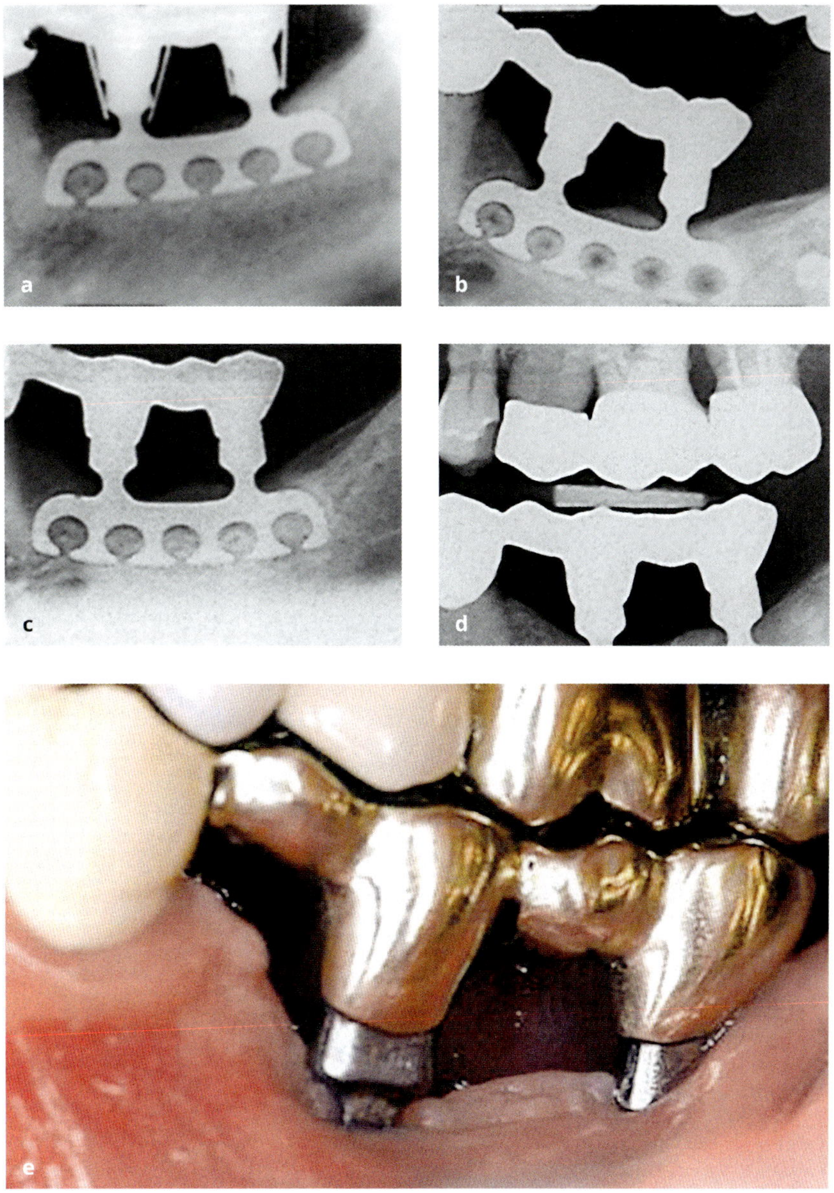

Figs 6-5a–e Monitoring the longevity of a blade-type implant that remained successful for at least 21 years. **(a)** After implant placement. **(b)** Four years later; peri-implant bone stability can be observed. **(c)** Six years later, the situation was stable. **(d)** The last bitewing radiograph, which was taken 21 years after implant placement, did not reveal the full extent of the implant. However, around the neck of the distal abutment, and the mesial surface of the mesial abutment, stability of the alveolar bone could be observed. **(e)** The clinical picture reveals peri-implant tissues with moderate inflammation.

Table 2 Success criteria according to Albrektsson et al[3]

- Implants must be immobile
- No indication of peri-implant radiolucency
- The mean annual vertical bone loss should not exceed 0.2 mm after their first year of function and 0.1 mm per year thereafter
- Absence of inflammation, pain, neuropathy, or paresthesia
- The success rate after 5 years should reach 85%; after 10 years it should be 80%

Clearly, bone loss was expected around blade and subperiosteal implants. This explained why bone loss that reached one-third of the implant's height 5 years after placement was considered acceptable. In addition, a connective tissue capsule was formed around the implant; consequently, some mobility was acceptable and expected. If it reached 1 mm, the restoration was considered successful. Of course, with current knowledge, such extensive bone loss confirms a condition that is far from successful, while clinically detectable mobility is a reason for failed osseointegration.

After obtaining experience with the use of osseointegrated implants, Albrektsson et al[3] proposed a set of objective criteria for determining the success of implant systems (Table 2). These criteria were proposed to evaluate the efficacy of different implant systems; however, they have erroneously been used to evaluate single implants in recent decades (Fig 6-6).

The reference to peri-implant radiolucency concerned the continuous lucent zone observed in blade-type implants, where there was connective tissue encapsulation, radiographically depicting radio-

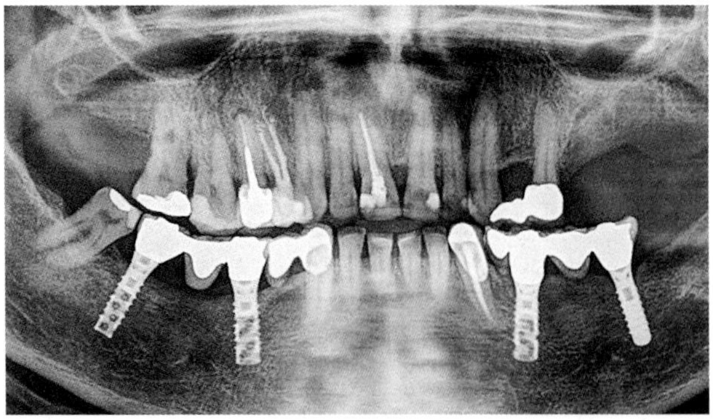

Fig 6-6 Radiograph of a patient with implants in positions 45, 47, and 34, 28 years after placement (case of Dr A. Vilos†).

Table 3 Success criteria according to Buser et al[4]

- Absence of persistent subjective discomfort (pain, foreign body sensation, or insensitivity)
- Absence of recurrent peri-implant inflammation with suppuration
- Lack of mobility
- Absence of continuous radiolucency around the implant
- Possibility of implant-supported restoration placement

lucency. Percentages of 85% and 80% for the 5-and 10-year periods, respectively, were considered acceptable without any scientific evidence for the values. Although reported as success rates, they obviously referred to survival. Today, a significant number of implant systems are available. It is imperative that the clinician seeks scientific documentation dating back at least 5 to 10 years to support the safety and efficacy of the implant.[3]

A few years later, Buser et al[4] presented success criteria for the ITI dental implant system, as the Straumann implant system was known in the 1990s (Table 3). The lack of objectivity is apparent in these criteria. The only indirect quantitative criterion is the absence of mobility. Peri-implant inflammation was evaluated only if it coexisted with suppuration, not to mention loss of attachment, depth of peri-implant pockets, or radiographic evidence of bone loss. The only criterion regarding peri-implant bone loss included was the presence of continuous radiolucency around the implant, which meant complete loss of osseointegration. This extreme view is inadequate to evaluate success and in contrast to the view expressed a few years later during the joint symposium of the National Institutes of Health and the American Academy of Periodontology (AAP) in 1997. This view argued that a successful implant should not show any peri-implant radiolucency. However, an important criterion was mentioned for the first time, which concerned the possibility of placement of an implant-supported restoration.[5]

In 2000, the AAP proposed a set of criteria to determine success, trying to gather as much information as possible to make the evaluation process maximally objective[6] (Table 4). While this proposal included quantitative criteria for the degree of bone loss considered acceptable, no reference was made to criteria used for the diagnosis of peri-implantitis, such as peri-implant pocket depth (PPD) and bleeding on probing (BOP). Finally, the reference to the satisfaction of the criteria for the clinician and the patient does not define a measurable way of determining what is acceptable in terms of function or esthetics of the prosthetic reconstruction.

To correct the vagueness and shortcomings of these attempts to establish success criteria, a group at the University of Bern, Bern, Switzerland proposed the criteria presented in Table 5 and Figs 6-7a, b.

It is clear, as will be discussed in Chapter 7, that recording the initial clinical measurements and obtaining initial reference radiographs, as well as keeping patient records, are prerequisites for evaluating the success of a particular implant. Any implant that does not meet these criteria but that is still functioning should be considered as "surviving".

At this point, the need for global acceptance of specific success criteria should be highlighted. For the same group of patients or implants, different success rates may arise depending on the criteria chosen by the clinician or research team (Fig 6-8).

The term "failure" refers to the loss of an implant. However, sometimes it describes the first episode when the performance or function of the implant falls below a predetermined and clearly defined level, based on quantitative criteria. Considering

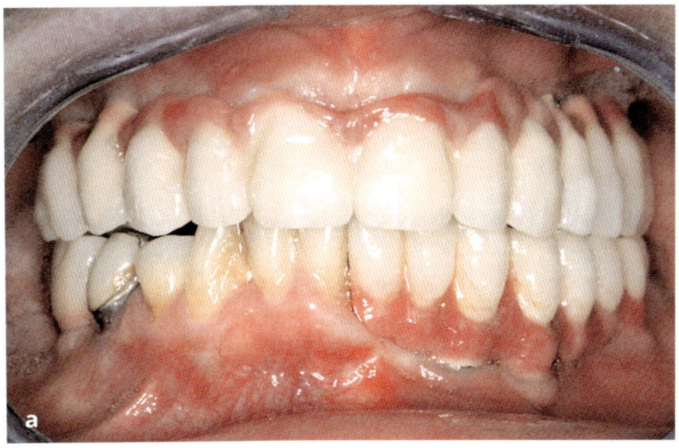

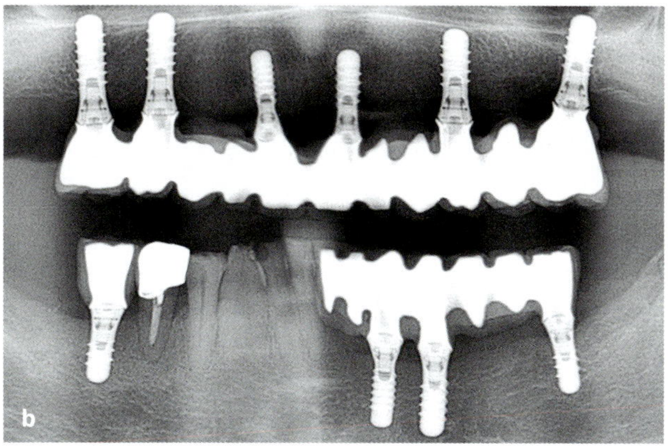

Figs 6-7a, b Clinical and radiographic images of a patient with a fixed cross-arch implant-supported prosthetic reconstruction in the maxilla, and an implant-supported crown on the right and a partial denture on the left in the mandible. The implants operated in biologically and functionally acceptable conditions, meeting the patient's esthetic needs for 8 years. The implants were characterized as successful.

Table 4 AAP criteria for implant success[5,6]

- Absence of persistent signs or symptoms such as pain, inflammation, neuropathy, paresthesia, or injury to vital anatomic structures
- Lack of mobility
- Absence of continuous peri-implant radiolucency
- Insignificant progressive bone loss less than 0.2 mm per year after the expected and physiologic bone remodeling that takes place during the first year after functional loading
- Satisfaction of both the dental practitioner's and the patient's criteria regarding the implant-supported restoration

Table 5 Success criteria set out by the University of Bern, Bern, Switzerland[7]

- Absence of implant mobility
- Absence of continuous peri-implant radiolucency
- Absence of persistent signs or symptoms (pain, inflammation, neuropathy, paresthesia, or injury to vital anatomic structures)
- After the first year of surgery, vertical bone loss should not exceed 0.2 mm per year
- Absence of peri-implant pockets ≥ 5 mm with BOP
- Fulfillment of the objective esthetic specifications and objective requirements of the patient

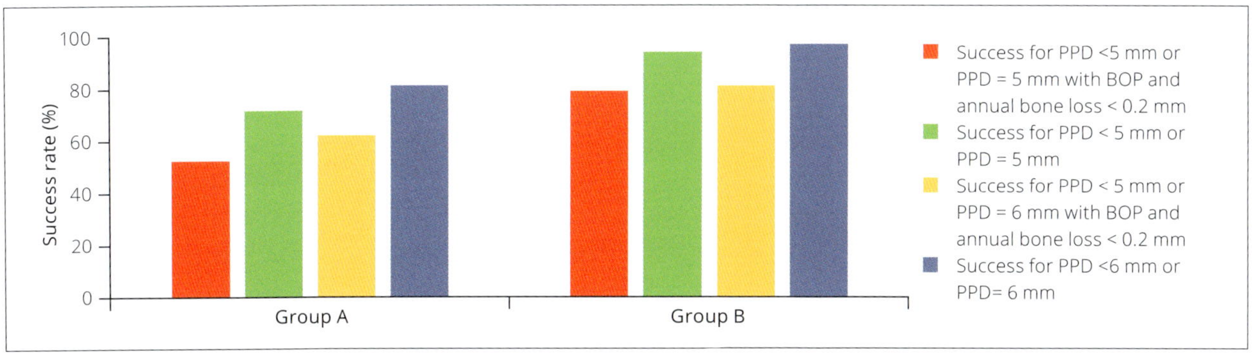

Fig 6-8 Implants in patients with a history of periodontitis (group A) and in periodontally healthy patients (group B). Clinical measurements of periodontal pocket depth (PPD) and BOP were performed, as well as radiographic measurements of bone loss after 10 years of function. For the same implants, success rates differed depending on which criteria were chosen and how strict they were. However, regardless of the definition of success, it was statistically significantly lower for implants placed in patients with a history of periodontitis (modified by Karoussis et al.[7]).

the fact that the term "failure" has prevailed to describe implant loss, it is more appropriate to speak of "complications" to describe the aforementioned conditions.

Implant complications and failures are classified into three categories:

- Biologic: the inability to achieve or maintain osseointegration.
- Mechanical: technical problems such as implant fracture, loosening of the retaining screw of the prosthetic reconstruction or transmucosal abutment, fracture of the restoration, coating material.
- Complications or failures related to the patient: esthetic, psychologic, or phonetic aspects.[8]

Biologic complications may include peri-implant mucositis or peri-implantitis. The development of one of these diseases does not necessarily mean that the implant will fail, but these are conditions that certainly must be treated. They indicate an increased risk for future failure and should therefore be diagnosed at an early stage. If the appropriate treatment is applied, peri-implant tissues may be brought to a healthy state. Identification of the risk factors involved in a biologic complication is of extreme value as the best treatment is prevention. Two conditions still need to be clarified regarding the failure of an implant.[9] Failures may be categorized into those related to the inability to achieve osseointegration before functional loading, and implant losses after successful initial osseointegration. The terms used to describe these are early and late failures, respectively.

Early failures may arise due to smoking, the presence of uncontrolled diabetes mellitus, inexperience on the part of the clinician, contamination of the recipient area, the inability to achieve initial stability, incorrect surgical handling, premature exercise of uncontrolled occlusal forces, or flap tear during regenerative procedures. Regarding the implant placement process, factors that may be involved are overheating of the bone during preparation of the implant bed, insufficient water spray, worn cutting tools, and eccentric movements of the cutting tool. Early failures are rare and low rates of 1% to 2% have been reported.[10–14]

Late failures occur due to the loss of osseointegration along the entire length and perimeter of the implant. The most usual cause of late failures is peri-implantitis, and less often implant fracture.

Survival rates vary depending on the type of implant-supported prosthetic reconstruction. A series of thorough systematic reviews concluded that the survival rate of dental implants 5 years after placement is 90.1% where a mixed restoration has been performed, 95.4% where a prosthetic reconstruction is purely implant-supported, and 96.8% for single implant crowns. Ten years after placement, this number may be reduced to 82.1%, 92.8%, and 96.3%, respectively. It is worth mentioning that these percentages are lower than the survival rate of natural teeth for the same period of time, even those that have undergone dental treatment, treatment of periodontitis, or prosthetic reconstruction. Although dental implant treatment has become more widely accepted in recent decades, the cost remains high, so, it is clear that there is still a need for significant improvement of the predictability of implant treatments.[10-16]

Consequently, the factors influencing the outcome of implant therapy are of great interest and have been classified into parameters relating to the patient, the anatomy of the edentulous area, and the type and properties of the implant. The former include factors such as smoking, history of periodontitis, systemic diseases, and history of previous radiation therapy. In addition, the success and survival rate of implants in deficient areas has been studied extensively after the application of various regenerative techniques, such as guided bone regeneration and sinus floor elevation.[17]

Regarding the characteristics of the implant, a field of interest is surface treatment and morphology at the macro-, micro-, and nano-level.[18]

The factors that determine the success of osseointegration are:

- biocompatibility of the implant material;
- implant design;
- careful handling by and appropriate training of the clinician;
- proper planning of temporary and transitional prosthetic reconstruction;
- avoidance of uncontrolled functional loading before osseointegration is achieved;
- satisfactory quality of bone tissue;
- absence of inflammation at the implant recipient site;
- control, establishment, and maintenance of periodontal health before implant placement.

References

1. Misch CE, Perel ML, Wang HL, et al. Implant success, survival, and failure: the International Congress of Oral Implantologists (ICOI) Pisa Consensus Conference. Implant Dent 2008;17:5–15.
2. Schnitman PA, Shulman LB. Recommendations of the consensus development conference on dental implants. J Am Dent Assoc 1979;98:373–377.
3. Albrektsson T, Zarb G, Worthington P, Eriksson AR. The long-term efficacy of currently used dental implants: a review and proposed criteria of success. Int J Oral Maxillofac Implants 1986;1:11–25.
4. Buser D, Weber HP, Lang NP. Tissue integration of non-submerged implants. 1-year results of a prospective study with 100 ITI hollow-cylinder and hollow-screw implants. Clin Oral Implants Res 1990;1:33–40.
5. van Steenberghe D. Outcomes and their measurement in clinical trials of endosseous oral implants. Ann Periodontol 1997;2(1):291–298.
6. Research, Science and Therapy Committee of the American Academy of Periodontology. Position Paper Dental Implants in Periodontal Therapy. J Periodontol 2000;71(12):1934–1942.
7. Karoussis IK, Salvi GE, Heitz-Mayfield LJA, Brägger U, Hämmerle CHF, Lang NP. Long-term implant prognosis in patients with and without a history of chronic periodontitis: a 10-year prospective cohort study of the ITI Dental Implant System. Clin Oral Implants Res 2003;14:329–339.
8. Hanif A, Qureshi S, Sheikh Z, Rashid H. Complications in implant dentistry. Eur J Dent 2017;11:135–140.
9. Charyeva O, Altynbekov K, Zhartybaev R, Sabdanaliev A. Long-term dental implant success and survival—a clinical study after an observation period up to 6 years. Swed Dent J 2012;36:1–6.
10. Pjetursson BE, Tan K, Lang NP, Brägger U, Egger M, Zwahlen M. A systematic review of the survival and complication rates of implant-supported fixed partial dentures (FPDs) after a mean observation period of at least 5 years. Clin Oral Implants Res 2004;15:625–642.
11. Lang NP, Pjetursson BE, Tan K, Brägger U, Egger M, Zwahlen M. A systematic review of the survival and complication rates of fixed partial dentures (FPDs) after an observation period of at least 5 years. II. Combined tooth—implant—supported FPDs. Clin Oral Implants Res 2004;15:643–653.
12. Tan K, Pjetursson BE, Lang NP, Chan ESY. A systematic review of the survival and complication rates of fixed partial dentures (FPDs) after an observation period of at least 5 years. Clin Oral Implants Res 2004;15:654–666.
13. Pjetursson BE, Thoma D, Jung R, Zwahlen M, Zembic A. A systematic review of the survival and complication rates of implant-supported fixed dental prostheses (FDPs) after a mean observation period of at least 5 years. Clin Oral Implants Res 2012;23(suppl 6):22–38.
14. Pjetursson BE, Brägger U, Lang NP, Zwahlen M. Comparison of survival and complication rates of tooth-supported fixed dental prostheses (FDPs) and implant supported FDPs and single crowns (SCs). Clin Oral Implants Res 2007;18(suppl 3):97–113.
15. Moraschini V, Poubel LA, Ferreira VF, Barboza Edos S. Evaluation of survival and success rates of dental implants reported in longitudinal studies with a follow-up period of at least 10 years: a systematic review. Int J Oral Maxillofac Surg 2015;44:377–388.
16. Lekholm U, Gunne J, Henry P, et al. Survival of the Brånemark implant in partially edentulous jaws: a 10-year prospective multicenter study. Int J Oral Maxillofac Implants 1999;14:639–645.
17. Esposito M, Hirsch JM, Lekholm U, Thomsen P. Biological factors contributing to failures of osseointegrated oral implants. (I). Success criteria and epidemiology. Eur J Oral Sci 1998;106:527–551.
18. Papaspyridakos P, Chen C-J, Singh M, Weber H-P, Gallucci GO. Success criteria in implant dentistry: a systematic review. J Dent Res 2012;91:242–248.

7 Diagnosis of Peri-Implant Disease

Diagnosis of peri-implantitis is based on several criteria. Diagnostic methods complement one another, and the clinician should be able to assess all available diagnostic information so that a proper diagnosis of the condition of the peri-implant tissues may be ascertained.

I. CLINICAL EXAMINATION

The information obtained and recorded from the clinical examination is as follows:

- bleeding on probing (BOP);
- peri-implant pocket probing depth and peri-implant clinical attachment level;
- suppuration and exudation on probing;
- implant stability.

7.1 BOP

BOP is the main pathognomonic clinical finding to diagnose inflammation of peri-implant tissues. To avoid false positive measurements, the application of excessive probing pressure should be avoided. Such a force should not exceed 0.3 N. Bleeding on light probing with a periodontal probe is indicative of the presence of peri-implant inflammation at the bottom of the sulcus or pocket:

- Probing depth of at least 5 mm, without bleeding, may still indicate peri-implant health.
- Probing depth < 5 mm with BOP is characteristic of peri-implant mucositis.
- Probing depth ≥ 5 mm makes the comparison of the situation with the initial measurements of sulcus depth and radiographic examination essential to verify either the presence of peri-implant mucositis or peri-implantitis (Figs 7-1a–c).

Absence of BOP has a highly negative prognostic value, not only for teeth but also for implants. It is an index of the absence of peri-implant inflammation and, as a result, indicates the stability of the condition of peri-implant tissues. On the other hand, the presence of BOP of the peri-implant sulcus may pose a significant risk for the development of peri-implantitis if peri-implant mucositis is not treated early. However, the extent to which BOP is correlated with future peri-implant loss of attachment is subject to debate.[1]

In the past, the presence of BOP did not constitute a reliable prognostic indicator of peri-implantitis progression; the view that prevailed at the time was that only the absence of BOP could be used as an indicator for stability of the peri-implant condition.[2] However, recent studies in patients with implants that responded to a maintenance care program drew the conclusion that there was indeed a progression of peri-implantitis in patients who did not comply with the recall care program after monitoring for

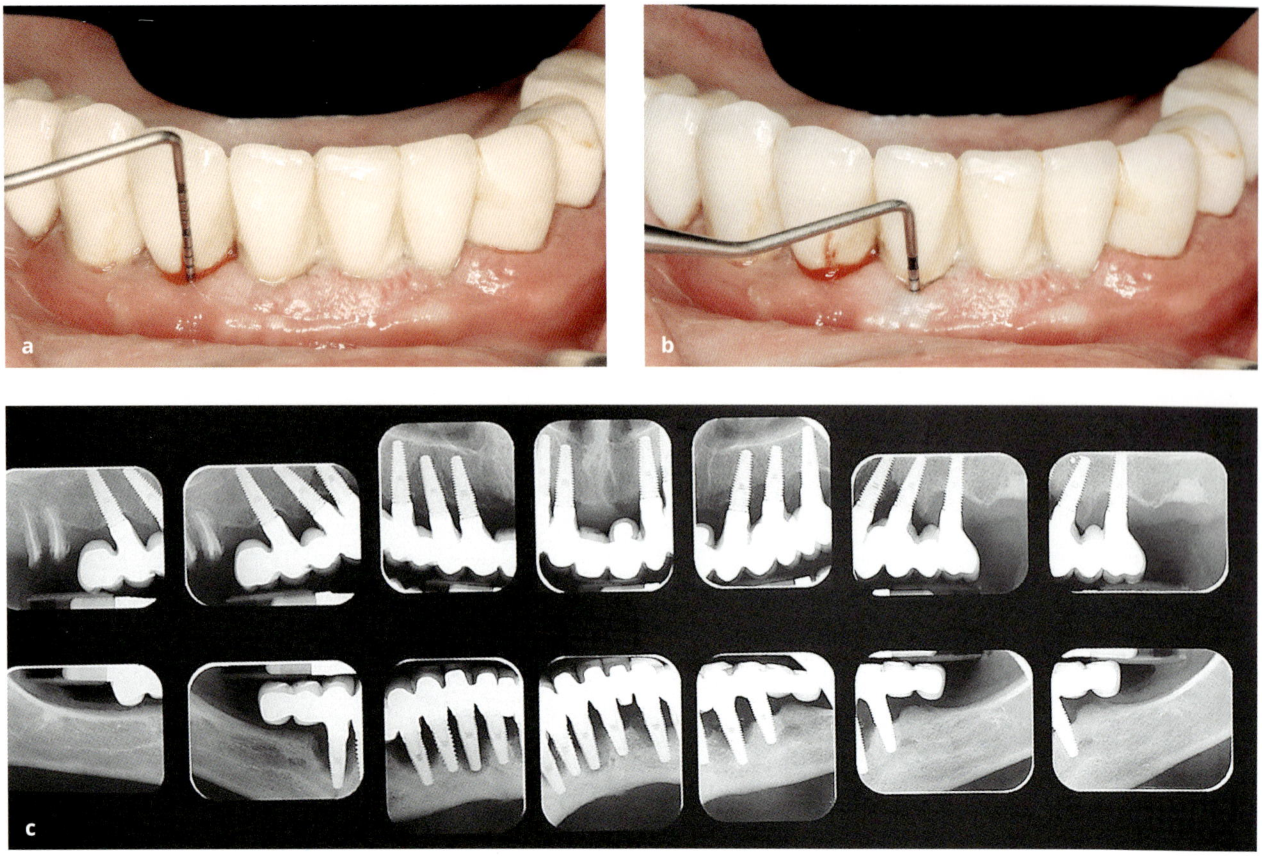

Figs 7-1a–c BOP is a diagnostic criterion of inflammation. Combined with probing depth and radiography, a diagnosis of peri-implant mucositis or peri-implantitis can be made. The treatment of this case is presented in Figure 15-1.

2 years. It is remarkable how BOP in more than 50% of recalls has more than 50% sensitivity and 100% specificity for peri-implant sites. Moreover, BOP in the peri-implant sulcus at two consecutive recalls during the maintenance care phase has a greater positive predictive value in peri-implant than in periodontal sites. In other words, the greatest indication for peri-implant stability comes from the absence of BOP. This may be ensured with the application of oral hygiene and patient compliance with a personalized maintenance care program.[3]

7.2 Peri-implant probing depth and clinical attachment

The term "probing" is defined according to the soft tissue attachment in natural dentition. At the implant surface, however, a true attachment is only mediated by the junctional epithelium, with hemidesmosomes and the basement membrane. For the supracrestal fibers of connective tissue, the term is only used incorrectly because those fibers do not really insert into the implants. Instead, they are simply aligned alongside or angularly in relation to the implant, while some come into simple contact with the implant surface. In any case, they do not form a true biologic attachment (Fig 7-2).

The use of a periodontal probe is essential for diagnosis as probing of the peri-implant sulcus or pocket may lead to accurate assessment of the probing attachment level. At the same time, probing may be used to assess inflammation (Figs 7-3a, b).

The peri-implant sulcus is a narrow space between the free peri-implant mucosa and the surface of the implant reconstruction. The depth of the peri-implant sulcus or pocket is defined as the distance between the crest of the peri-implant mucosa and the bottom of the peri-implant sulcus or pocket. The peri-implant clinical attachment level is defined as the distance between the implant neck, that being the reference point, and the bottom of the peri-implant sulcus or pocket.

For a valid comparison, measurements should be performed at different time points (recalls) so that differences in the depth of the peri-implant sulcus or pocket may be assessed. Recording all measurements is essential. Only by keeping extensive records can an early diagnosis of peri-implantitis be established. The initial measurements, which are taken right after placement of the final reconstruction, are used as the reference.[4]

The depth of the gingival crevice reaches up to 3 mm, whereas the peri-implant sulcus reaches up to 4 mm in a state of homeostasis. Deepening of the gingival crevice to more than 3 mm may constitute a divergence from the physiologic state. When it comes to implants, the peri-implant sulcus may be deeper than 4 mm without implying the presence of a peri-implant pocket. A depth of 5 mm or more may still be compatible with peri-implant health under conditions where there is no inflammation. Such depths are frequently encountered in the esthetic zone or at sites where peri-implant tissue thickness is greatest (Figs 7-4a–d and 7-5).

In the case of peri-implant health and when the applied force and angle during probing are correct, the edge of the periodontal probe reaches the apical part of the junctional epithelium, the length of which is approximately 2 mm in a state of homeostasis.

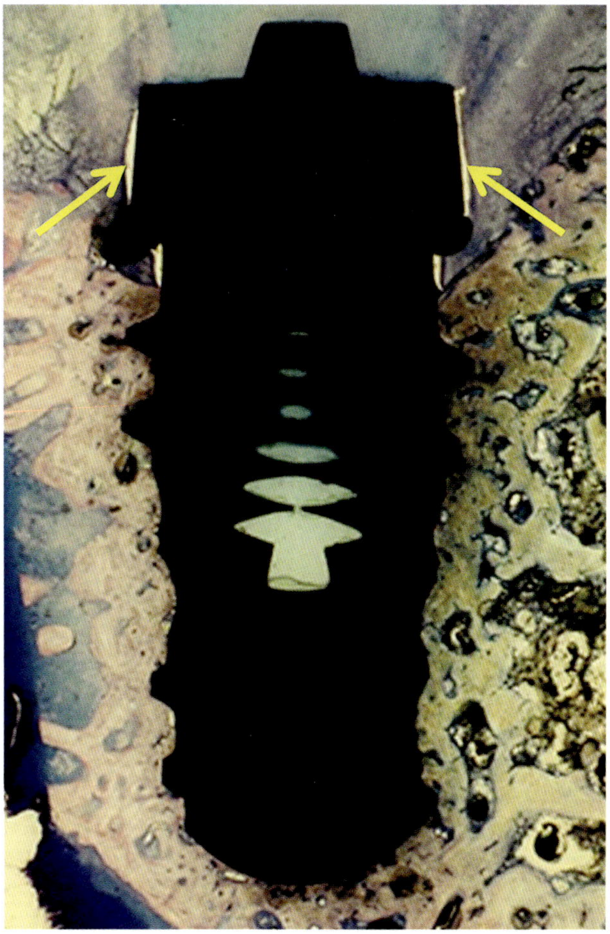

Fig 7-2 Histologic sample from a dog, where an implant and its relationship with the peri-implant tissues can be seen long after functional loading. The absence of fibers that insert into the implant surface creates a blank space (white areas, yellow arrows) during sample sectioning for the histologic examination.

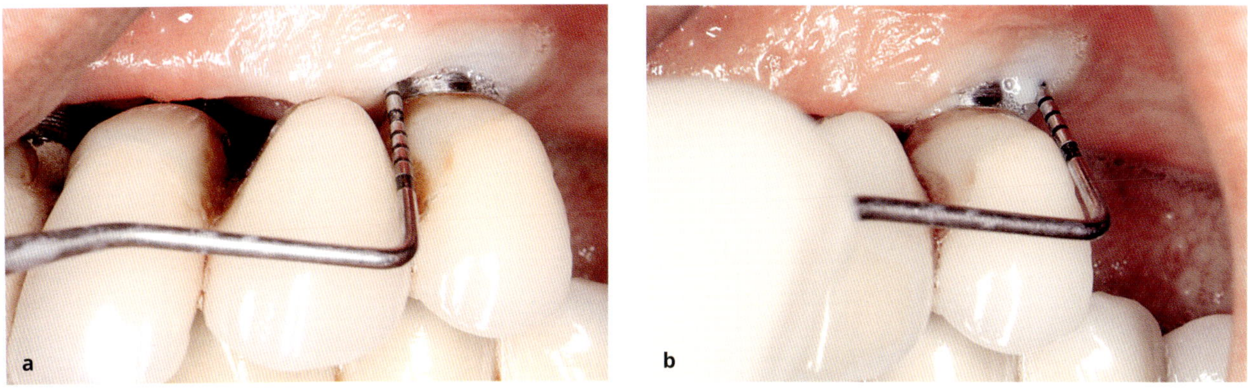

Figs 7-3a, b Using a periodontal probe, loss of the peri-implant tissue attachment can be noted, as well as the depth of the peri-implant pockets and bleeding or suppuration on probing.

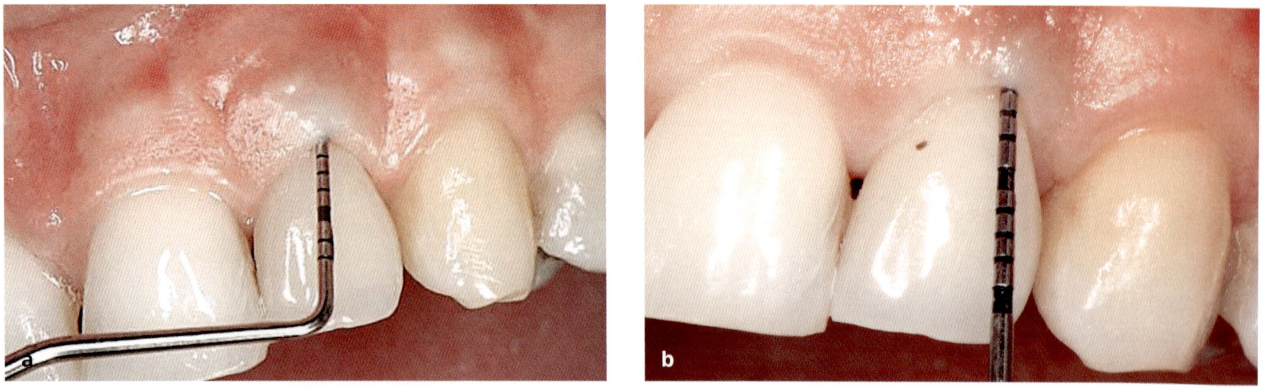

Figs 7-4a, b It is important to keep an archive of clinical measurements. For implant no. 22, a 6-mm-deep peri-implant crevice was recorded on the patient's file right after placement of the restoration. **(a)** Four years after implant placement, a probing depth of 6 mm can be seen. **(b)** Seventeen years after implant placement, there is still a 6-mm probing depth on implant no. 22. This is not a pocket because the implant was deliberately placed more apically for esthetic reasons. There is a small alteration (recession) of the gingival margin of teeth nos. 21 and 23.

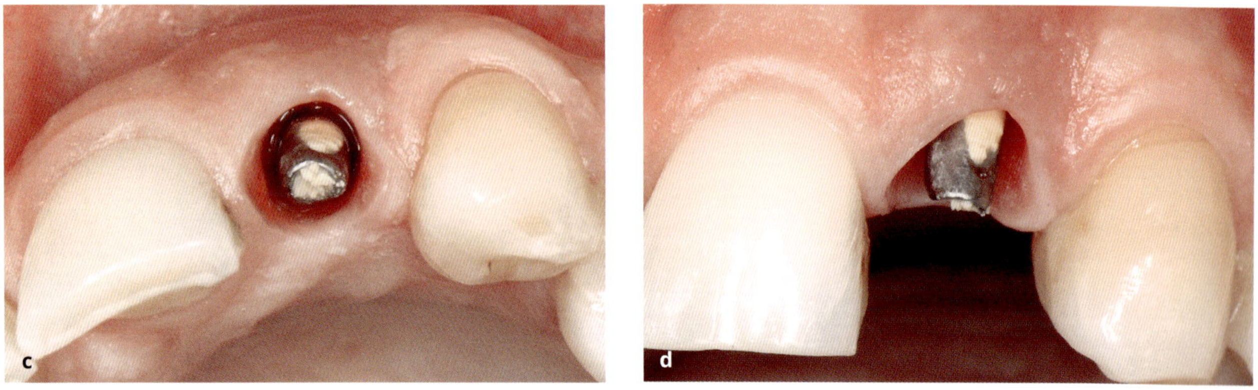

Figs 7-4c, d After removal of the crown, the healthy peri-implant mucosa in the peri-implant crevice can be observed.

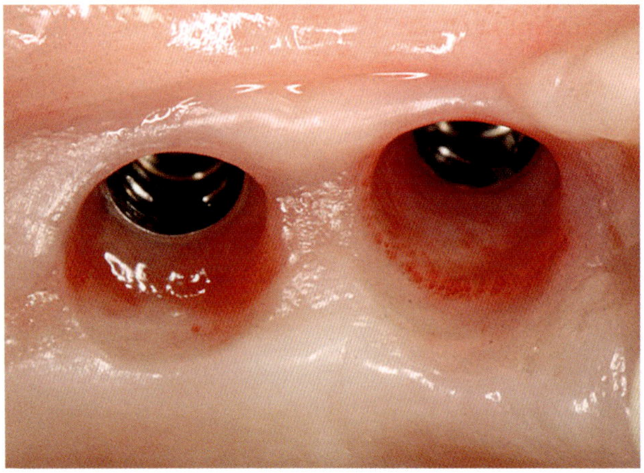

Fig 7-5 Greater magnification of Fig 7-3, where the absence of inflammation can be seen around the implants that were placed in a site with thick mucosa, thus creating deep crevices from the beginning. Small capillaries can be observed as they show through the junctional epithelium of the peri-implant crevices.

Should forces exceed 0.15 N, the periodontal probe will penetrate the peri-implant connective tissue. The same is true for cases where peri-implant inflammation is present. The greater the severity of inflammation, the greater the insertion depth of the periodontal probe. Considering that peri-implant connective tissue fibers do not attach to the implant surface, resistance of the peri-implant connective tissue to penetration of the probe is weaker than that of the supracrestal connective tissue of surrounding teeth. Thus, even the slightest degree of peri-implant inflammation might allow deeper insertion of the periodontal probe into the peri-implant connective tissue.[5,6] This explains why a peri-implant pocket depth of 5 mm or less measured with a periodontal probe, with the concomitant absence of BOP, indicates peri-implant health.

It is also clear why, in cases where the depth is equal to or greater than 5 mm with concomitant BOP,

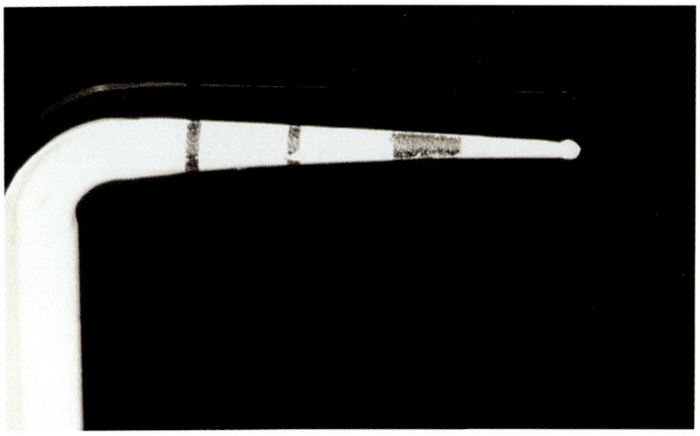

Fig 7-6 In the past, probing of peri-implant pockets was only done with plastic probes. It is now common knowledge that the implant surface is not negatively affected by nontraumatic contact with metal instruments.

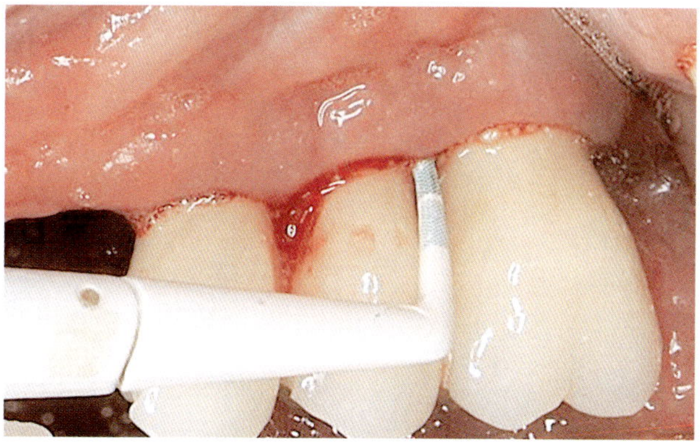

Fig 7-7 Plastic periodontal probe using standard force.

this could be an indication for peri-implantitis; hence, that site should be examined further. In such cases, the record of previous measurements may be very useful.

Probing of the peri-implant sulcus and pocket does not cause trauma when executed with a metal or plastic periodontal probe using a slight force of approximately 0.15 N (or at least up to 0.25 N) (Figs 7-6 and 7-7).[7]

An integral part of the initial treatment plan is the design of an appropriate implant restoration, as the peri-implant sulcus or pocket depth and clinical attachment levels are often difficult to assess. Implant restorations that lack the appropriate anatomic design and have an excessively bell-shaped structure force the use of a periodontal probe with a greater angle with regard to the long axis of the implant. Moreover, they make the application of proper oral hygiene extremely challenging, thereby increasing the risk of the development of peri-implantitis. Finally, clinical measurements may be made difficult by the morphological peculiarities of the implant itself, such as exposed threads, platform switching, or even surface roughness.

Over the years, platform switching has been a controversial topic. Although suggested by several implant manufacturers, probing of the peri-implant sulcus is practically impossible. Those in favor of this implant design believe that it provides greater stability at the marginal peri-implant bone level because achieving biologic width is easier. In a recent systematic review and meta-analysis of 22 clinical studies, bone resorption around the implant neck was on average 0.49 mm when platform switching was applied. On the other hand, for an implant–abutment connection of the same diameter, the mean bone resorption was 1.01 mm (Figs 7-8 and 7-9a, b).[8]

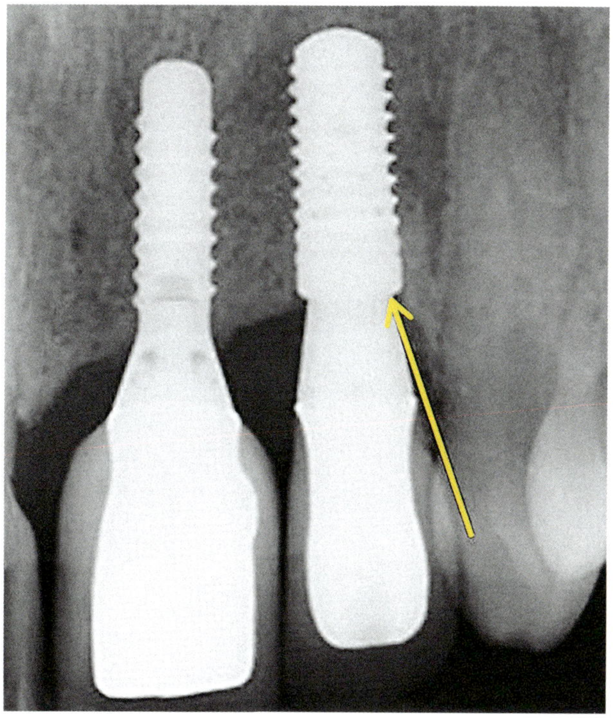

Fig 7-8 A radiograph is the only means to evaluate bone destruction in cases where platform switching has been selected; even if there is bone destruction due to peri-implantitis, insertion of the periodontal probe should stop when it reaches the neck of the implant (yellow arrow).

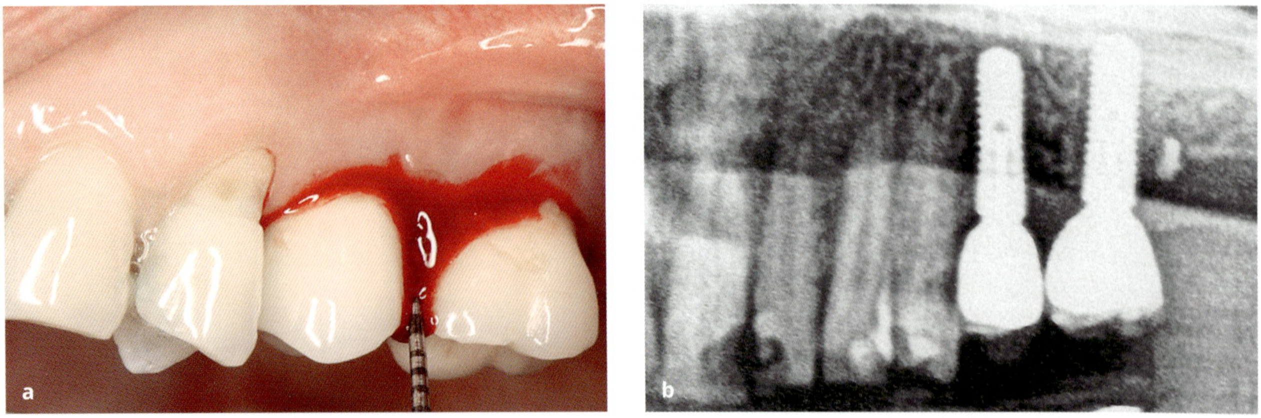

Figs 7-9a, b BOP is a diagnostic criterion of inflammation. Insertion of the periodontal probe, however, is blocked due to platform switching. Only radiographic examination can establish the diagnosis of peri-implantitis because this is the only examination that can reveal bone destruction.

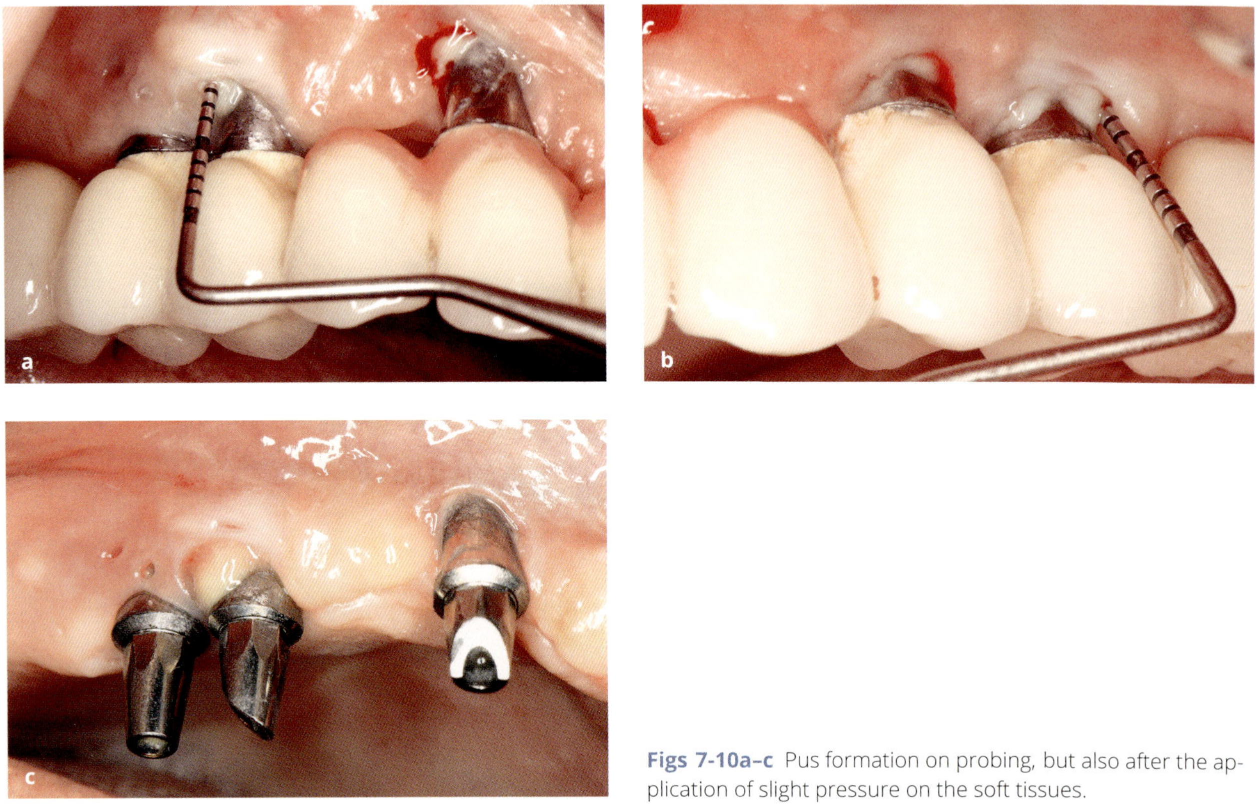

Figs 7-10a–c Pus formation on probing, but also after the application of slight pressure on the soft tissues.

7.3 Suppuration and exudation on probing

Suppuration or exudation from the peri-implant sulcus or pocket is usually observed during or right after probing, and constitutes a significant sign of peri-implant inflammation. Pus is a product of tissue destruction and consists mainly of dead microorganisms and immune cells. Exudation usually indicates a high concentration of inflammatory cells in peri-implant tissues, including multinuclear neutrophils, as well as dead microorganisms and host cells. Suppuration on probing of peri-implant tissues has been associated with severe peri-implant inflammation (Figs 7-10a–c and 7-11).

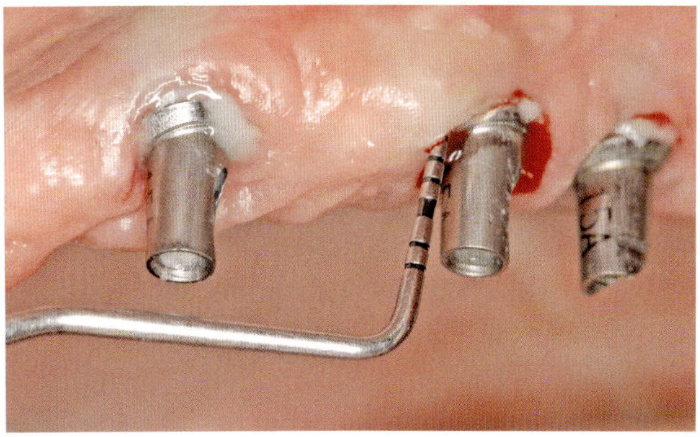

Fig 7-11 Pus formation and BOP of a peri-implant pocket indicate that a radiographic examination is required immediately.

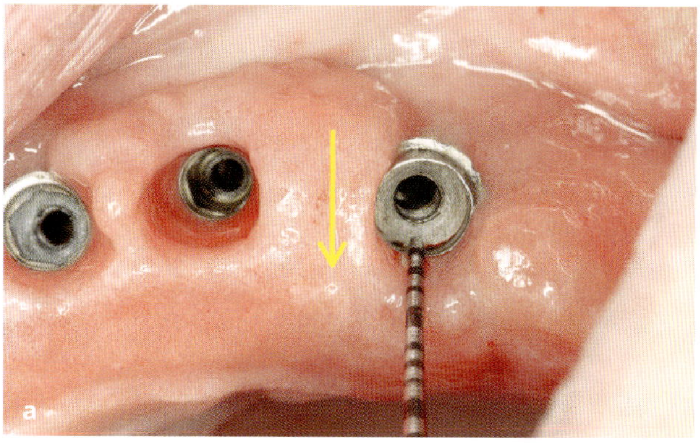

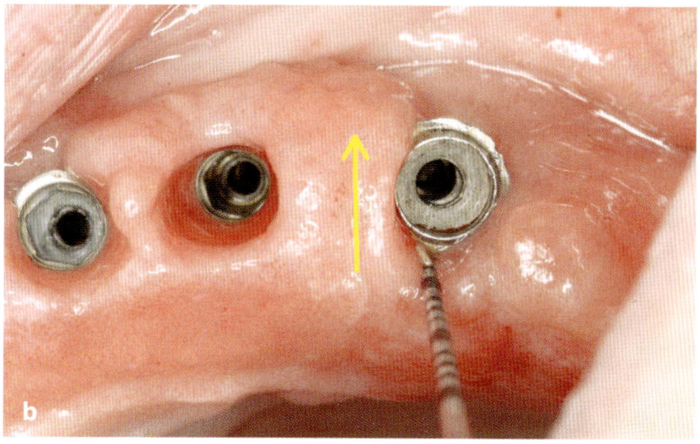

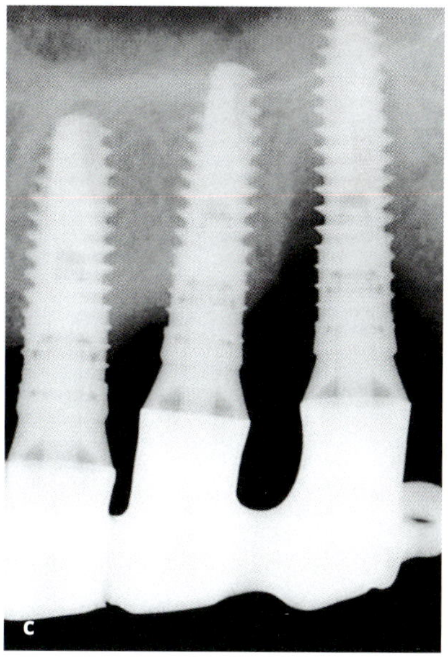

Figs 7-12a–c (a and b) Implant mobility that is present only in cases of complete loss of osseointegration. The implant position changes depending on the direction of the force used (yellow arrows). **(c)** On the radiograph, bone destruction that extends to the most apical threads of implant 25 may be observed.

7.4 Implant stability

To properly evaluate the absence of implant mobility, it is necessary to remove the superposed prosthesis so that a false recording of mobility of a detached restoration can be avoided (Figs 7-12a–c and 7-13a–d). Implant mobility is a diagnostic element that proves the complete loss of osseointegration, which may be attributed to the final stage of peri-implantitis, implant fracture, or the early inability to achieve osseointegration. This clinical criterion cannot be used for the diagnosis of peri-implantitis at an early stage because there are many cases where the implant does not present with mobility, even if the greatest portion of the supporting bone has been lost. Only 1 to 2 mm of bone support may remain intact and still make the implant stable. For this reason, it is a mistake to assess implant mobility to diagnose peri-implantitis (Figs 7-14 and 7-15).

Moreover, redness and edema of the peri-implant mucosa are indicative signs of peri-implant inflammation, which could be either peri-implant mucositis or peri-implantitis (Figs 7-16a, b). However, neither redness nor edema are reliable diagnostic signs in most cases. The degree of keratinization and thickness of peri-implant tissues, which vary between patients but also between different sites in the same oral cavity, significantly affect the clinical picture of the color and volume of peri-implant tissues. As redness of the peri-implant mucosa depends on many factors, such as its thickness and degree of keratinization, it is possible that at a site with increased thickness of keratinized peri-implant tissues, there will not be any redness despite the underlying presence of inflammation. On the other hand, a healthy site could be mistaken as red due to a lack of keratinized tissues (Fig 7-17).

Moreover, color is evaluated using different subjective criteria by different examiners and is, of course, affected by the color of the implant abutments. Titanium abutments give the peri-implant

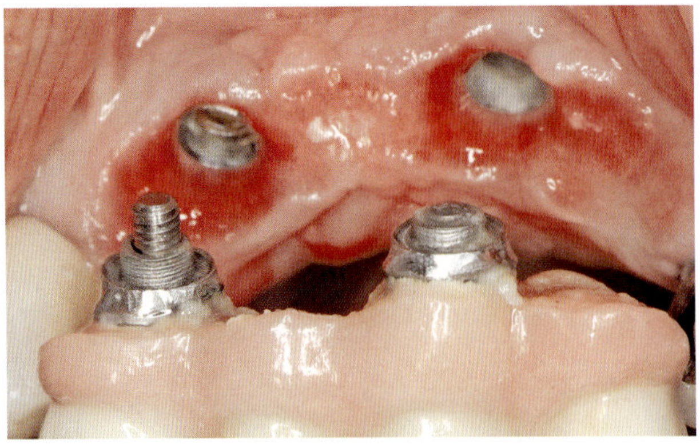

Fig 7-13a The patient complained about implant mobility. Unscrewing of the prosthesis revealed significant accumulation of biofilm and an inflammatory clinical situation in the peri-implant crevices. This was caused by ineffective oral hygiene, implant fracture, an absence of maintenance care, and fracture and loosening of the fixation screws that occurred over a long time.

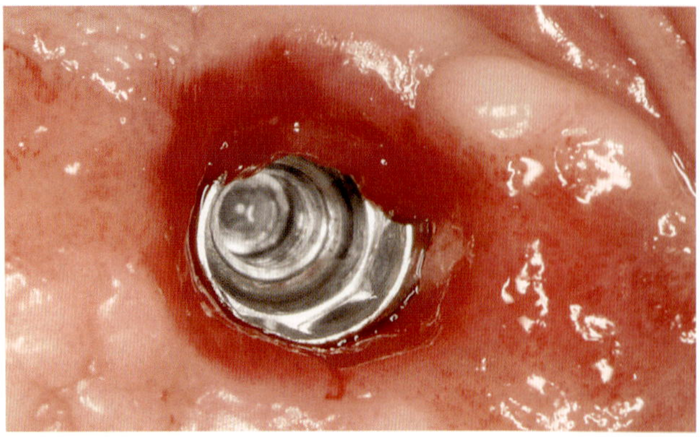

Fig 7-13b Mucosal hyperplasia that has claimed the abutment seat at the intact implant. This is a case where a technical complication (fracture of the implant and fixation screw) led to a biologic complication (peri-implant mucositis).

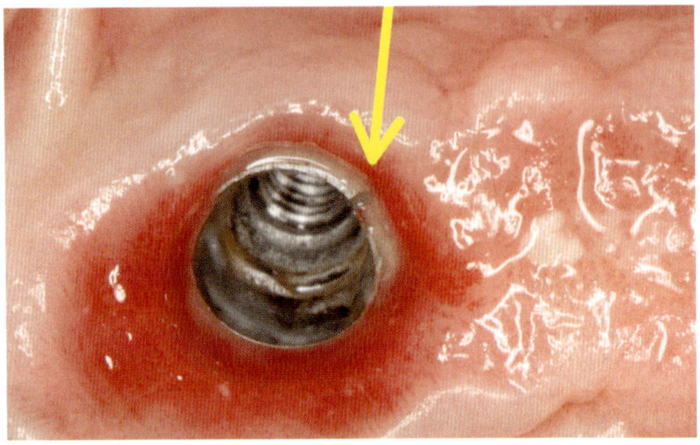

Fig 7-13c Line of the implant fracture (yellow arrow).

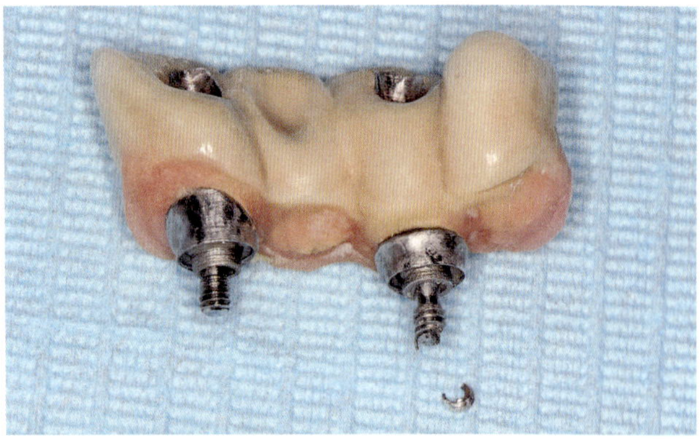

Fig 7-13d Fracture of the fixation screw.

mucosa a gray shade, whereas zirconia abutments result in a whitish shade.

Regarding the increased volume of soft peri-implant tissues, comparison to the initial situation can only be achieved by the clinician who treated the patient, especially when they have the initial photographs from that site. An increase in the volume of the peri-implant mucosa may be due to tissue edema, but it may also be due to other reasons, such as specific drugs or the poor fitting of a removable prosthesis.

The production of a dull sound on percussion is an indication of disturbance or even loss of osseointegration, whereas a clear metallic sound is normal. Even though such a clinical sign may provide important information in some cases where osseointegration has failed, it does not offer any information regarding peri-implantitis. For this reason, it cannot be used as a diagnostic criterion. Lastly, resonance frequency analysis has not been shown to provide information with regard to the diagnosis of peri-implantitis.

Peri-implant mucositis and peri-implantitis are not painful for the patient. Should a patient report pain, the possibility of final-stage peri-implantitis should be examined, which, if present, will also reveal implant mobility. Furthermore, excessive loading may lead to loss of osseointegration in rare cases. Careful evaluation for the possible presence of a foreign body inside the peri-implant sulcus or pocket should also be performed (Figs 7-18a, b).

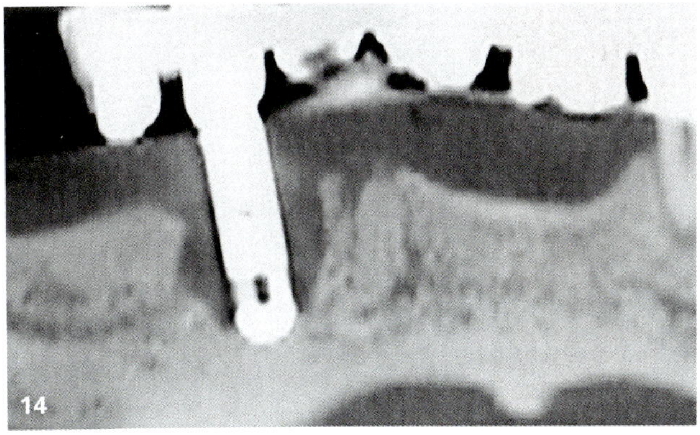
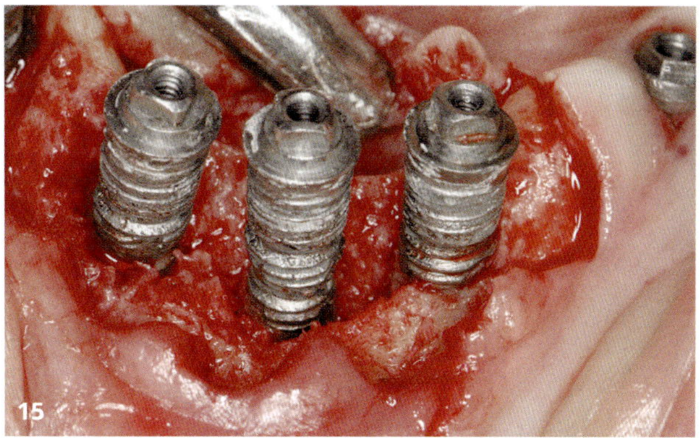

Figs 7-14 and 7-15 Mobility is not a diagnostic index for the presence of peri-implantitis. Both the implant depicted on the radiograph in Fig 7-14 and the implants in Fig 7-15, despite the significant bone destruction, do not present any degree of mobility.

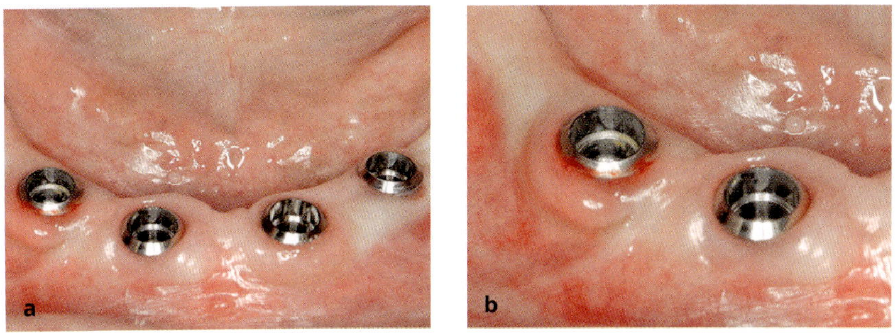

Figs 7-16a, b **(a)** Clinical image of peri-implant tissues. **(b)** Cautious evaluation at a higher magnification reveals the first signs of inflammation, which are redness and edema in the soft tissues of the distal implant.

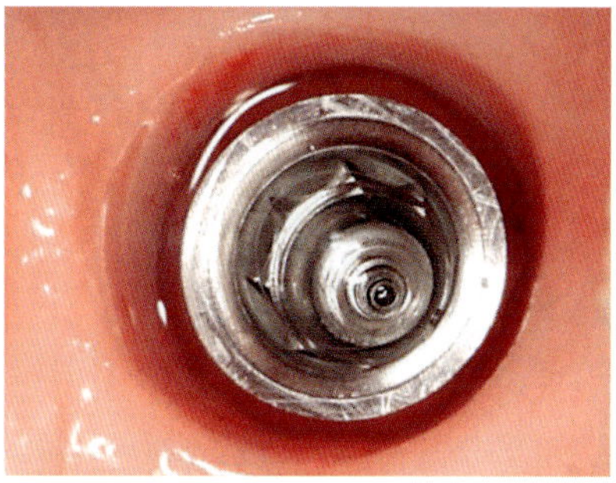

Fig 7-17 Clinical image of healthy peri-implant tissue after unscrewing the crown and the implant abutment. The bright pink color is associated with peri-implant health and the presence of a thick phenotype with abundant keratinized mucosa.

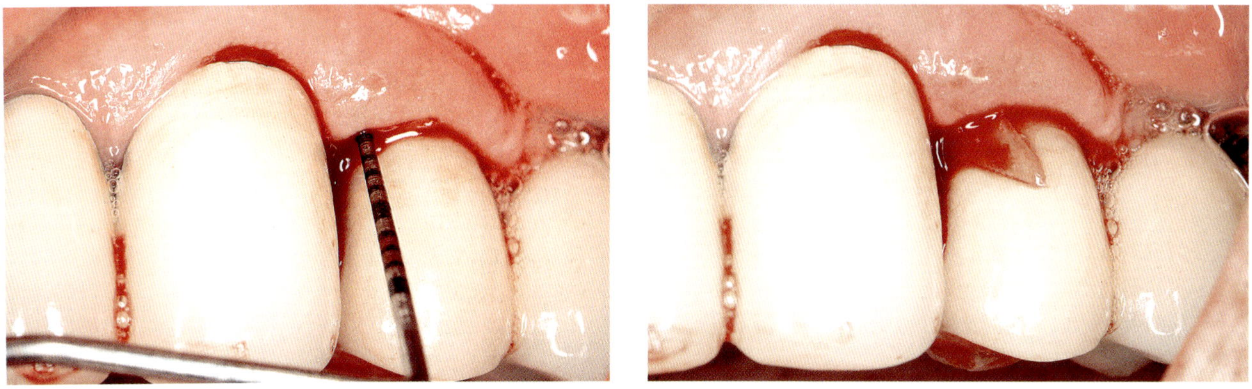

Fig 7-18a, b **(a)** The patient who had these implants for 12 years complained about edema and slight pain around no. 24. Clinically, there was inflammation and BOP, although the depth of the peri-implant crevice had increased. **(b)** A slight "scaling" movement with the periodontal probe caused the exit of a foreign body from the peri-implant crevice, which was blamed for this symptomatology and clinical image.

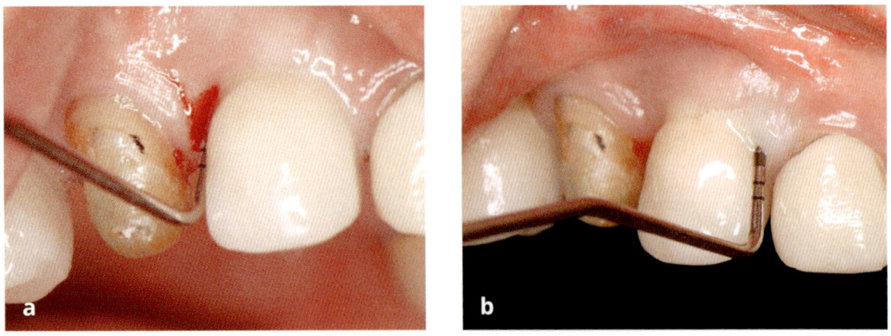

Figs 7-19a, b 9-mm-deep peri-implant pockets, bleeding and suppuration on probing.

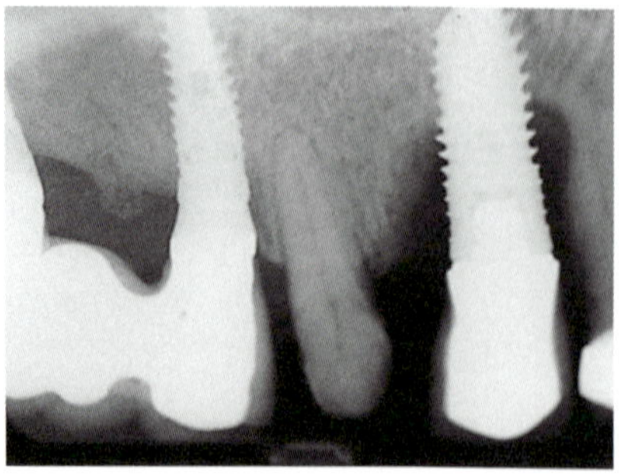

Fig 7-19c The radiograph reveals severe bone loss around implant no. 13.

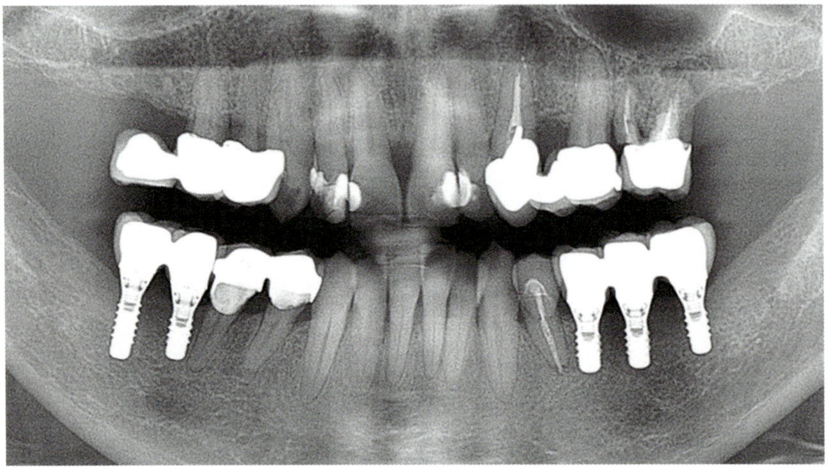

Fig 7-20a Radiographic image of a patient after placement of implant-supported restorations.

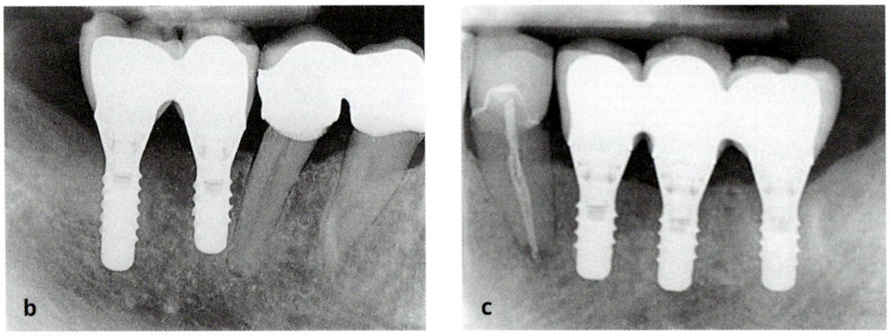

Figs 7-20b, c Radiographic images of the same patient 5 years after placement of the implant-supported restorations. Comparison of the two radiographs reveals the long-term stability of the osseointegration.

II. RADIOGRAPHIC EXAMINATION

Radiographic examination is an irreplaceable part of the diagnostic procedure for peri-implantitis and is always evaluated in combination with the existing clinical findings (Figs 7-19a–c).[9]

Radiographs are the most important diagnostic measure in cases where platform switching has been performed. A positive correlation between radiographic bone loss and the peri-implant pocket or attachment loss has been established. Radiographic examination is used to record, compare, and study changes in peri-implant bone over time. The reference is the radiograph, which is taken right after the placement of the final restoration (baseline), using the neck of the implant as a stable landmark for the comparative evaluation of measurements (Figs 7-20a–c and 7-21a, b).

Radiographic data gathered before placement of the restoration must not be used as a reference due to the changes that occur as bone remodeling be-

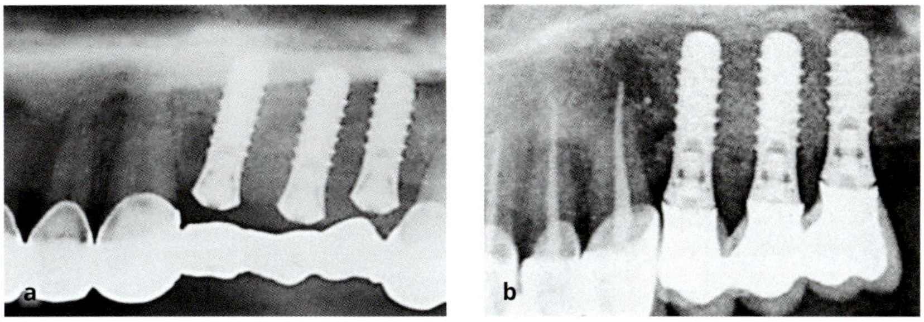

Figs 7-21a, b (a) Radiographic image of a patient after implant placement. **(b)** Radiographic image of the same site 15 years later. Note the slight alteration in the height of the bone crest, which, in combination with the absence of inflammation, is not a sign of peri-implantitis **(b)** Alteration of the height of the bone crest can be attributed to the bone remodeling process after placement of the implant reconstruction.

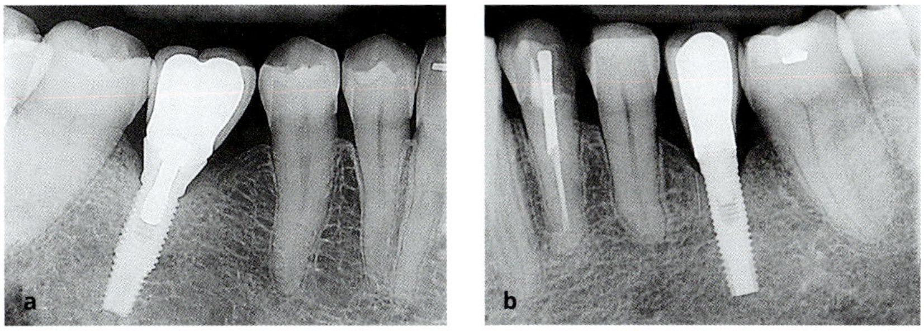

Figs 7-22a, b These implants were placed 12 years previously, deeper than the osseous crest. The present position of the peri-implant bone does not show angular defects because, after connecting an implant with the abutment, bone remodeling took place as natural formation of the biologic width.

tween implant placement and placement of the final restoration takes place (Figs 7-22a, b).

Over the past decades, it has become acceptable and expected for a change in the margin of the alveolar bone to occur at about 1.5 mm in the first year of functional loading and at 0.2 mm per year subsequently. As mentioned in Chapter 6, these values were described for the first time and without any scientific evidence by Albrektsson et al. The fact that bone loss even at a rate of 0.2 mm per year may be expected raises questions. Frequently, patients present with little or no bone loss over the years, provided they regularly follow a maintenance care program. Taking a radiograph after placement of the prosthetic appliance is recommended.

To summarize, the clinician must perform a radiographic examination following the guidelines below with regard to the placement and prosthetic restoration of implants:

- examination should be carried out immediately after surgical placement of the implants;
- examination should be performed to evaluate the fit of the implant abutments;
- examination should be performed straight after placement of the implant restoration so that the radiograph may be used as a reference;
- examination should be carried out 1 year after functional loading because the greatest changes in peri-implant bone are noted over this period;
- examination should be carried out during maintenance care, when there is BOP or suppuration on probing, as well as an increase in the probing depth of peri-implant crevices or pockets ≥ 6 mm;
- during maintenance care, when there are no clinical signs of pathology, a radiographic evaluation every 2 to 3 years may be recommended (Figs 7-23a–d).

Not only during initial placement, but also during maintenance care, the radiographic evaluation of implants and peri-implant tissues must include adjacent teeth that may affect the implant site, such as periodontally compromised teeth and teeth with residual periapical pathology after endodontic treatment. Lastly, radiographic depiction of a constant and visible radiopaque line that surrounds the implant represents osseointegration failure and is accompanied by implant mobility. Sometimes, in conventional radiologic techniques, narrow and circumferential radiopacity may be noted, without endosseous damage, while clinically there are no signs of pathology. This is an optical phenomenon attrib-

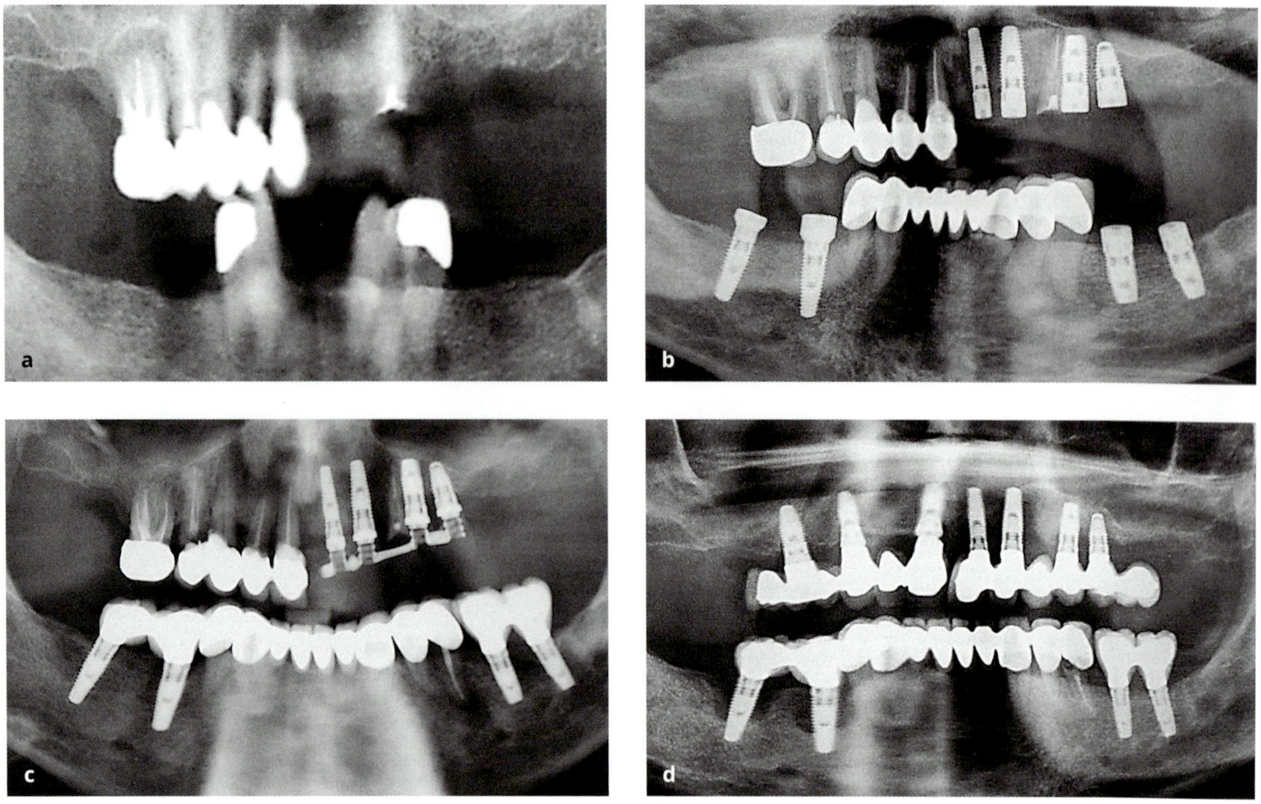

Figs 7-23a–d Record keeping with radiographic and clinical data for the long-term monitoring of patients. **(a)** Initial image, **(b)** image taken immediately after implant placement in the mandible, **(c)** after completion of the implant reconstruction, and **(d)** 10 years later. During that time, the patient was not consistent in their adherence to the maintenance care program. In combination with the clinical findings, the presence of peri-implantitis is established.

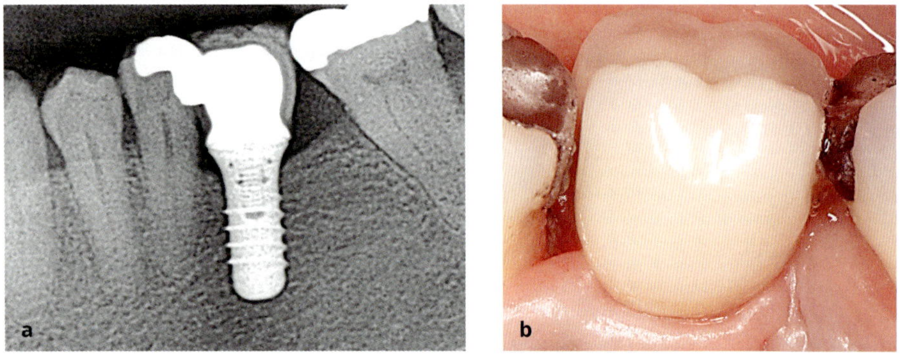

Figs 7-24a, b **(a)** A continuous radiolucent zone around the implant may be observed, with a Mach band effect. **(b)** The clinical image confirms the health of the peri-implant tissues (no signs of pocket formation, absence of bleeding).

utable to the '"enhancement" of contrast that the human eye performs when observing elements with different shades of gray. Specifically, the dark zone is perceived as darker and the light zone as even lighter. This phenomenon is called the "Mach band effect" and takes its name from the German physicist Ernst Mach (1838–1916) who first described it (Figs 7-24a, b).[10]

For the radiologic evaluation of peri-implantitis, conventional techniques such as panoramic and periapical radiographs, computed tomography (CT) scans, and CBCT are successfully used.

7.5 Panoramic radiography

As panoramic radiography is the only radiologic examination that allows the concurrent depiction of all teeth, implants, and adjacent anatomic sites, it may be used as an initial diagnostic radiographic image. However, compared to other radiologic methods, it has significant restrictions. In many cases, there are superpositions, while the clarity of the depiction is not high; thus, small changes in the bone, on a vertical plane at the implant sites, cannot be detected. Sites with implants often appear distorted, especially in the maxillary and mandibular anterior region, making the thorough evaluation of implant sites difficult, if not impossible. Digital panoramic radiographs have significantly improved the pictorial precision of the technique. Moreover, panoramic radiography, like any conventional radiologic technique, allows the depiction of the peri-implant bone only at the distal and mesial aspects. This particular depiction method has low sensitivity but high specificity as far as the finding of a small amount of bone loss is concerned; for this reason, it does not contribute to the early diagnosis of peri-implantitis.[11]

7.6 Periapical radiography using the parallel cylinder technique

Conventional periapical radiography using a parallel cylinder or parallel cone is a reliable method to evaluate the dimensions and state of the peri-implant bone in the adjacent sites. With the assistance of a film packet or digital sensors and a holder, periapical radiographs are taken in such a manner that the beam is vertical to the implant's long axis. This technique, using of the same settings, makes it possible to take similar radiographs, which can then be compared. Compared to panoramic radiographs, periapical radiographs have higher accuracy, and much smaller changes in dimensions may be visualized (a degree of 2.5% to 10.0% for periapical radiographs versus 20.0% to 30.0% for panoramic radiographs. Like panoramic radiographs, periapical radiographs depict the height of the peri-implant bone only at the mesial and distal aspects of the implant. In clinical practice, taking periapical radiographs is the simplest radiologic method for the frequent evaluation of implants and peri-implant tissues during maintenance care (Figs 7-25a–g).[12]

	18	17	16	15	14	13	12	11	21	22	23	24	25	26	27	28
PPD p	/	---	---	/	5--	---	---	---	/	---	---	---	/	---	---	/
PPD b	/	---	---	/	5--	---	---	4-5	/	5--	---	---	/	-4-	---	/

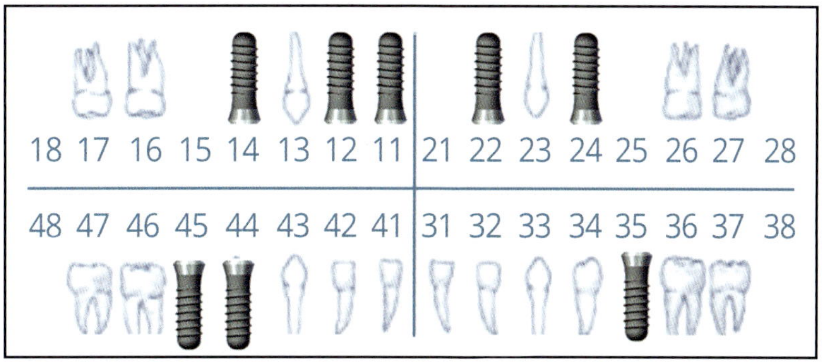

	48	47	46	45	44	43	42	41	31	32	33	34	35	36	37	38
PPD b	/	---	---	---	---	---	---	---	---	---	---	---	---	---	---	/
PPD l	/	---	-4-	---	---	4--	---	---	---	---	---	---	---	---	---	/

Fig 7-25a Chart of clinical measurements of the depth of peri-implant and periodontal crevices during the reconstructive phase of dentition (prosthetic rehabilitation). Crevices 1 to 3 mm deep are not recorded. Sites with BOP are shown in red.

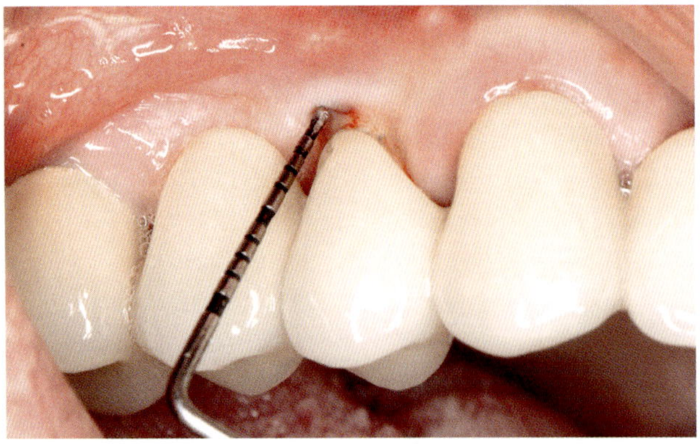

Fig 7-25b Measurement and recording of clinical parameters during the prosthetic rehabilitation phase.

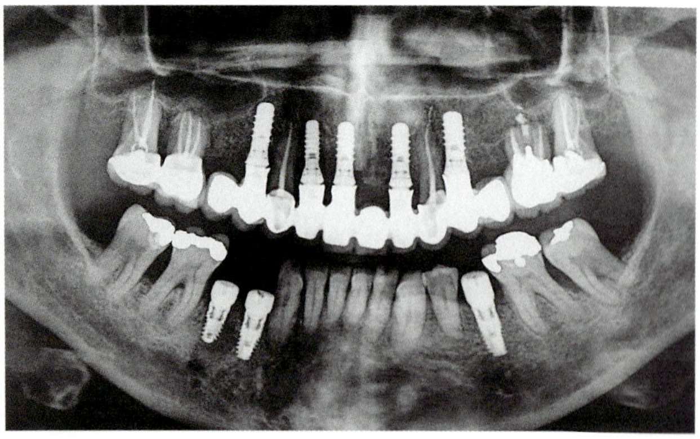

Fig 7-25c Taking a radiograph during the prosthetic rehabilitation phase is vital, not only to evaluate the fitting of the implant restorations, but also so it can be used as a reference point to be compared with future radiographs.

	18	17	16	15	14	13	12	11	21	22	23	24	25	26	27	28
PPD p		857	757		1188	755	778	565		777	656	857		855	956	
PPD b		767	855		9810	5-5	867	778		645	5-6	587		687	957	

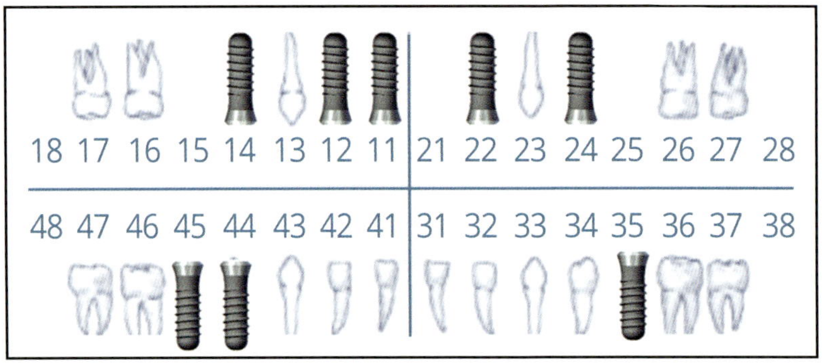

	48	47	46	45	44	43	42	41	31	32	33	34	35	36	37	38
PPD b		577	766	757	767	7-6	5--	544	445	5-4	545	646	775	657	1065	
PPD l		568	877	777	777	755	4-4	---	---	---	4-4	567	777	767	587	

Fig 7-25d Nine years after the initial clinical measurements, periodontitis and peri-implantitis were diagnosed with many pockets, the majority of which bled on probing.

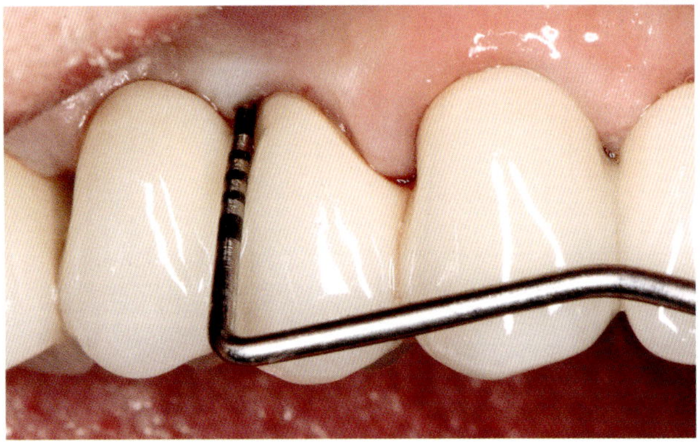

Fig 7-25e Measurement and recording of clinical parameters, after the patient returned to the practice 9 years after completion of the restoration.

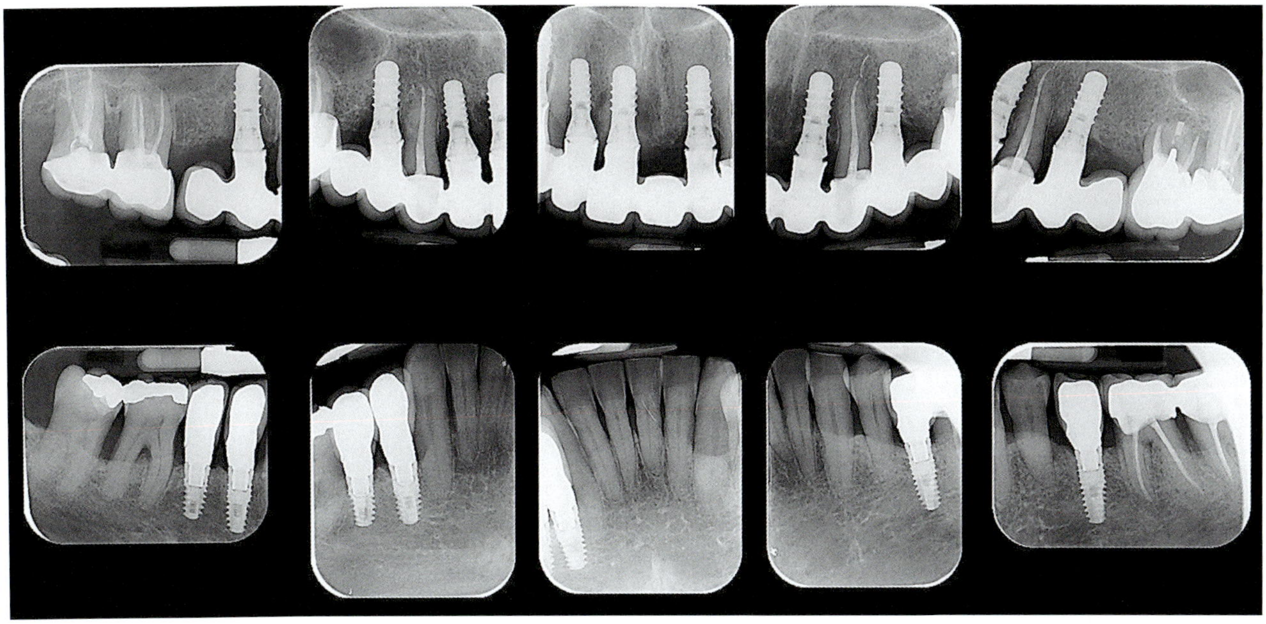

Fig 7-25f Comparison of the condition of the bone–implant contact, despite not being done using the same type of radiograph (initial panoramic radiograph), reveals the existence, degree, and extent of bone loss, for example, at implant no.14.

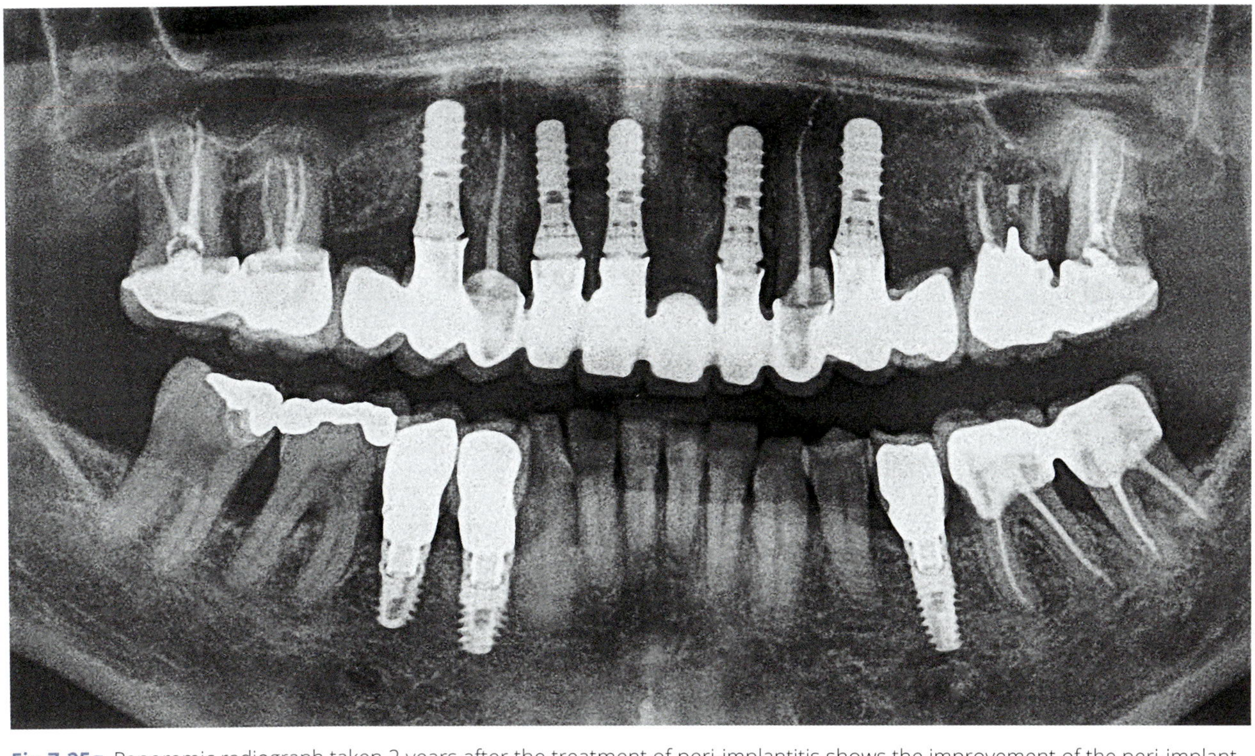

Fig 7-25g Panoramic radiograph taken 2 years after the treatment of peri-implantitis shows the improvement of the peri-implant bone condition at no. 14.

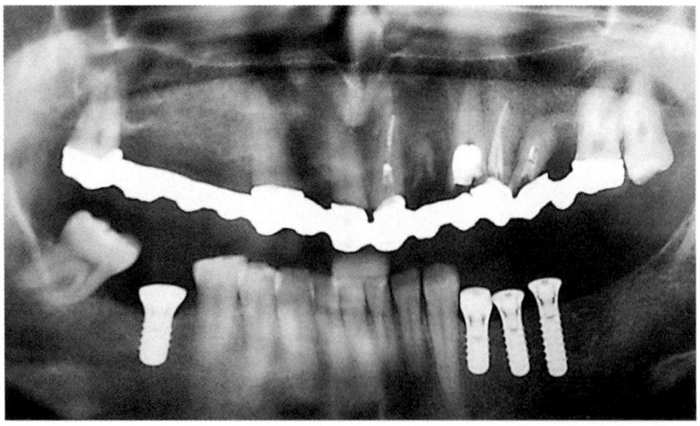

Fig 7-26a Radiographic image of a patient right after implant placement in the mandible.

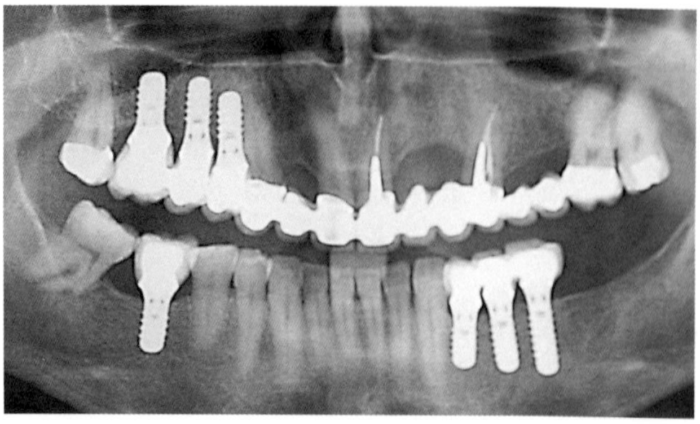

Fig 7-26b Panoramic radiograph of the patient 10 years after implant placement in the mandible and 9 years after full-arch maxillary rehabilitation.

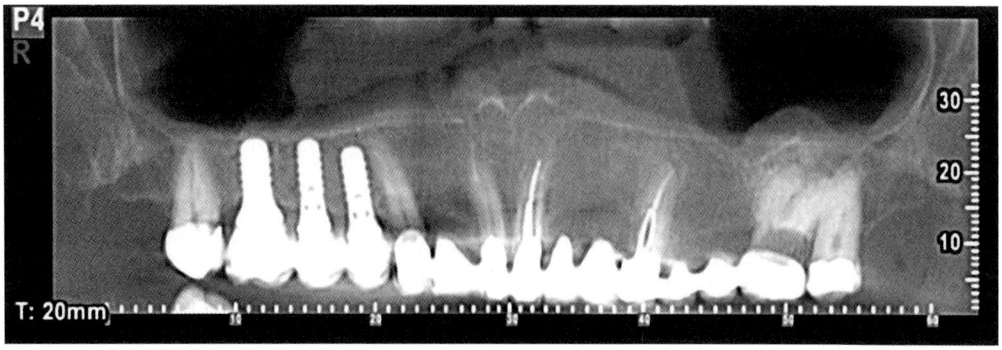

Fig 7-26c Fifteen years after implant placement in the maxilla, due to the extensive caries lesion on tooth 26, a CBCT scan was performed in the maxilla to evaluate the possibility of placing implants in that area.

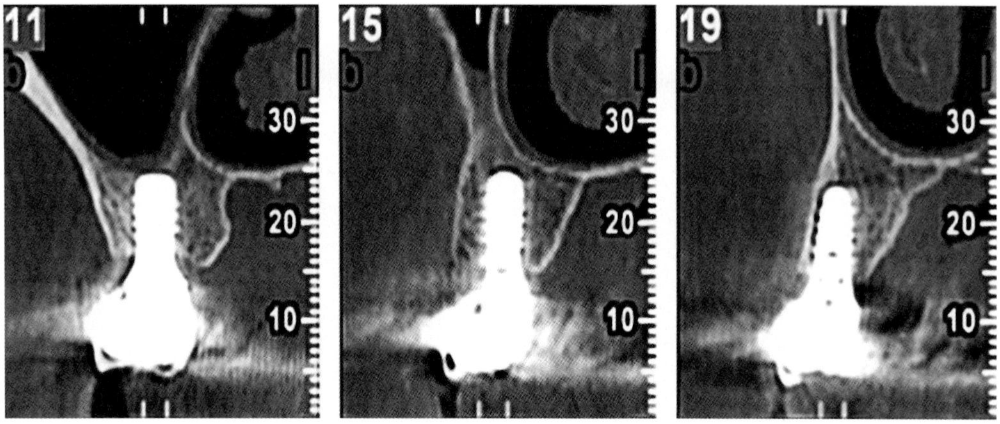

Fig 7-26d In the CBCT micrographs, the intact peri-implant alveolar bone, with no signs of bone destruction, may be observed 15 years after implant placement.

7.7 CT

The function of CT is based on the principle of creating transverse slices at a steady pace of 1 to 2 mm. Usually, it is used in the context of presurgical evaluation to achieve a better depiction of the osseous background. Less commonly, it is used during maintenance care. The main advantages of this radiologic method are the ability to yield the peri-implant bone in three dimensions and also depict the buccal and lingual or palatal alveolar plates, as well as produce a very detailed image (Figs 7-26a–d and 7-27a, b). CT can rarely be used for further evaluation of im-

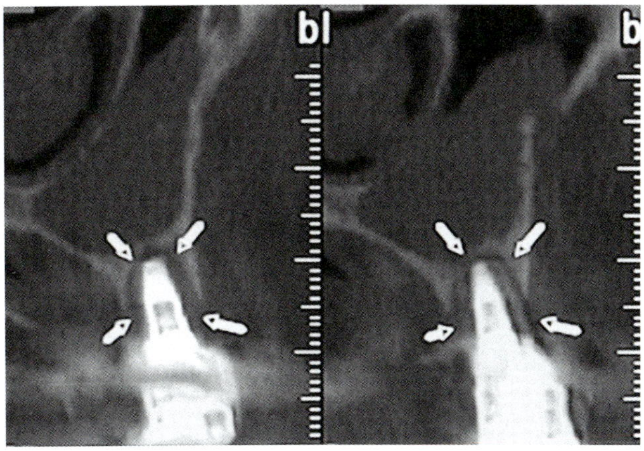

Fig 7-27a CBCT scan depicting the morphology of the bone and 3D bone destruction.

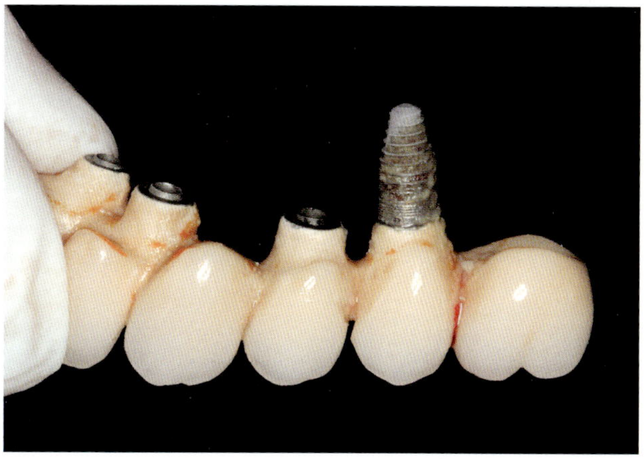

Fig 7-27b After unscrewing the prosthesis, implant no. 25 had completely lost its osseointegration. Fig 7-27 is the continuation of the case presented in Fig 7-23.

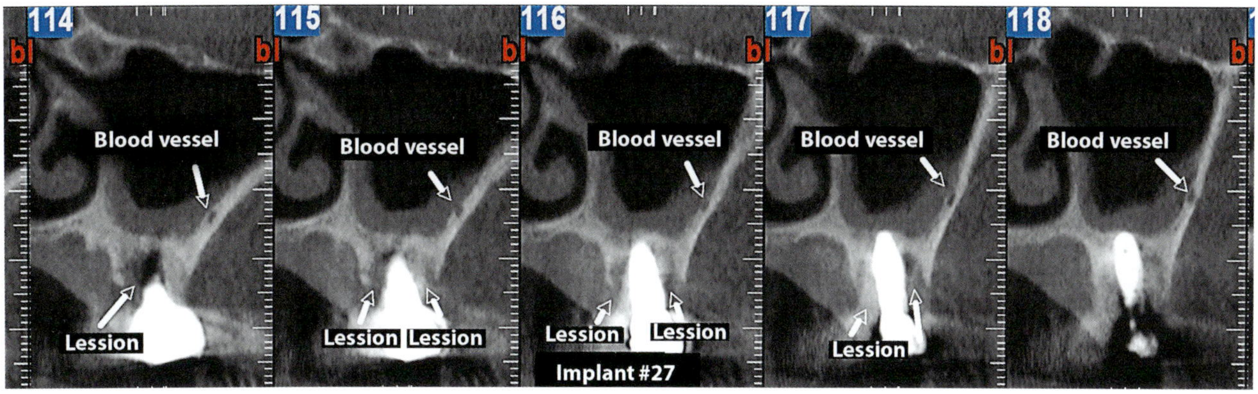

Fig 7-28 CBCT can be used to diagnose the degree of bone destruction and the morphology of peri-implant osseous lesions. In this case, the circumferential intraosseous lesion around implant no. 27 can be observed.

plants that present clinical signs of peri-implantitis (Fig 7-28) or to monitor the course of a therapeutic intervention, such as guided bone regeneration (Fig 7-29). A drawback of CT is the relatively high dose of radiation. The development and manufacture of new radiologic equipment have significantly reduced exposure time and radiation dose.

7.8 CBCT

This radiologic method can produce slices at different levels, in similar fashion to CT. It also requires much smaller radiation doses. The whole field of examination is irradiated with a single conical beam and with a single rotation around the patient's head.

Lastly, it allows the comparison and thorough depiction of hard and soft tissues of the oral and maxillofacial complex. The much smaller distortion and artifact formation at areas with metallic elements make it the most suitable diagnostic tool for the diagnosis of peri-implant bony lesions.[13]

III. LABORATORY EXAMINATIONS

7.9 Microbiologic testing

As a complementary way to diagnose peri-implant diseases, microbiologic testing may be used. For the qualitative and quantitative report of micro-

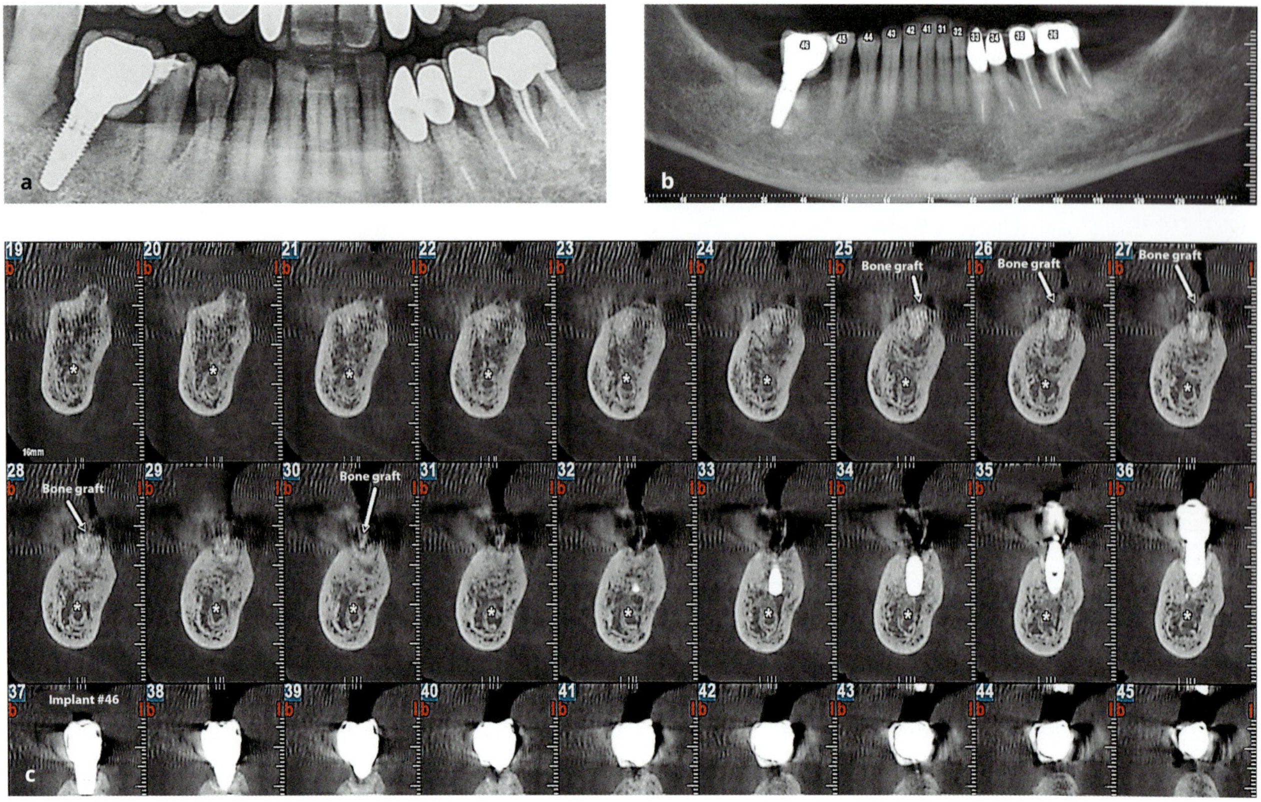

Figs 7-29a–c CBCT, combined with a clinical examination, may confirm the success of a regenerative technique. **(a)** Bone destruction and exposure of many threads of implant no. 46. **(b)** Filling of the peri-implant lesion at no. 46, as well as filling of the post-extraction socket of no. 47, can be observed 2 years after guided bone regeneration with demineralized freeze-dried bone allograft and collagen membrane placement. **(c)** Cross-sectional views confirm the filling of the lesions with bone.

organisms found in the peri-implant pocket, modern microbiologic methods such as DNA–DNA hybridization, gene detection, and polymerase chain reaction are used. These techniques are complemented with traditional microscopic techniques, such as dark-field or phase-contrast microscopy and microbiologic cultures. These microbiologic techniques are used to detect a possible increase in periodontal pathogens: *Porphyromonas gingivalis*, *Aggregatibacter actinomycetemcomitans*, *Prevotella intermedia*, and *Treponema denticola*. An increase of certain populations of microorganisms has been associated with a heightened risk of further attachment loss in periodontitis. An increase in the populations of the aforementioned presumptive periodontal pathogens is associated with a higher risk of peri-implant bone destruction. Thus, microbiologic examinations not only contribute to the diagnosis of peri-implantitis, but also improve the positive predictive value of the clinical and radiologic examinations (Figs 7-30a, b).[14,15]

7.10 Analysis of peri-implant crevicular fluid and saliva

There is an association between the condition of periodontal tissues and the levels of several biochemical markers of inflammation in the gingival crevicular fluid. Biochemical markers associated with disease progression are interleukin-1β and interleukin-6, prostaglandin E_2, collagenase, elastase, myeloperoxidase, β-glucuronidase, aspartate aminotransferase, several glycosaminoglycans, and growth factors such as tumor growth factor-β, platelet-derived growth factor, and tumor necrosis factor-α. Many studies have shown an association between the levels of biochemical markers of inflammation and the condition of peri-implant tissues. Moreover, some associations with inflammation mediators found in saliva have been studied; their collection is much easier.[16]

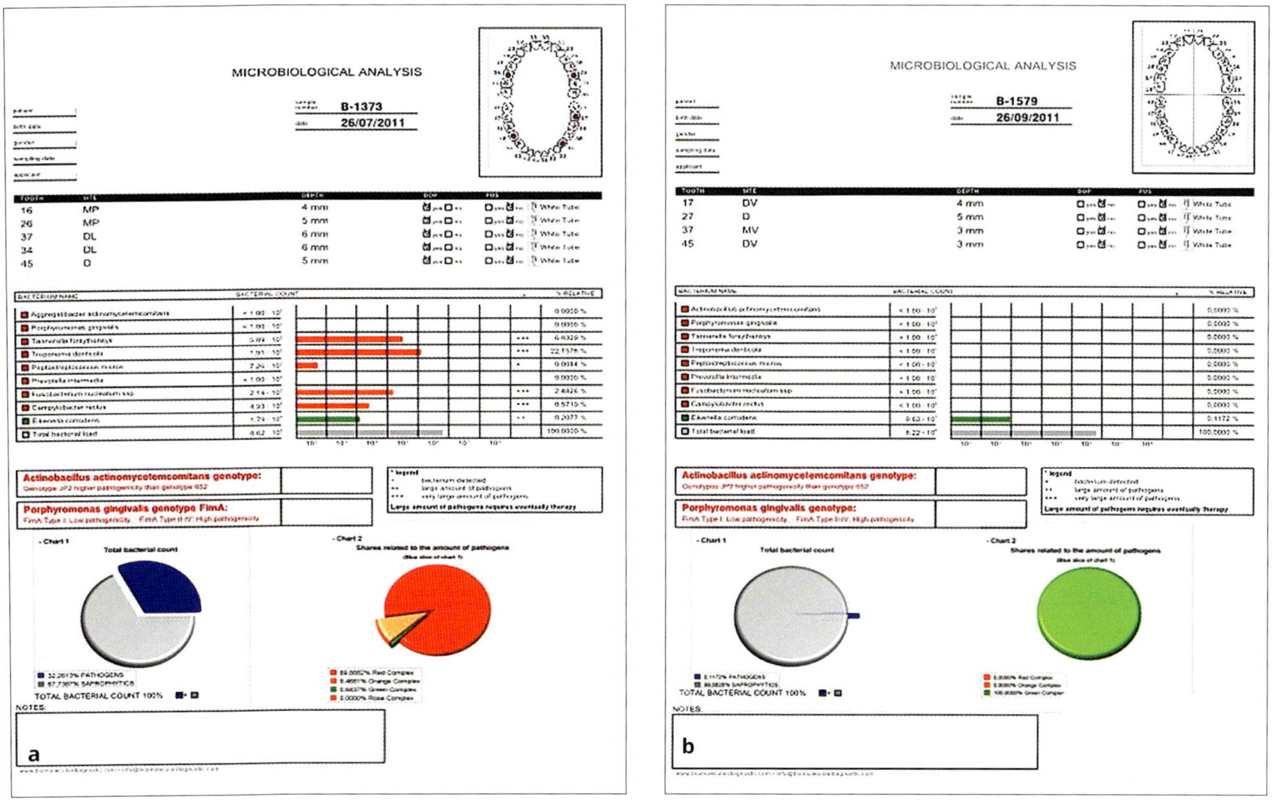

Figs 7-30a, b Microbiologic examinations showing the presence of periodontal pathogens in the peri-implant pockets. **(a)** Before and **(b)** after the initial phase of therapy for the treatment of peri-implantitis.

According to recent data, a lack of detection of the aforementioned biochemical markers is indication of the health of peri-implant tissues. Nevertheless, specific microbiologic examinations or biochemical analyses have yet to be developed.[17]

References

1. Muñoz V, Duque A, Giraldo A, Manrique R. Prevalence of peri-implant disease according to periodontal probing depth and bleeding on probing: a systematic review and meta-analysis. Int J Oral Maxillofac Implants 2018;33:e89–e105.
2. Lang NP, Adler R, Joss A, Nyman S. Absence of bleeding on probing. An indicator of periodontal stability. J Clin Periodontol 1990;17:714–721.
3. Hashim D, Cionca N, Combescure C, Mombelli A. The diagnosis of peri-implantitis: a systematic review on the predictive value of bleeding on probing. Clin Oral Implants Res 2018;29(suppl 16):276–293.
4. Romandini M, Berglundh J, Derks J, Sanz M, Berglundh T. Diagnosis of peri-implantitis in the absence of baseline data: a diagnostic accuracy study. Clin Oral Implants Res 2021;32:297–313.
5. Ericsson I, Lindhe J. Probing depth at implants and teeth. An experimental study in the dog. J Clin Periodontol 1993;20:623–627.
6. Lang NP, Wetzel AC, Stich H, Caffesse RG. Histologic probe penetration in health and inflamed peri-implant tissues. Clin Oral Implants Res 1994;5:191–201.
7. Lindhe J, Meyle J. Peri-implant diseases: consensus report of the Sixth European Workshop on Periodontology. J Clin Periodontol 2008;35:282–285.
8. Santiago JF Jr, Batista VE, Verri FR, et al. Platform-switching implants and bone preservation: a systematic review and meta-analysis. Int J Oral Maxillofac Surg 2016;45:332–345.
9. Naveau A, Shinmyouzu K, Moore C, Avivi-Arber L, Jokerst J, Koka S. Etiology and measurement of peri-implant crestal bone loss (CBL). J Clin Med 2019;8:166.
10. Nielsen CJ. Effect of scenario and experience on interpretation of mach bands. J Endod 2001;27:687–691.

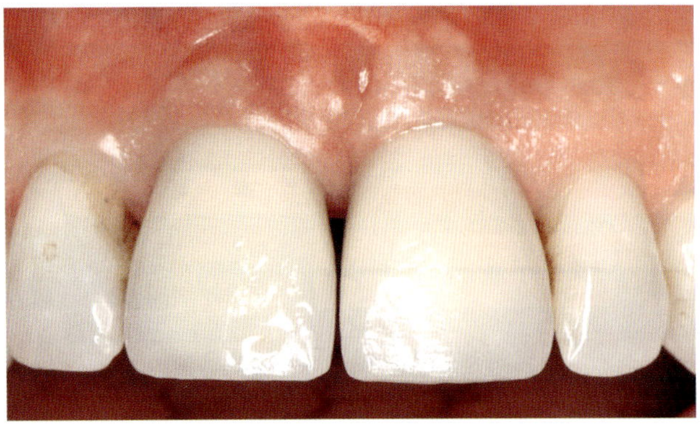

Fig 8-5a Clinical picture of implants in the two central incisor sites 14 years after placement of no. 11 and 10 years after placement of no. 21.

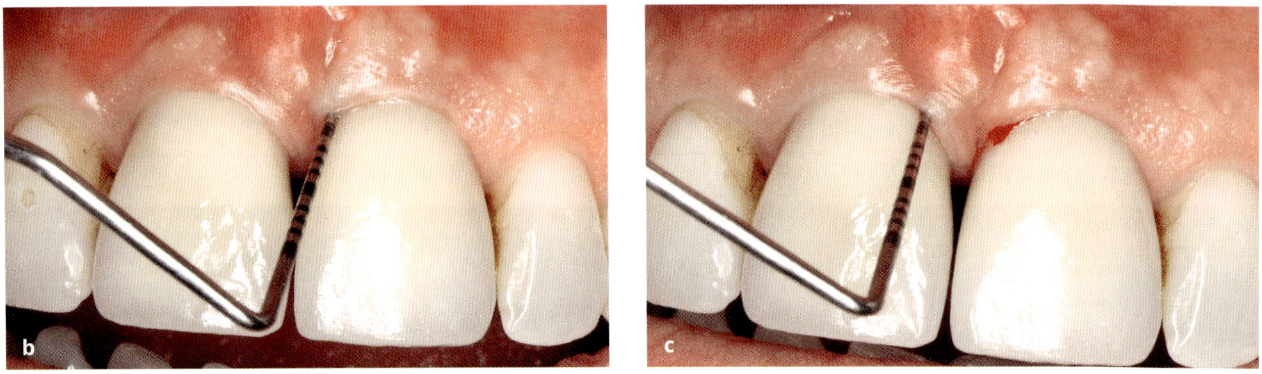

Figs 8-5b, c Probing reveals the presence of a peri-implant sulcus and absence of pockets.

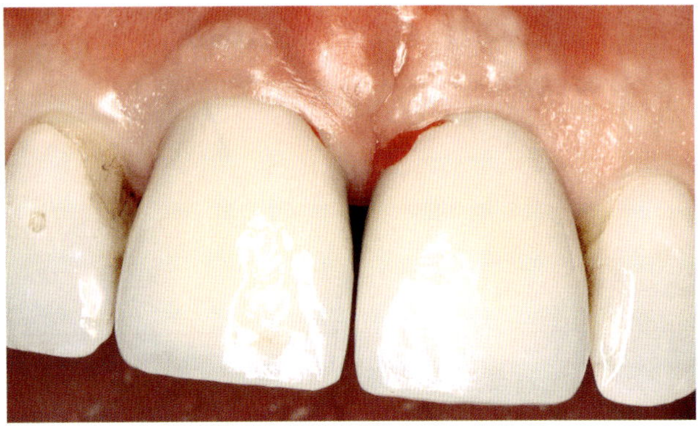

Fig 8-5d BOP confirms the diagnosis of peri-implant mucositis.

8.3.1 Step A

In this case, the patient has peri-implant mucositis. Step A of the CIST protocol is carried out, ideally with the implementation of the GBT protocol (Figs 8-5a–i).

The detailed therapeutic approach for peri-implant mucositis is described in Chapter 9. Special emphasis is placed on strengthening the guidelines and practicing effective oral hygiene. It is important to check whether or not the presence of a dental biofilm is due to the patient's inconsistency in administering oral hygiene or to a difficulty that may arise from poor design or poor adaptation of the implant restoration. If this is the case, then all that is needed is to correct the restoration and provide the prosthesis with the required morphology and adaptation(s).

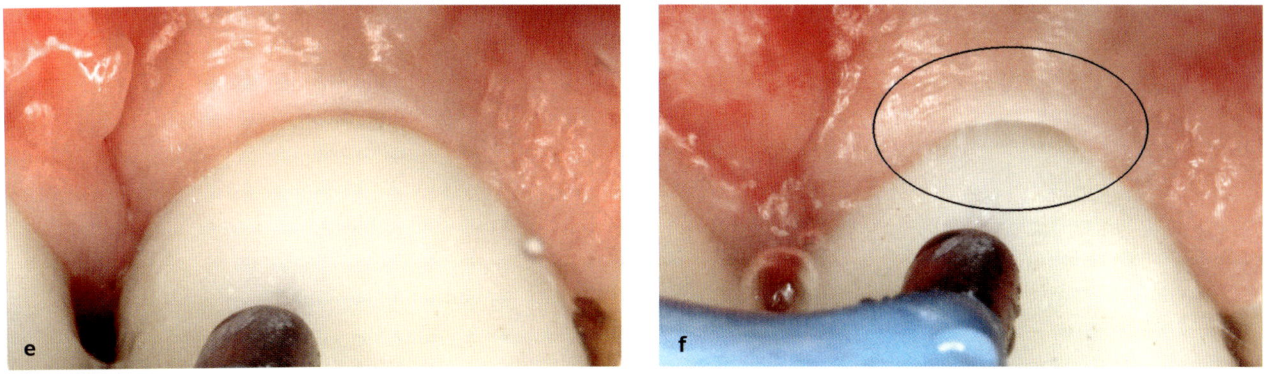

Figs 8-5e, f AIRFLOW removed microbial deposits up to 4 mm subgingivally. In **(f)**, the pressure from the ejected spray repels the mucosa, effectively widening the entrance to the sulcus. In this patient, steps A and B of the modified CIST protocol were applied.

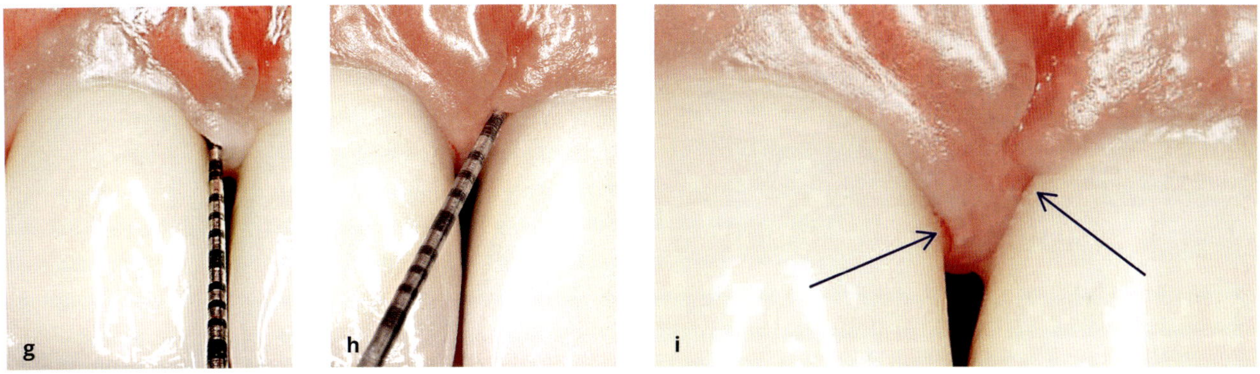

Figs 8-5g–i Four weeks after treatment, periodontal probing does not cause bleeding. Note the impressions made by the probe (blue arrows).

8.4 Clinical case 3

Clinical examination and disclosure of biofilm on teeth and implants reveal accumulation of dental biofilm or calculus deposits (or both) around the implants. During probing, a pocket depth of 5 mm or greater is recorded, as well as BOP and even suppuration. Periapical radiography does not yet reveal bone loss. Probing pocket depth is interpreted either as a consequence of deeper implant placement or as a result of inflammatory overgrowth of the peri-implant mucosa.

8.4.1 Steps A and B

In this case, the patient has peri-implant mucositis. Step A is carried out, ideally together with the application of the GBT protocol, and step B is added. This consists of providing 1% chlorhexidine gel for topical application twice daily, after removal of bacteria during oral hygiene procedures, for 3 to 4 weeks. In the case of pockets with a depth of 5 mm or greater, further bactericidal treatment with a laser may be indicated (Figs 8-6a–e).[6]

8.5 Clinical case 4

Clinical examination and disclosure of biofilm on teeth and implants reveal the accumulation of dental biofilm or calculus deposits (or both) around the implants. A probing pocket depth greater than 5 mm is recorded, as well as BOP or even suppuration. Periapical radiographs reveal some bone loss.

8.5.1 Steps A, B, C, and D

In this case, the patient has early-stage peri-implantitis. According to the original protocol, steps A and B are applied and step C is added; this consists of ad-

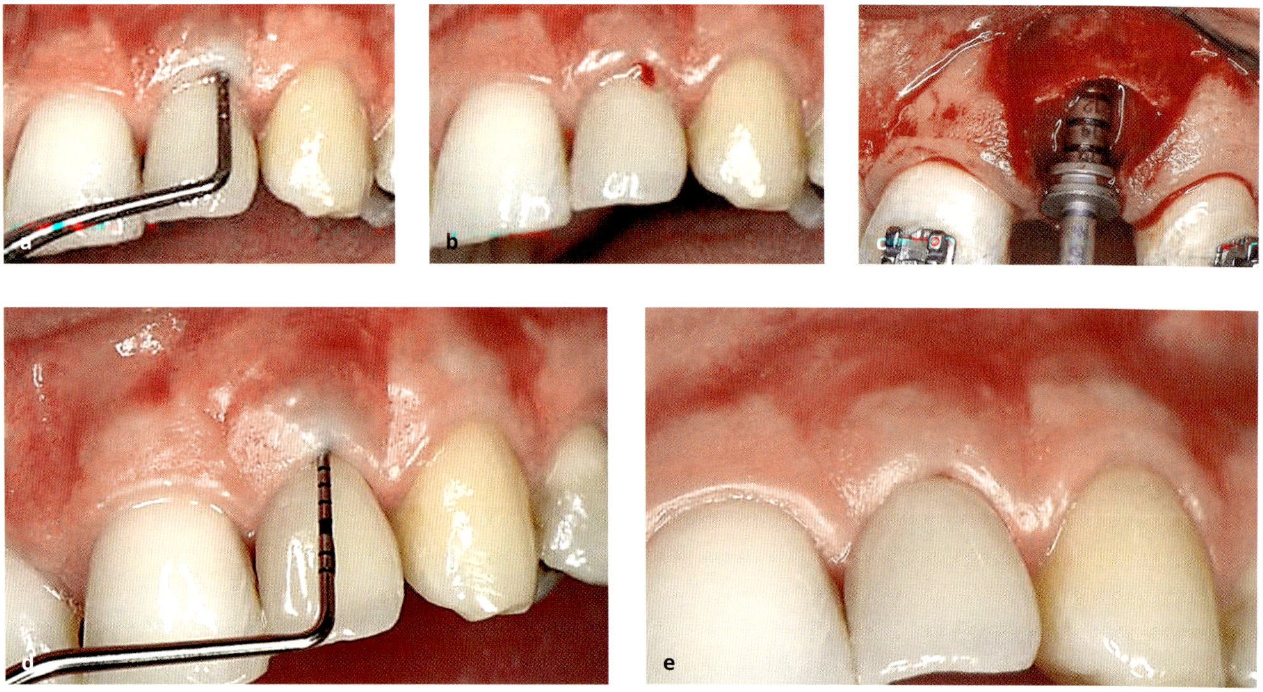

Figs 8-6a–e **(a and b)** Probing of a 6-mm peri-implant pocket that bled on probing 4 years after placement of implant no. 22. **(c)** The implant was inserted quite deep, resulting in a deep peri-implant sulcus. **(d)** Four weeks after treatment, no signs of inflammation were observed. **(e)** Impressions made with the periodontal probe without causing bleeding. These are images of the patient presented in Fig 7-4, showing peri-implant health 17 years after implant placement.

ministering systemic or local antibiotics suitable for the treatment of anaerobic periodontal pathogens (Fig 8-1). Over the last decade, literature that examined the potential of antibiotics in improving clinical parameters showed that short-term reductions in the population of periodontal pathogens and BOP are expected, although these results do not last in the long term. There is no significant improvement in probing pocket depth and clinical attachment level. In addition, the differences observed in microbial populations after antibiotic administration are smaller compared to those that occur after surgical treatment. For this reason, the first modification of the classical protocol (Fig 8-2) incorporated step C as part of step D. That is, after steps A and B, the clinical guideline is to administer perioperative antibiotics and use a surgical technique immediately. Therefore, steps A, B, C, and D should be used. The technique is selected according to the morphology of the bony defects, as described in Chapter 10, and the whole procedure is speeded up. Changing anatomic conditions (eg, pocket depth, morphology of bony defects, exposure of implant threads) will help the patient in the application of daily effective oral hygiene measures, while also helping the clinician to successfully maintain the therapeutic outcome in the long term after treatment of peri-implantitis (Figs 8-7a–j).

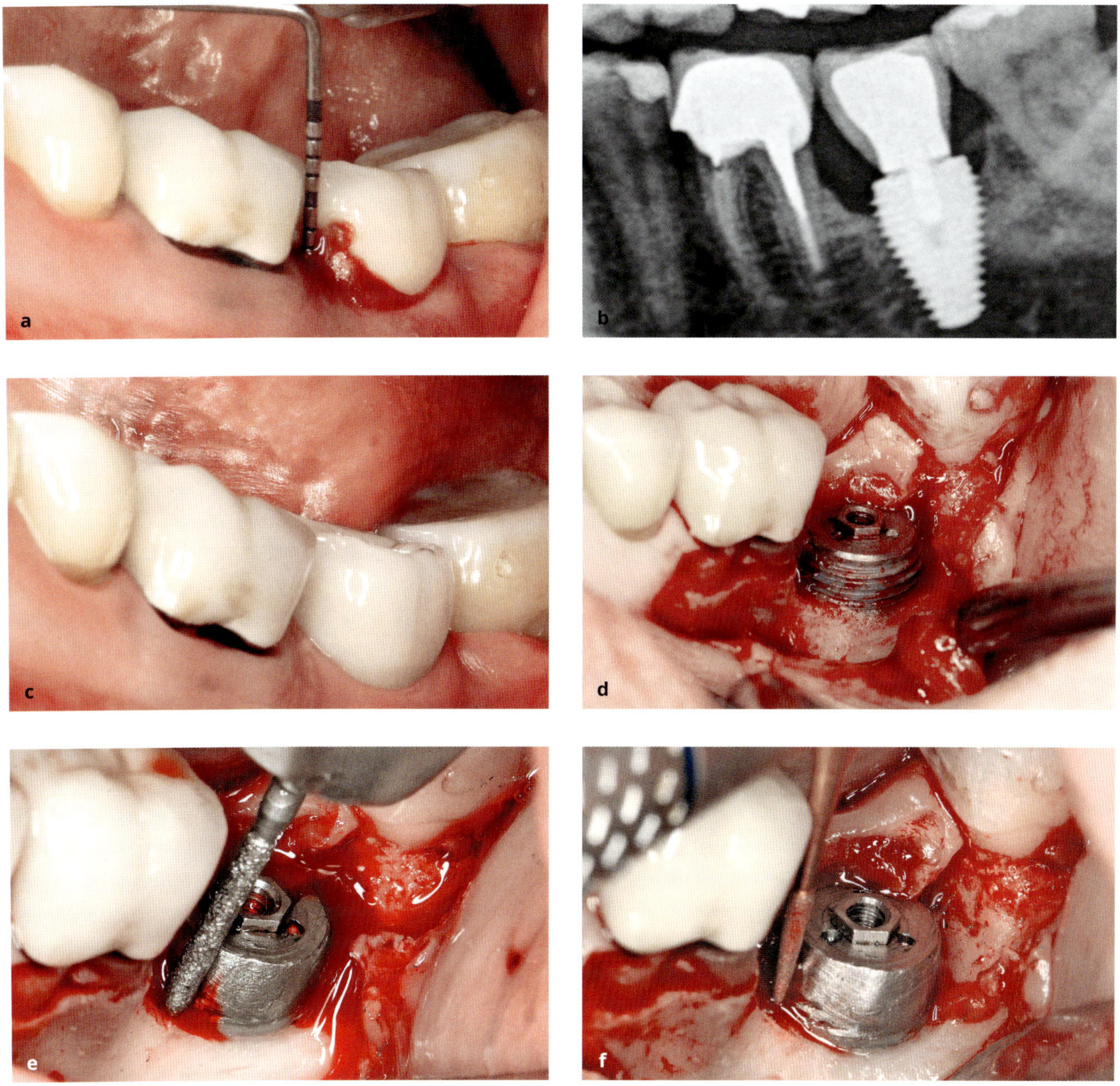

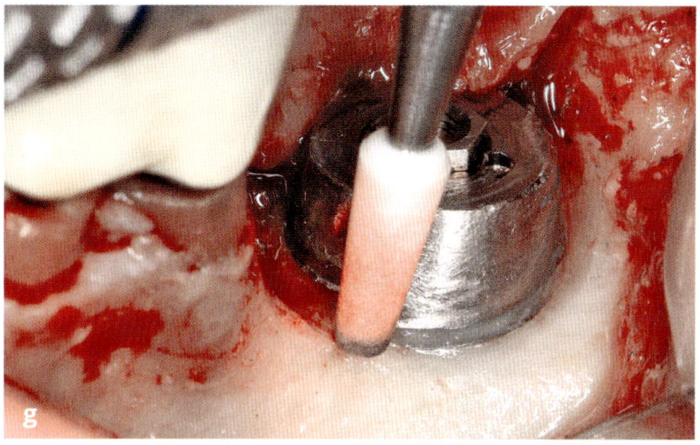

Figs 8-7a–g **(a)** Clinical picture of peri-implantitis. Peri-implant pockets and bleeding on probing are detected. **(b)** The radiograph shows bone loss and the characteristic circumferential defect configuration. **(c)** One month after applying steps A and B and before surgical treatment. **(d)** After raising the flap, and under perioperative antibiotics (amoxicillin 1 g three times daily for 5 days), the exposed implant threads can be seen due to bone loss. **(e to g)** Implantoplasty was applied using diamonds with different roughnesses; the process can be completed with Arkansas burs. Finally, bone surgery is carried out and the flaps are thinned if apical reposition is required to eliminate the pockets.

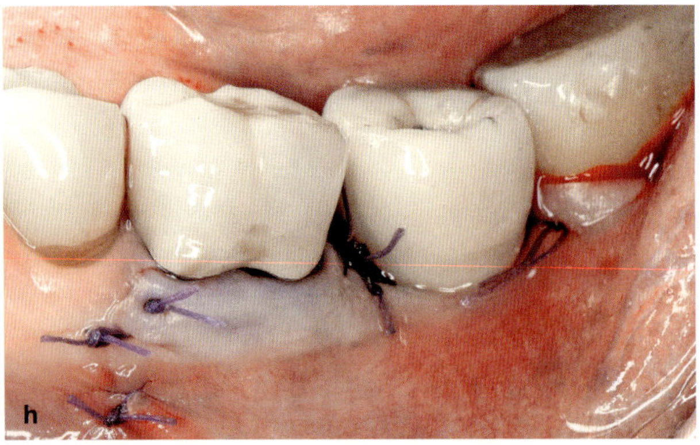

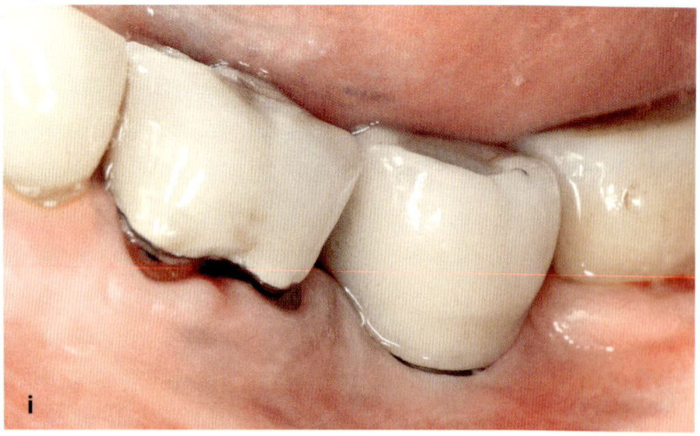

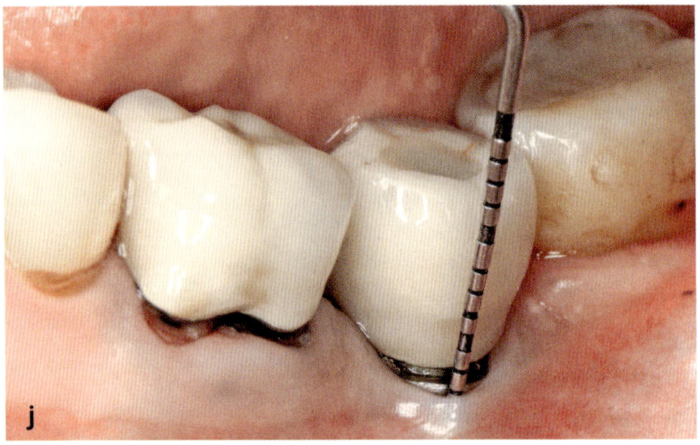

Figs 8-7h–j **(h)** After suturing. **(i)** Clinical image 3 months after surgery and **(j)** 6 months after surgery.

The decision to perform surgery is independent of the depth and morphology of the bony defect. The type of technique selected differs according to the existing clinical and radiographic findings (Figs 8-8a–x).

The current modification of the CIST protocol replaced the general guidelines on "mechanical removal of deposits" by implementing the GBT protocol for this purpose. The reasons for this change are discussed in Chapters 9 and 16.

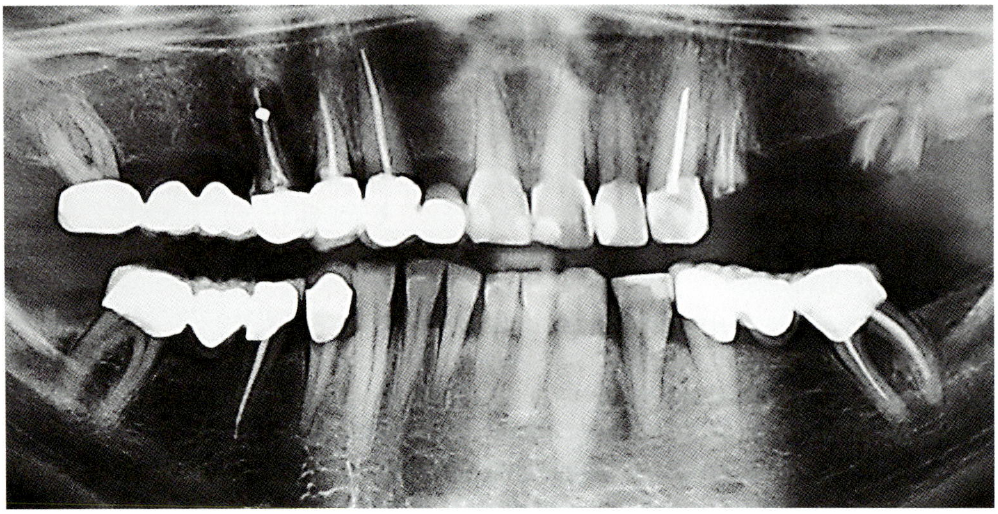

Fig 8-8a Radiographic image of a patient who decided to have implants for maxillary rehabilitation.

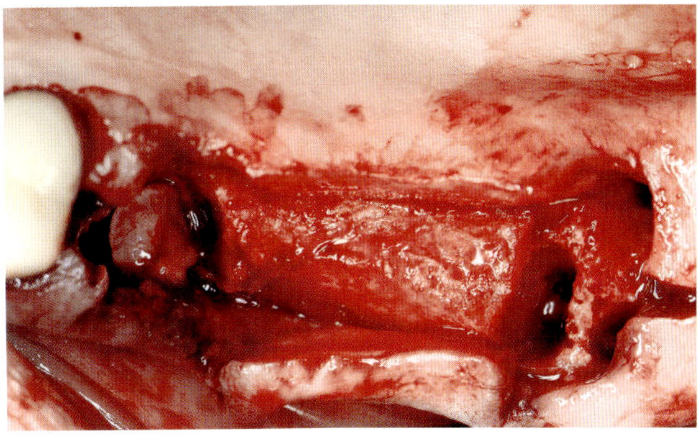

Fig 8-8b After tooth extraction, the alveolar ridge is prominent.

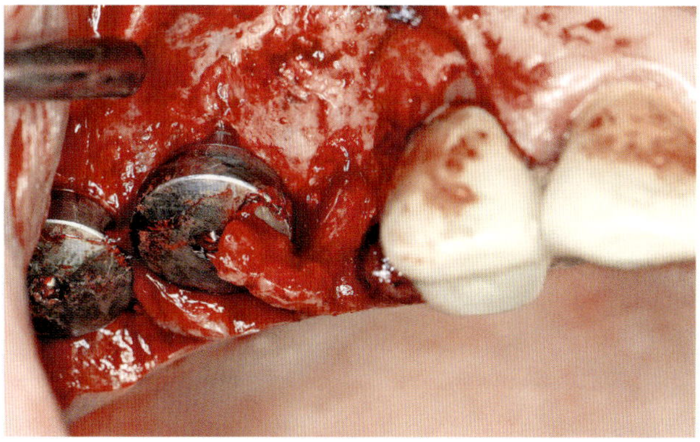

Fig 8-8c After implant placement in sites nos. 16 and 17 and preparation of the Palacci flaps for primary wound closure. Bone adequacy at the implant sites is also evident.

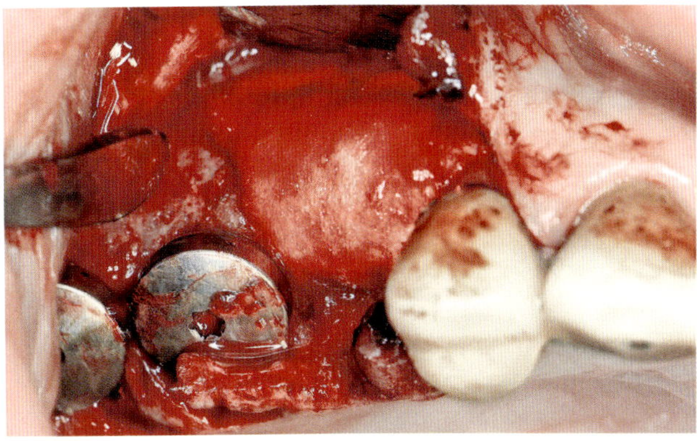

Fig 8-8d Placement of collagen membrane and bone graft for ridge augmentation.

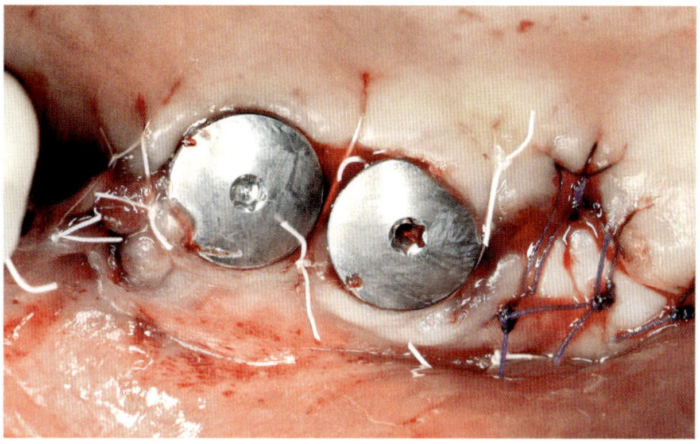

Fig 8-8e After suturing for primary wound closure.

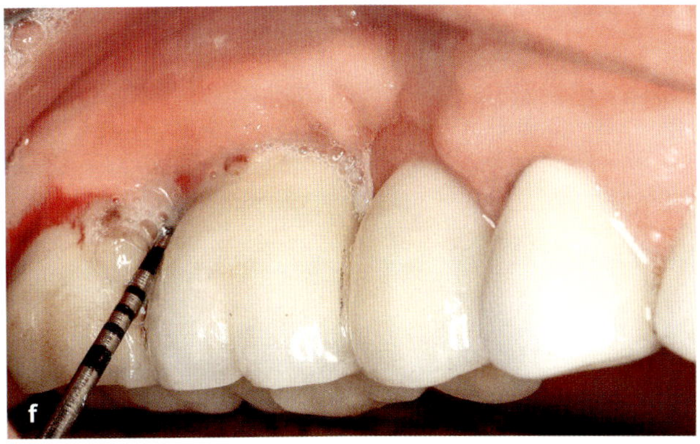

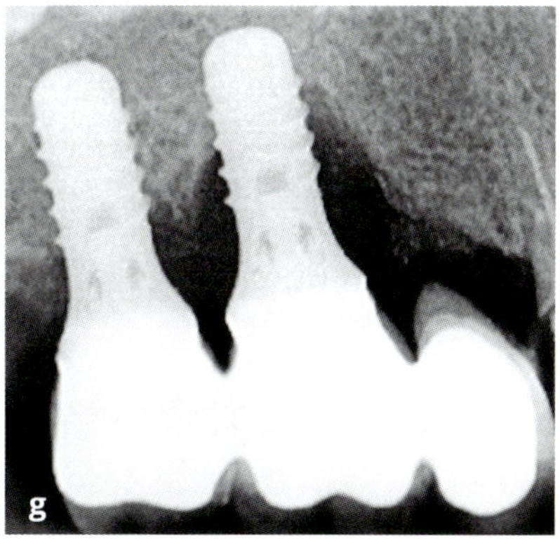

Figs 8-8f, g (f) Seven years after implant placement, during which time the patient failed to maintain the therapeutic result. Clinical examination revealed pockets, bleeding, and suppuration on probing. **(g)** Radiographic examination revealed significant bone destruction at implant no. 16 but less bone loss at implant no. 17.

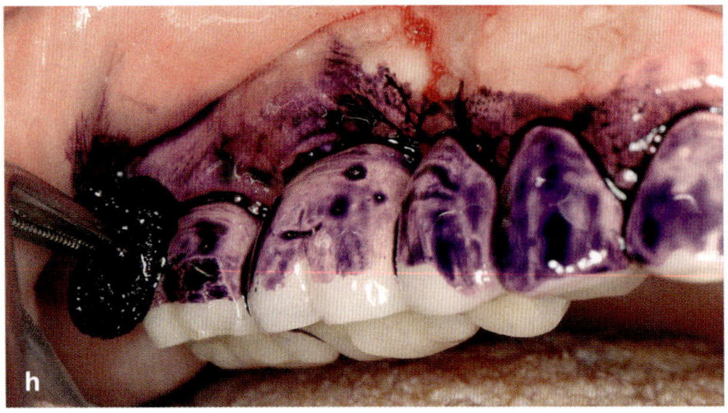

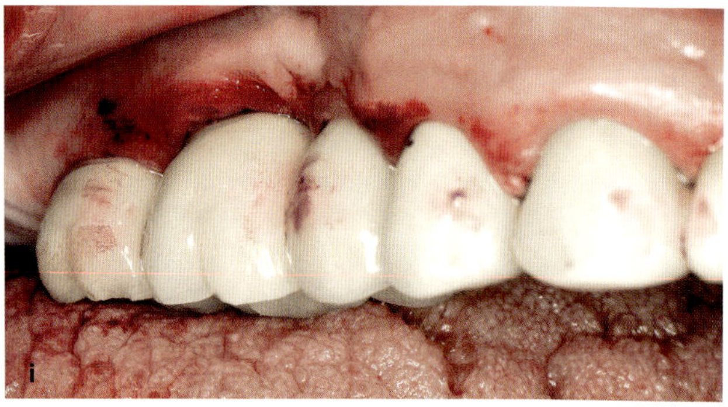

Figs 8-8h, i **(h)** The GBT protocol revealed the biofilm. **(i)** Areas with accumulated biofilm are apparent.

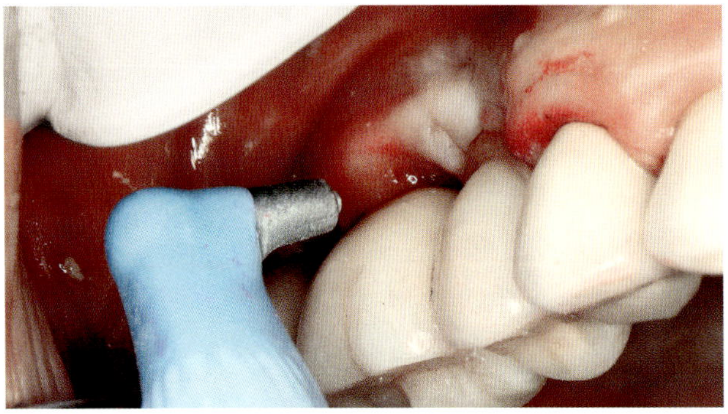

Fig 8-8j AIRFLOW application followed. In the image, the microbial communities discovered have already been removed and the direction of the spray beam to remove the microbial load up to 4 mm subgingivally can be seen.

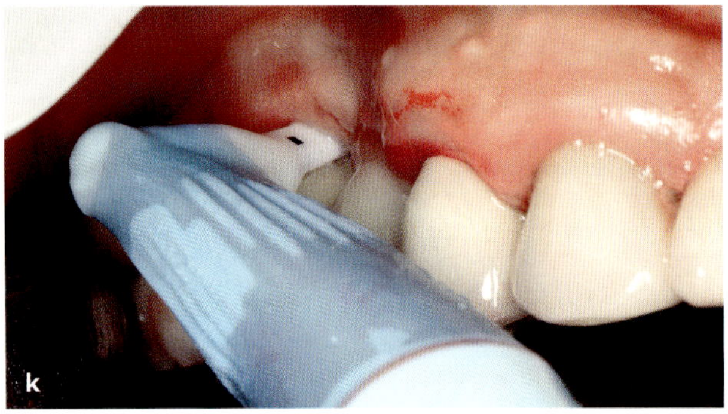

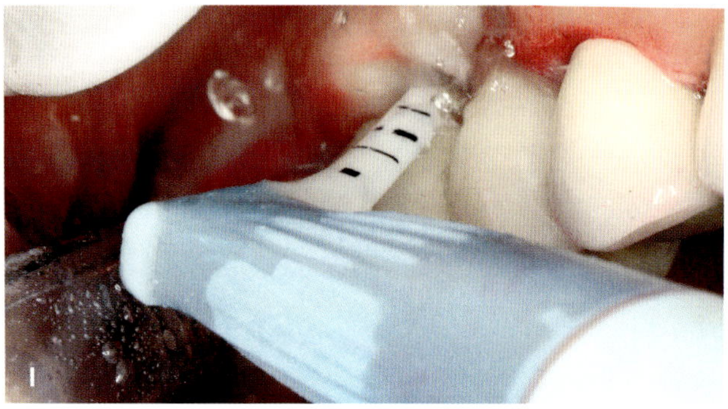

Figs 8-8k, l **(k)** Subgingival removal of deposits is achieved with PERIOFLOW. The entrance of the flexible nozzle at a depth of 9 mm can be seen. **(l)** The nozzle is moved in a vertical reciprocating direction.

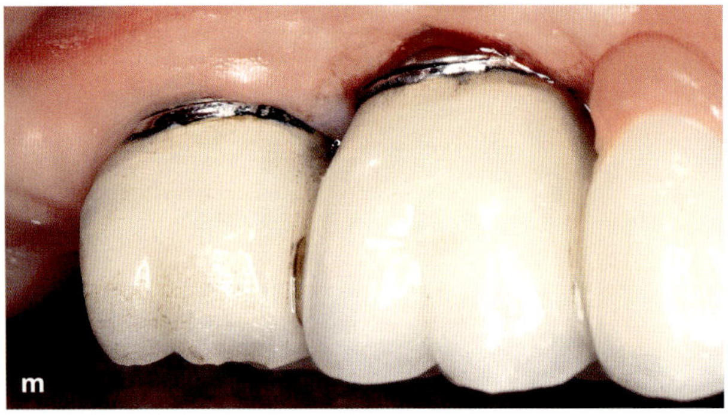

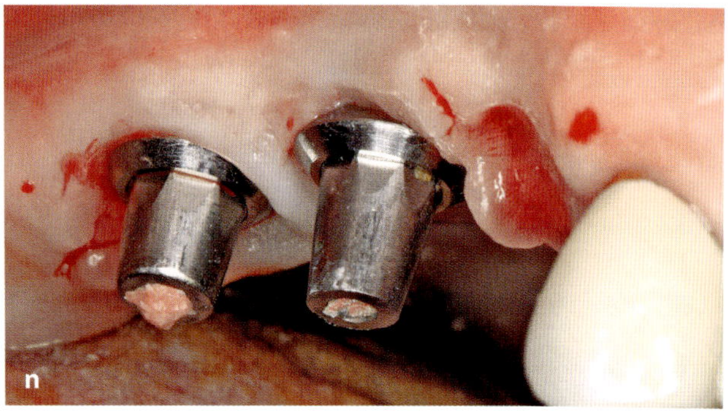

Figs 8-8m,n Seven weeks after GBT and 4 weeks after three 810-nm (1 W) diode laser sessions to achieve the required bactericidal effect. Before surgery for peri-implant bone regeneration, smaller pocket depths were detected; soft peri-implant tissue recession is evident.

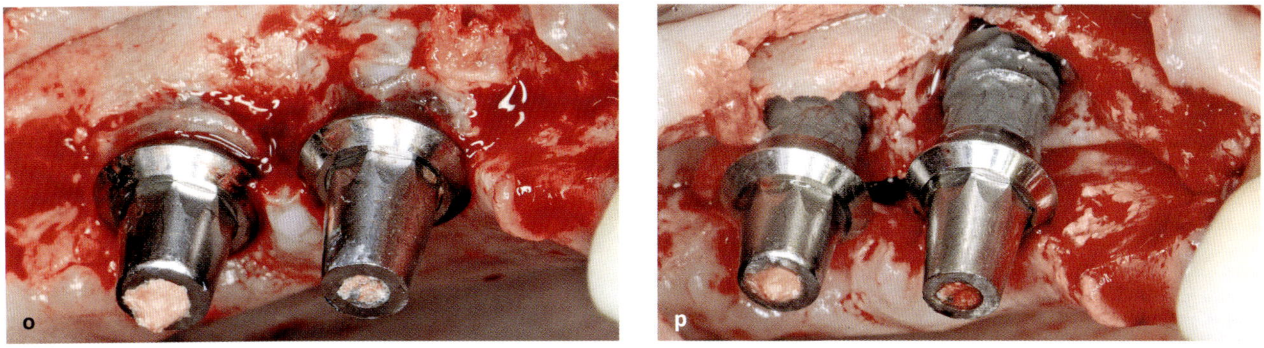

Figs 8-8o, p **(o)** After raising the full-thickness flap. **(p)** After removal of granulation tissue, the exposed surfaces of the implants are evident due to bone destruction.

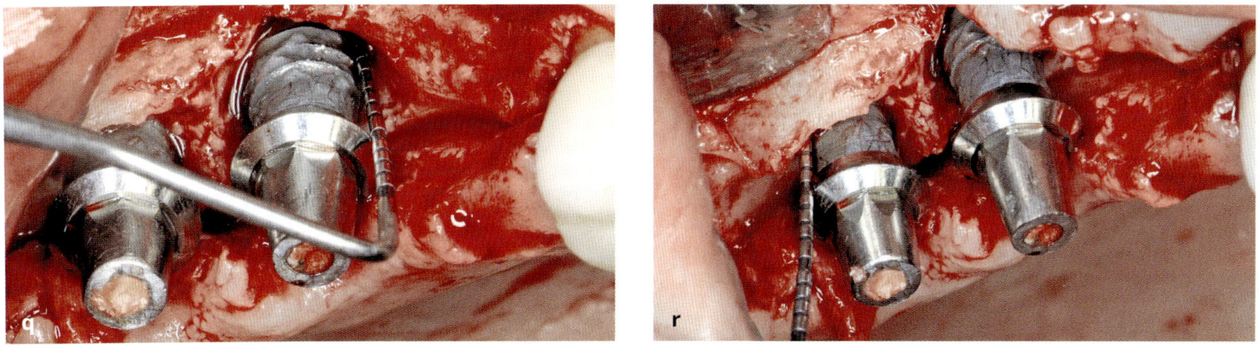

Figs 8-8q, r **(q)** The depth of the intrabony defect reaches 6 mm at implant no. 16. **(r)** At implant no. 17, the depth of the intrabony defect is less than 2 mm.

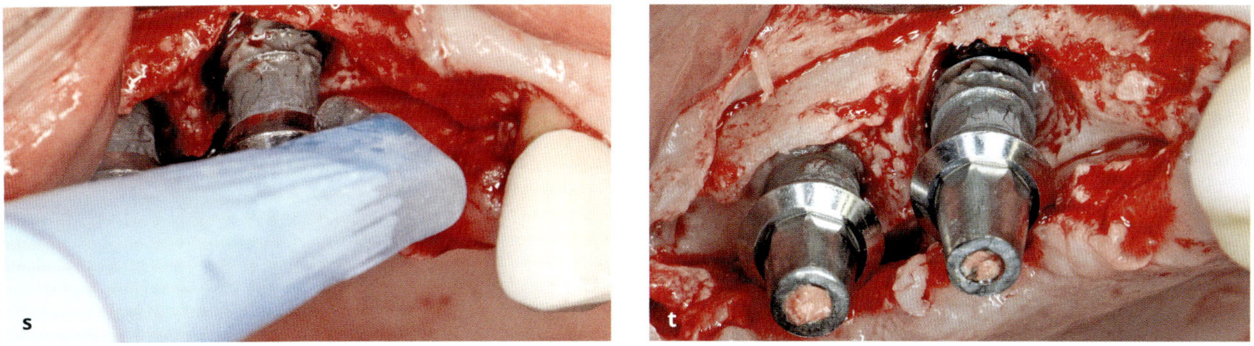

Figs 8-8s, t **(s)** Removal of the deposits from the implant surface with AIRFLOW and erythritol. **(t)** After removal of the deposits from the implants.

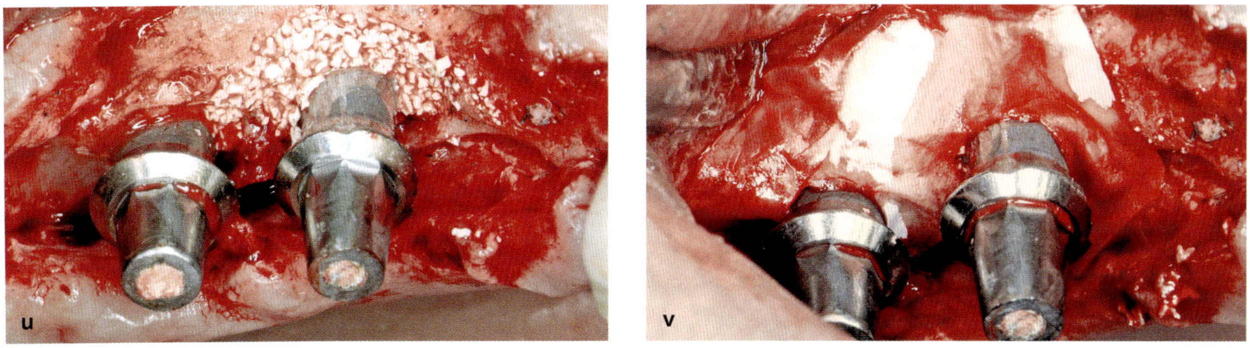

Figs 8-8u, v **(u)** Implantoplasty at the threads located coronally to the bone crest, filling the intrabony defect with a xenograft. **(v)** Placement and adaptation of the collagen membrane for guided bone regeneration.

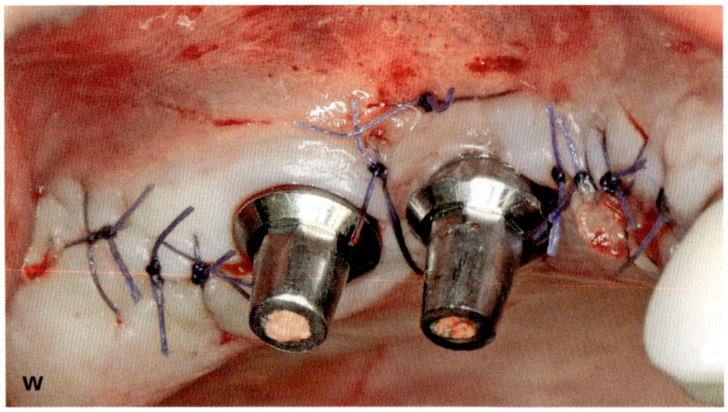

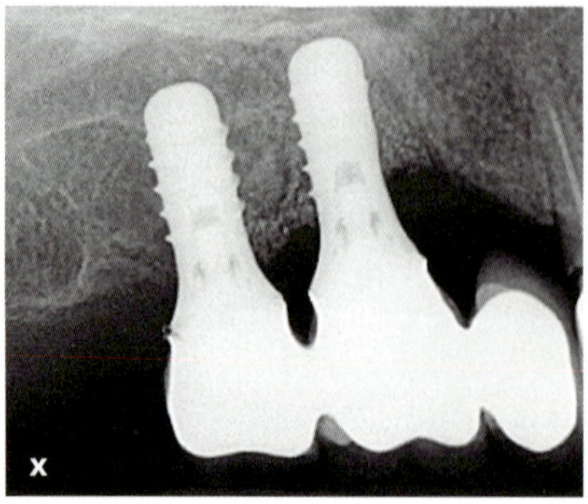

Figs 8-8w, x (w) After suturing for primary wound closure. **(x)** Five months later, filling of the intrabony defect with bone graft is observed radiologically.

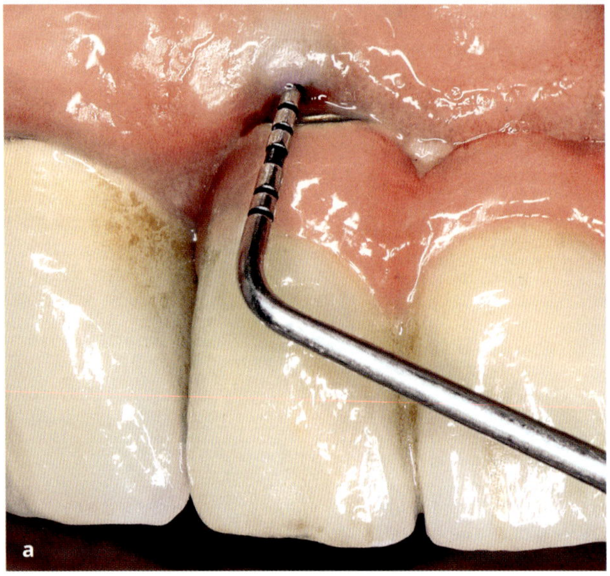

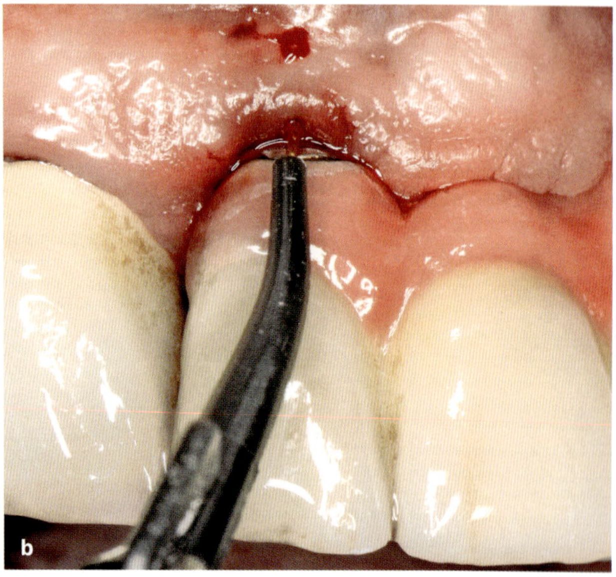

Figs 8-9a, b The laser provides bactericidal treatment and simultaneously activates the cellular healing processes, eliminating inflammation more quickly and successfully. Microbial populations recolonize after 6 months; however, in cases of peri-implantitis, it is incorrect to schedule the next recall session later than 3 months.

Another major difference in the current modification is the use of lasers to treat peri-implantitis before or during surgery for implant surface decontamination and granulation tissue removal (Figs 8-9a, b).[7–9]

8.6 Clinical case 5

According to the original protocol, this case presents a clinical situation similar to that of case 4, but with bone loss that has led to a deep crater (> 2 mm). According to the current modification of the CIST protocol (Fig 8-3), this case is treated like clinical case 4 using steps A, B, C, and D (Figs 8-10a–y).

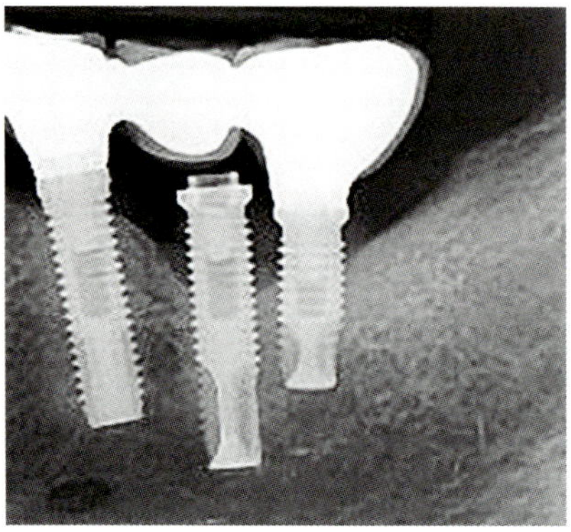

Fig 8-10a Radiographic image of a patient with peri-implantitis 8 years after implant placement.

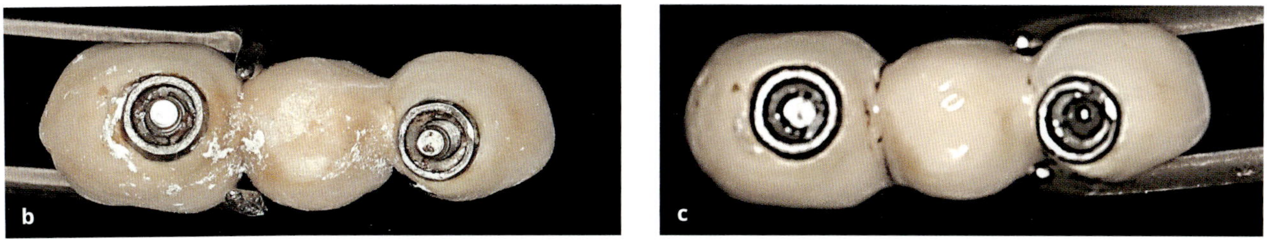

Figs 8-10b, c **(b)** After unscrewing the partial denture. Abundant biofilm deposits can be seen. **(c)** After removal of deposits with AIRFLOW using erythritol.

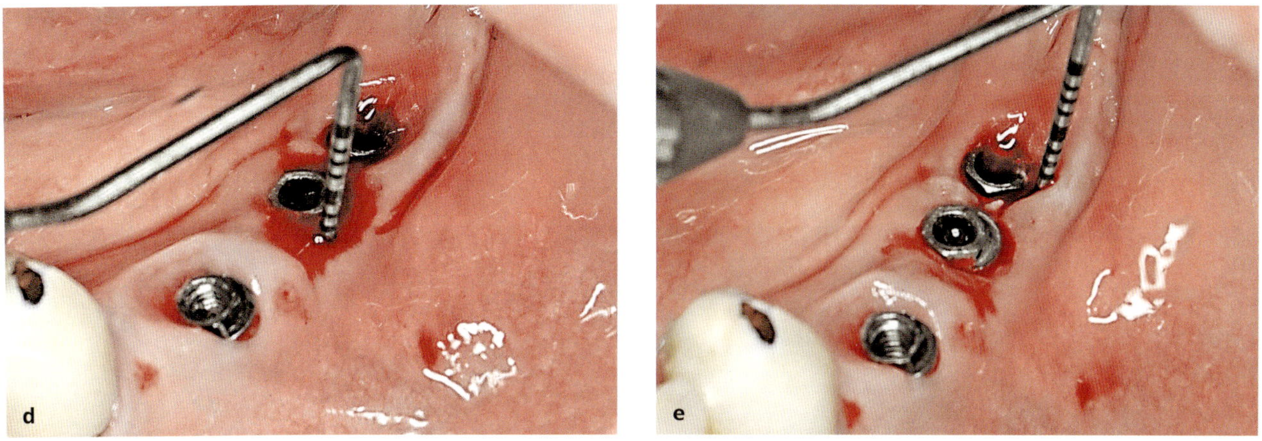

Figs 8-10d, e Probing revealed deep pockets.

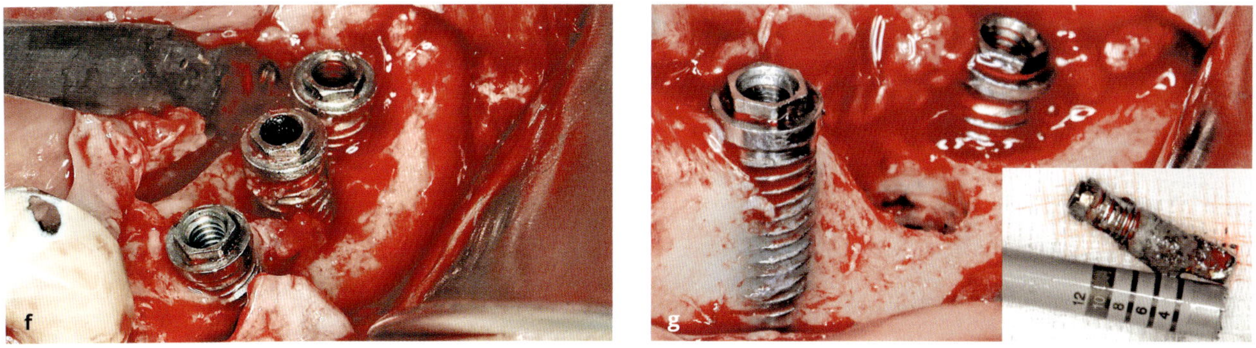

Figs 8-10f, g **(f)** After raising the flap, the middle implant was extracted because its presence would have made it impossible to perform effective oral hygiene on the last implant. The middle implant was also not used to support the partial denture. **(g)** After removal of the implant using a hollow cylindrical bur.

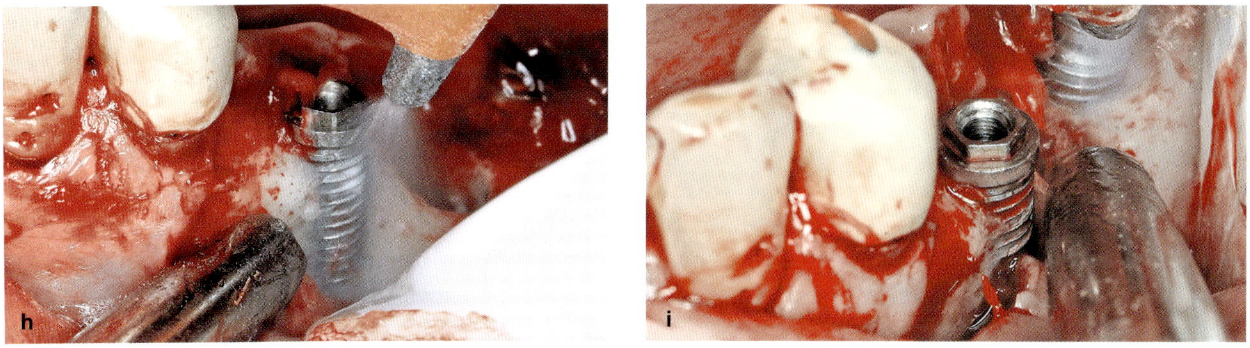

Figs 8-10h, i Removal of deposits with AIRFLOW and erythritol, being mindful not to direct the beam between the flap and bone, but using two powerful surgical suctions (metallic and broad, shown in white in **[h]**) to avoid facial emphysema.

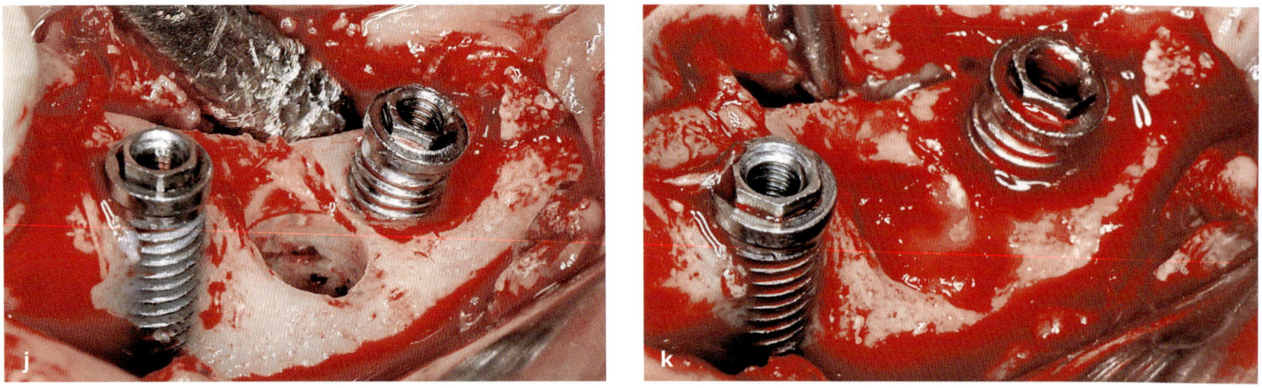

Figs 8-10j, k **(j)** The smooth surfaces of the implants can be seen after removal of the deposits. No implantoplasty was performed because the thickness of the titanium between the outer surface and the inner thread was low, with the risk of weakening its structure and the possibility of fracture. **(k)** Placement of a collagen plug in the prepared implant bed.

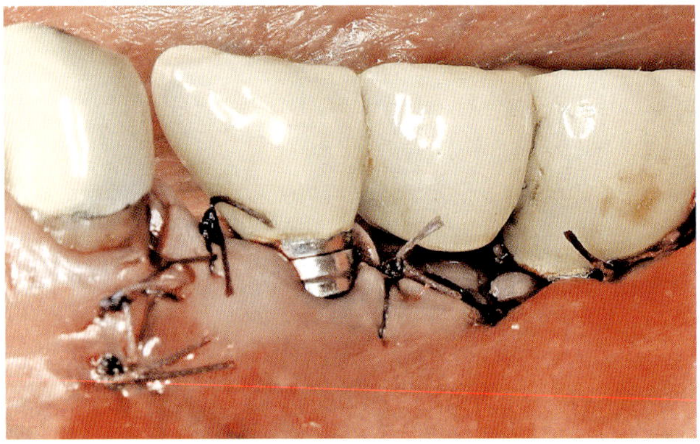

Fig 8-10l Suturing and apical flap repositioning.

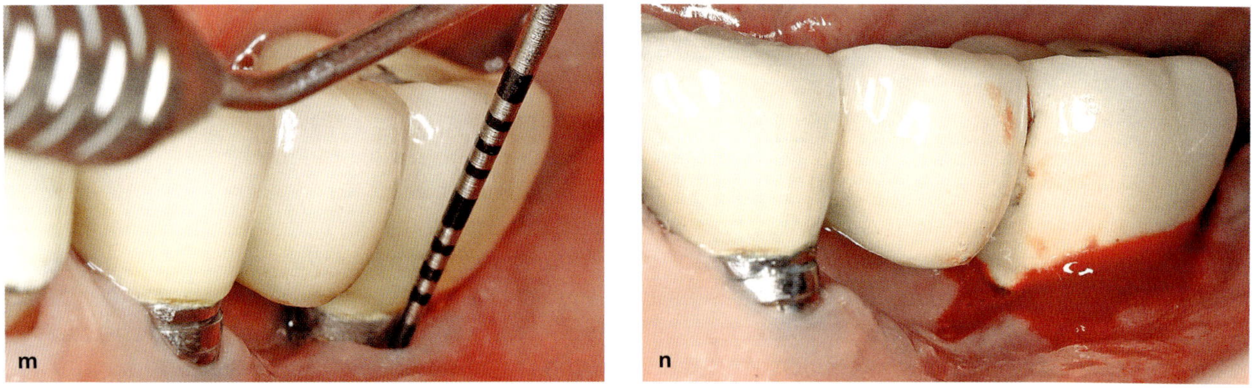

Figs 8-10m, n **(m)** Six months after surgery. Apical repositioning and establishment of a peri-implant sulcus can be seen. Extreme displacement and formation of a sulcus can be seen. **(n)** A return of inflammation can be observed.

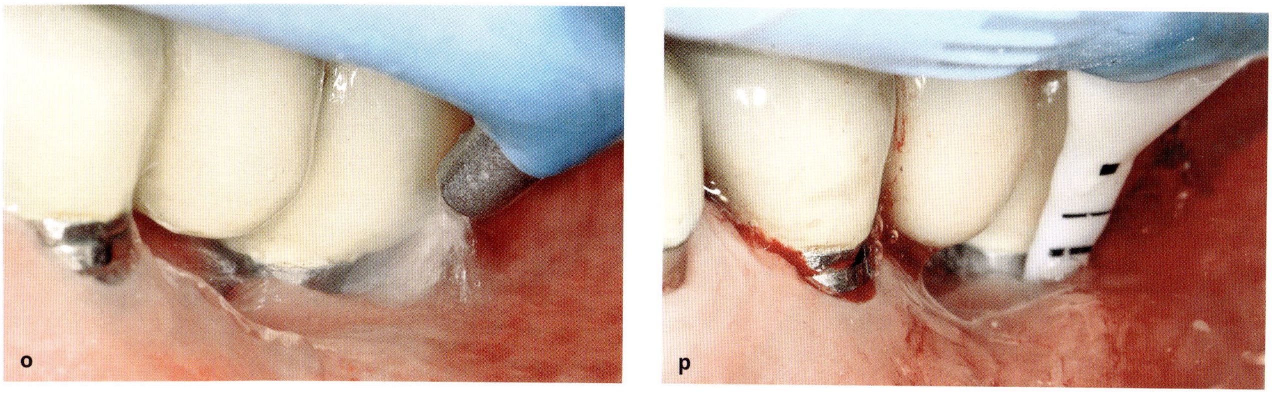

Figs 8-10o, p Implementation of the CIST protocol (steps A and B). AIRFLOW and PERIOFLOW handpieces, using erythritol.

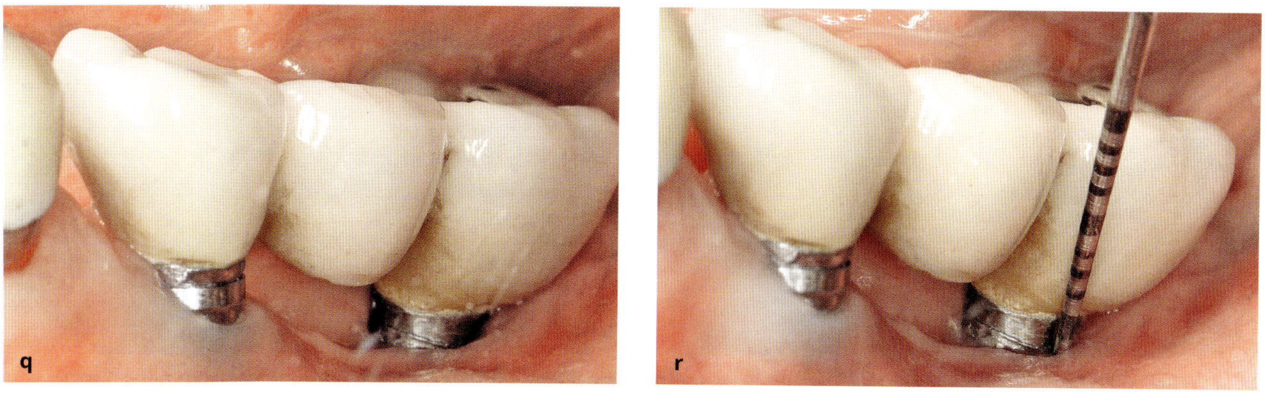

Figs 8-10q, r 1.5 years after surgery and with the patient complying with supportive periodontal therapy every 2 to 3 months, the area is maintained free of inflammation and pockets.

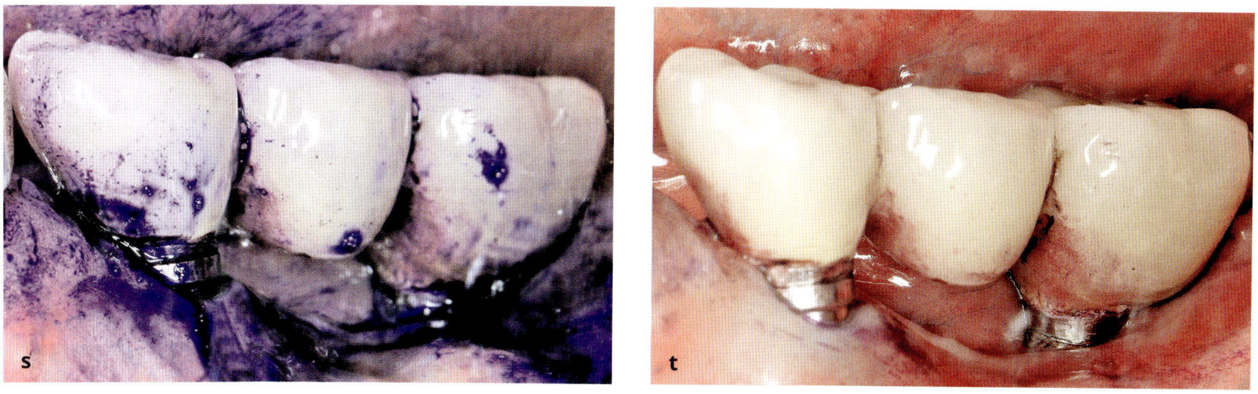

Figs 8-10s, t At each session, the GBT protocol is carried out to remotivate the patient in their oral hygiene and to guide them in the complete removal of microbial deposits to maintain oral health.

long-term implant prognosis may be expected, under biologically, functionally, and esthetically acceptable conditions.[6–8]

Diagnosis relies on bleeding occurring during the application of a mechanical stimulus. Bleeding on probing (BOP) is indicative of peri-implant mucositis.[9–12] If the force applied on probing exceeds 0.3 N, bleeding may be caused by mechanical trauma to the supracrestal connective tissue.[13] The presence of inflammation in the peri-implant tissues together with the absence of bone destruction lead to a diagnosis of peri-implant mucositis. In cases with BOP of a pocket of 4 mm or greater, a periapical radiograph is necessary to confirm the diagnosis of mucositis by excluding alveolar bone loss.[11,12] The clinical image of peri-implant mucositis is accompanied by redness of the peri-implant mucosa, edema, or suppuration. Clinical evaluation may be affected by tissue phenotype, smoking habits, forces applied to the probe, and the angulation and diameter of the periodontal probe.[5,14–17]

The depth of the peri-implant sulcus may differ from that of the gingival sulcus.[17] The position of the implant neck is determined during surgical placement.[11,12] Implant insertion in the esthetic zone usually requires a more apical placement of the implant to establish conditions that allow the mimicking of the morphology and emergence of a tooth.[18] Emphasis should be placed on taking a radiograph immediately after implant insertion and placement of the final restoration. Moreover, clinical measurements of the peri-implant sulcus depth during placement of the restoration are essential.[11,12]

The steps necessary to successfully diagnose and treat peri-implant mucositis (Figs 9-2a–f) are as follows[1,8,11,12,15,16,19]:

- disclosure of dental biofilm and demonstration of its presence to the patient;
- informing the patient about the role of biofilm, and the diagnosis and the risk for progression to peri-implantitis if mucositis is untreated;
- patient motivation, education, and training in the daily performance of effective oral hygiene. By disclosing the biofilm with a disclosing agent, its removal will be more efficacious than without disclosing it. With various oral hygiene practices, the disclosed biofilm has to be removed completely;
- application of air debriding decontamination using AIRFLOW (EMS Dental, Nyon, Switzerland) and erythritol if the peri-implant sulcus is up to 4 mm deep;
- application of complementary subgingival biofilm removal with PERIOFLOW (EMS Dental) and erythritol in sulci deeper then 4 mm;
- supplementary laser radiation with 810-, 940-, or 980-nm diodes or Er:YAG lasers (2,940 nm) in peri-implant sulci deeper than 4 mm;
- removal of calcified deposits with ultrasonics and special tips (PI, EMS Dental, Nyon, Switzerland) made of polyetheretherketone;
- rinsing the peri-implant sulci with a 01% to 0.2% chlorhexidine solution or 1% chlorhexidine gel;
- prescription of 1% chlorhexidine gel for home use for 3 to 4 weeks, twice daily, after mechanical biofilm removal;
- reevaluation after 4 weeks (Figs 9-3a–h). Typically, reevaluation after the treatment of gingivitis is performed after 2 weeks. However, longer periods than 3 weeks are necessary to establish mucosal health;
- if deemed necessary, surgical modification of the peri-implant mucosa to facilitate the insertion of mechanical means for oral hygiene or even reconstructive surgery to increase the width and thickness of keratinized mucosa;
- scheduling for the next maintenance care appointment (Figs 9-4a–h and 9-5a–h).

As mentioned in Chapter 8, two significant improvements are added to the cumulative interceptive supportive therapy (CIST) protocol:

- replacement of the guideline for mechanical debridement with the guideline for application of the guided biofilm therapy (GBT) protocol;[11,20]
- laser radiation to supplement the bactericidal effects (Figs 8-1 and 8-3).[21,22]

The sum of information for successful removal of the local etiologic factors (biofilms and calculus) is analyzed in Chapter 16. The advantages and disadvantages of several procedures suggested previously, as well as the detailed description and interpretation of the GBT protocol, is described in detail in Figs 9-6a–l.

The maintenance care phase concerns the period after active therapy for peri-implant mucositis or peri-implantitis. However, it primarily relates to the long-term maintenance of the outcome of initial implant therapy.[23] Clinicians are strongly advised to start its application immediately after the completion of therapy.

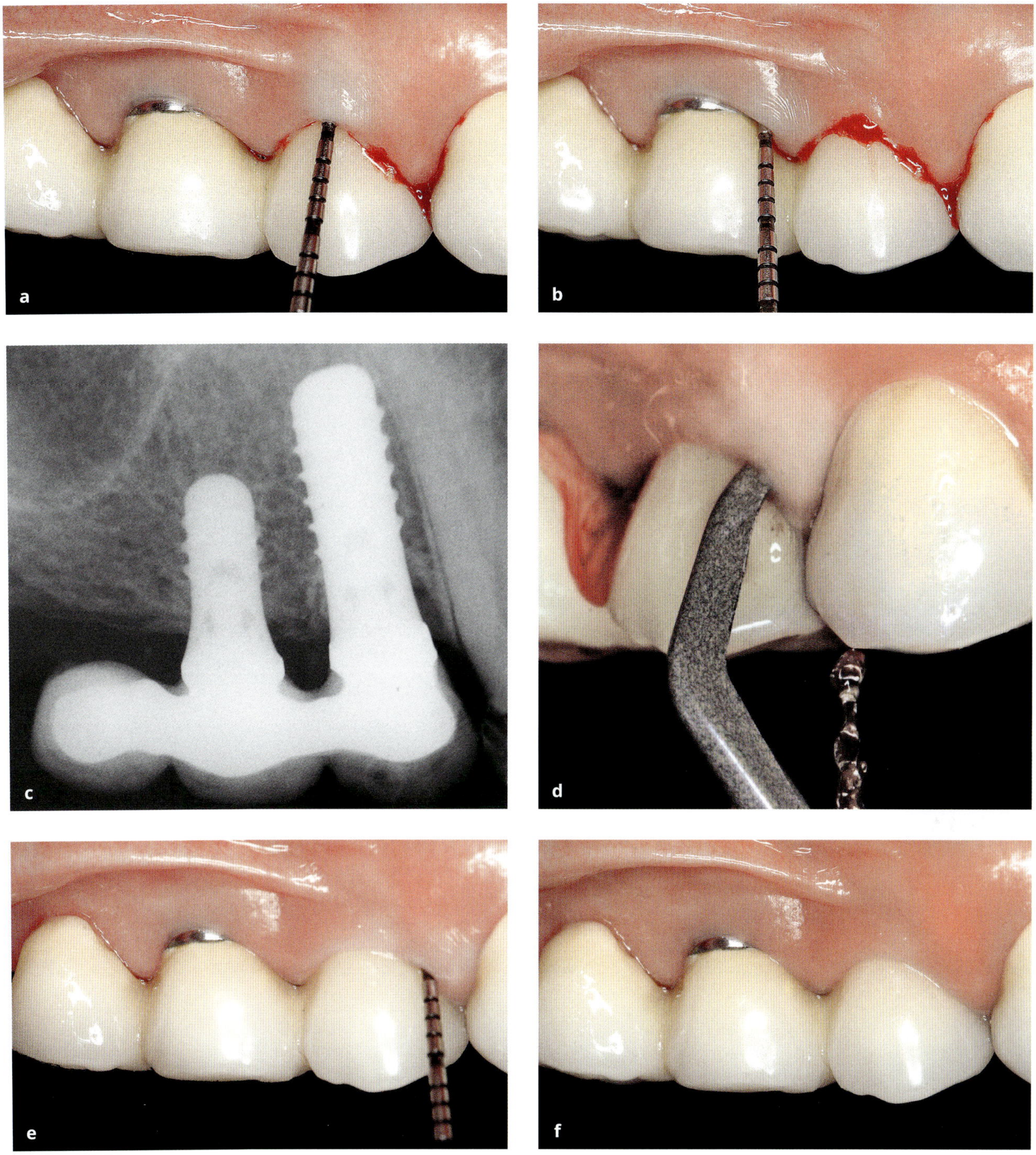

Figs 9-2a–f (a and b) Clinical images of peri-implant mucositis. There is inflammation of the soft tissues, without the presence of pockets. **(c)** The radiograph confirms the absence of bone loss. **(d)** Steps A and B of the CIST protocol are applied. The removal of deposits with a plastic ultrasonic tip may be seen. **(e)** Four weeks after therapy, during probing of the peri-implant sulcus. **(f)** The lack of bleeding after probing confirms the elimination of peri-implant inflammation.

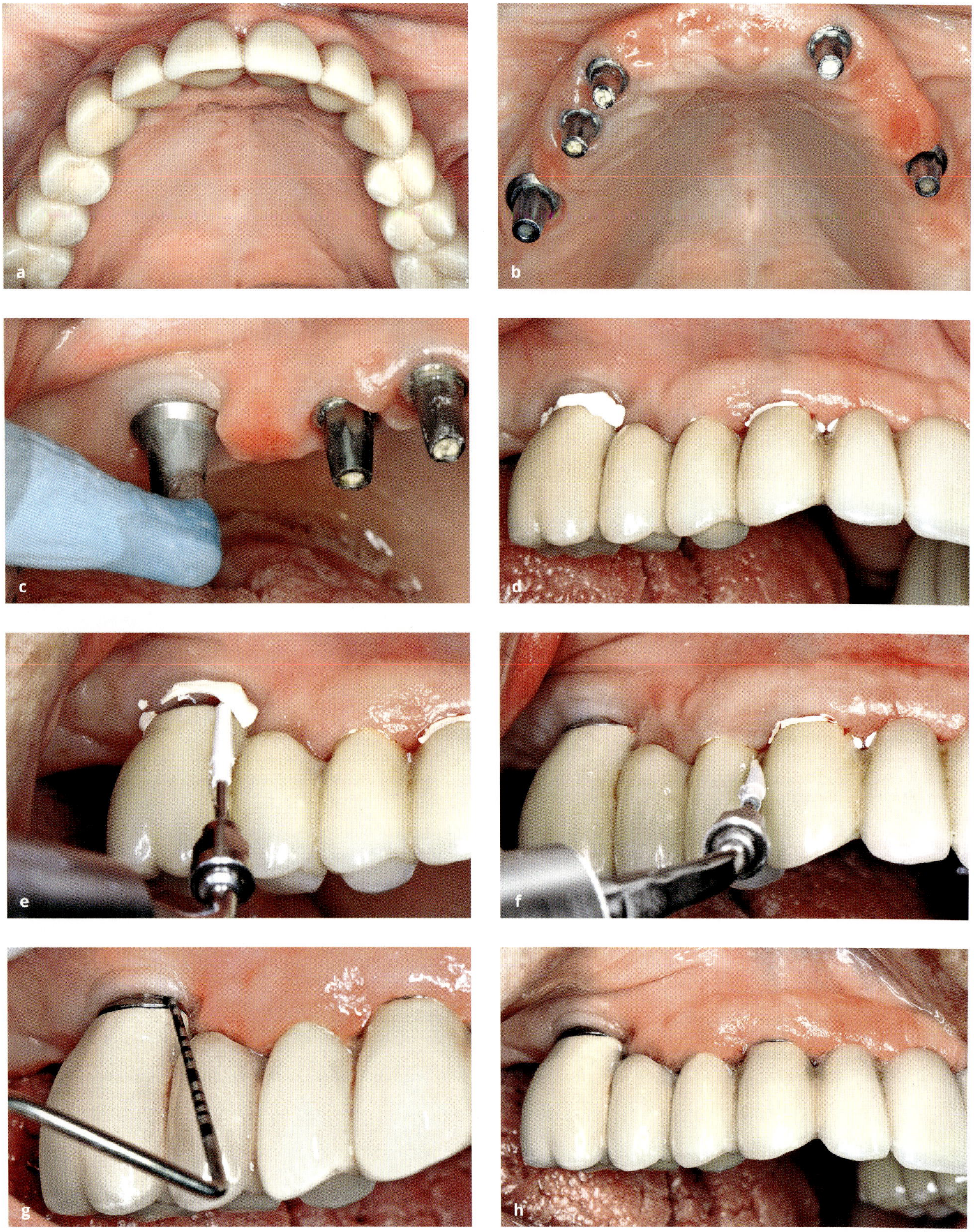

Figs 9-3a–h **(a)** Implant-supported fixed partial denture that was detached after 2 years of function. **(b)** Peri-implant mucositis due to delayed processing of the patient for supportive therapy, as well as the avoidance of interdental cleaning devices to prevent complete detachment of the prosthesis. **(c)** Biofilm removal with AIRFLOW and erythritol. **(d)** Excess cement can be seen after cementation with provisional cement. **(e and f)** Excess cement was removed with the PI tip (EMS Dental). **(g and h)** Four weeks after therapy, there was no BOP.

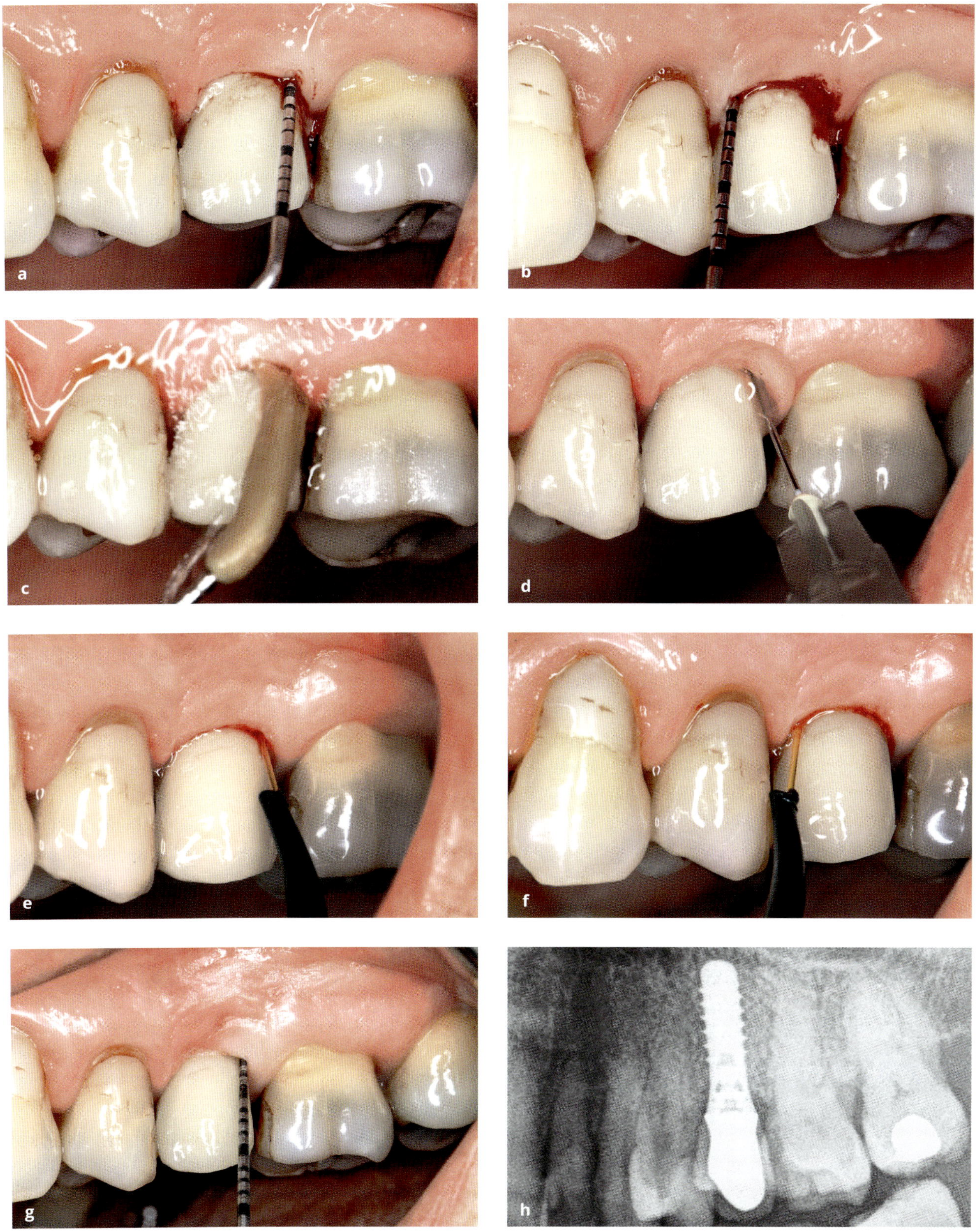

Figs 9-4a–h **(a and b)** BOP at implant no. 25, without the presence of pockets. The diagnosis is peri-implant mucositis. **(c)** Deposit removal with an ultrasonic tip. **(d)** Submucosal chlorhexidine irrigation. **(e and f)** 980-nm diode laser application (1 W) for bactericidal effect. **(g)** Four weeks after therapy, a healthy peri-implant sulcus could be probed. **(h)** Radiograph of the area reveals no bone destruction.

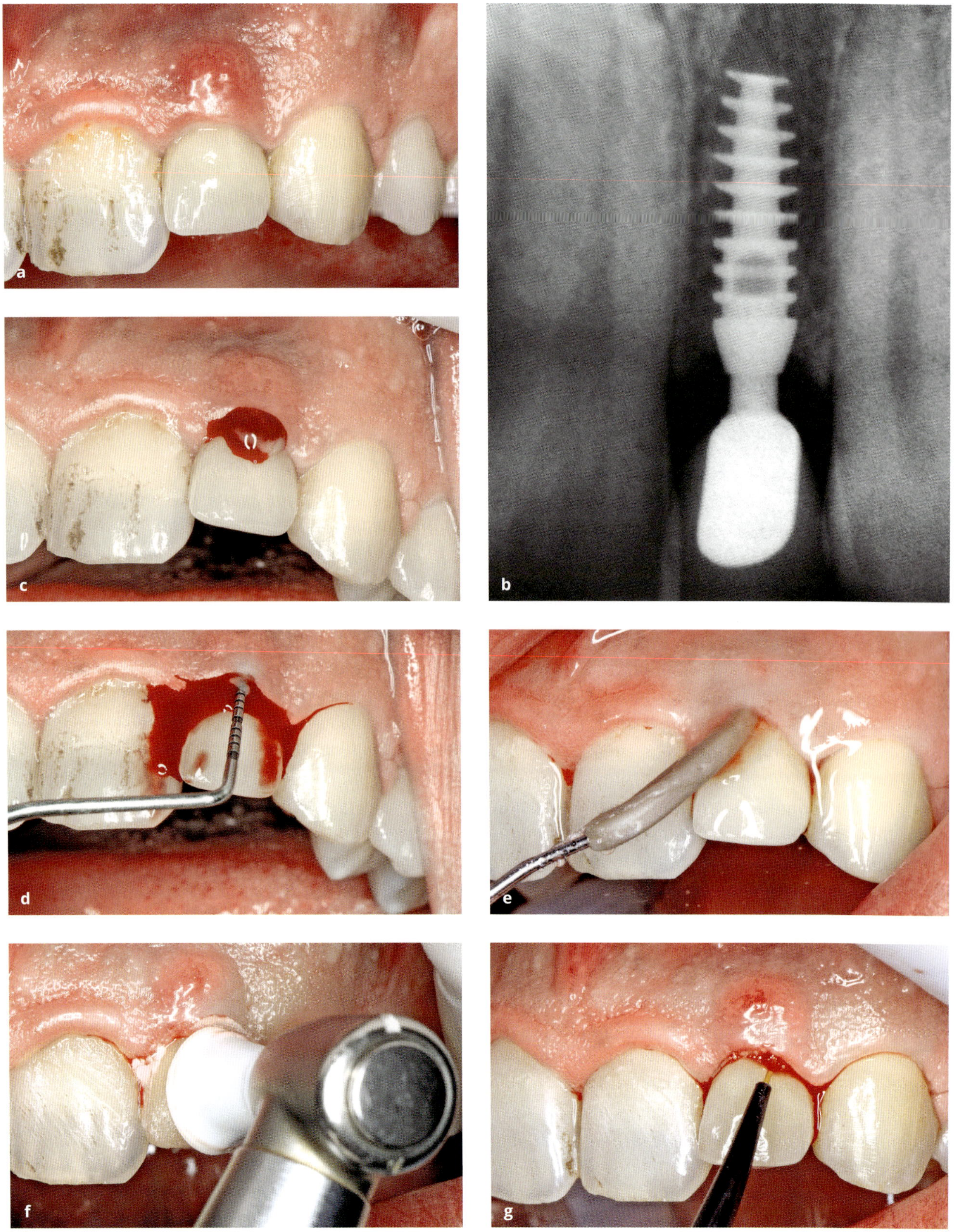
a
b
c
d
e
f
g

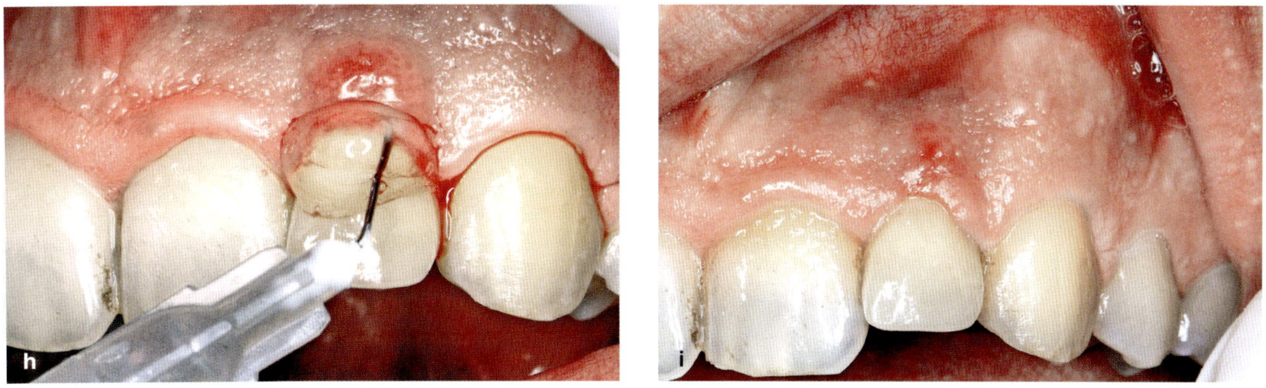

Figs 9-5a–i (a and b) Clinical and radiographic images of a patient 5 years after implant placement, which was performed at the age of 20. There was an increase in the volume of the soft tissues presenting a mucosal abscess. **(c)** Pressure on the peri-implant mucosa, apically to the overgrowth, led to the drainage of the abscess. **(d)** Probing revealed a deep peri-implant sulcus of 5 mm. **(e)** Removal of deposits with the use of a plastic ultrasonic tip. **(f)** Polishing with a rubber cup and fine-grained paste. **(g)** The area was irradiated with a 980-nm diode laser (1 W). **(h)** Submucosal irrigation with 1% chlorhexidine, which was prescribed to the patient for use at home for 4 weeks. **(i)** Two days later, when the patient attended for a checkup and oral hygiene instructions, significant reduction of the signs of inflammation could be seen.

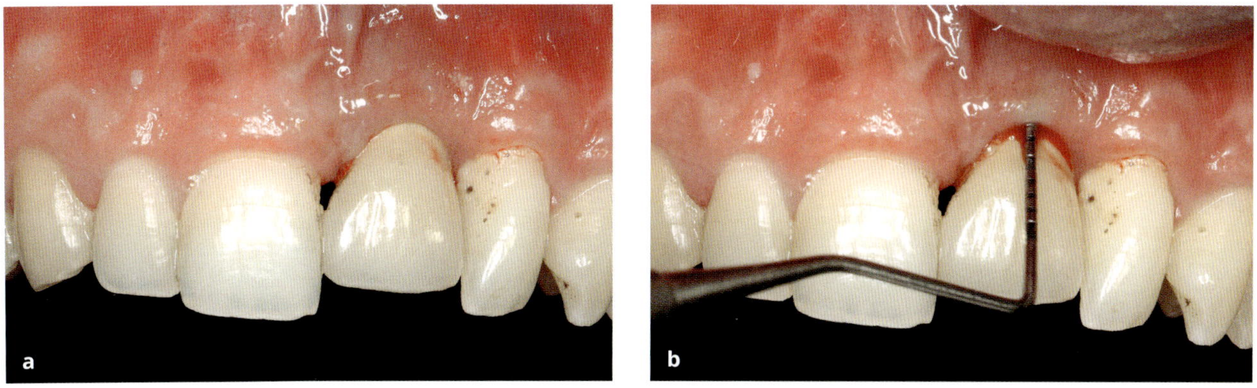

Figs 9-6a–c (a) Clinical image of a 29-year-old patient who had an implant placed in site no. 21 at the age of 17, before skeletal development was complete. This history was confirmed by the more coronal placement of the teeth compared to the crown on implant no. 21. The patient mentioned that when the implant-supported crown was initially placed, there was symmetry. **(b)** A pocket depth of 8 mm and BOP were observed. **(c)** The panoramic radiograph revealed an old-type implant (Frialit), which was positioned a great distance away from the imaginary line connecting the cementoenamel junctions of the adjacent teeth. This confirms that skeletal development was not complete when the implant was placed.

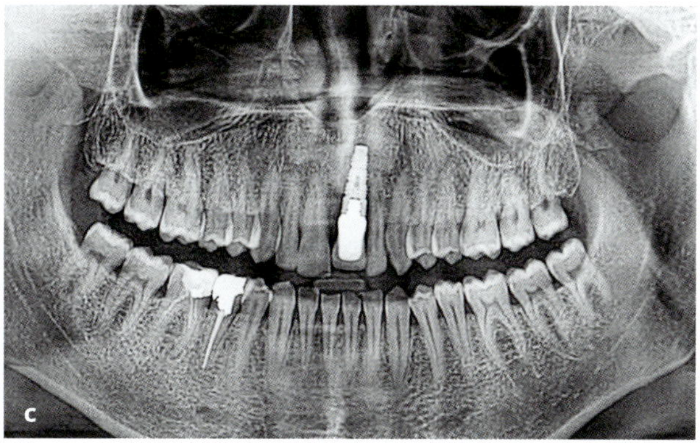

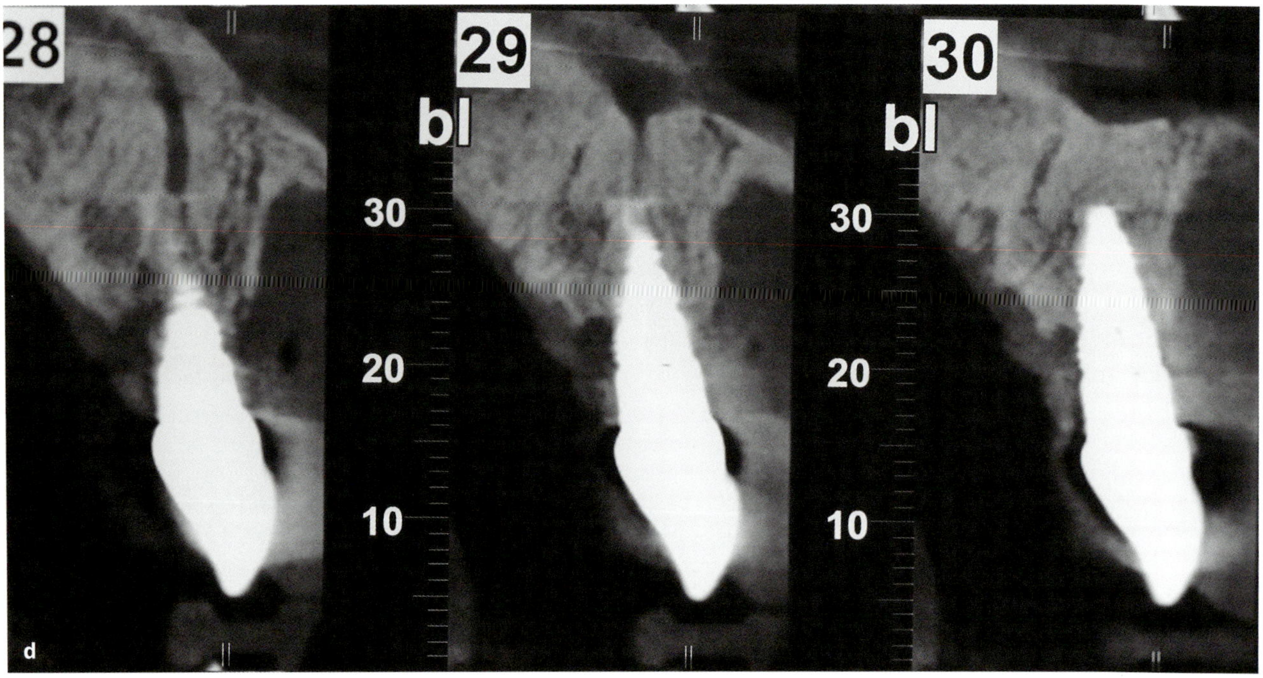

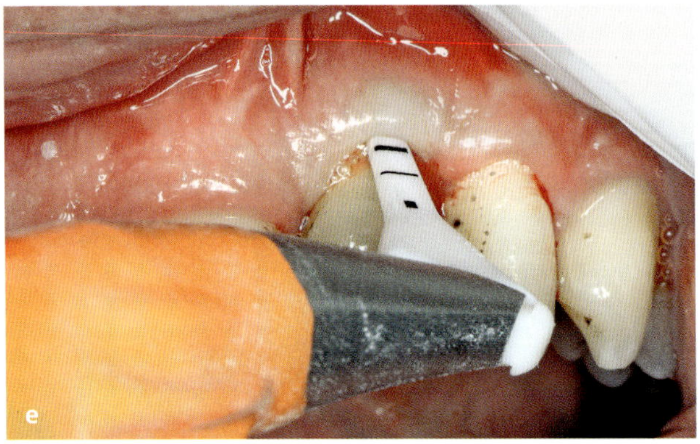

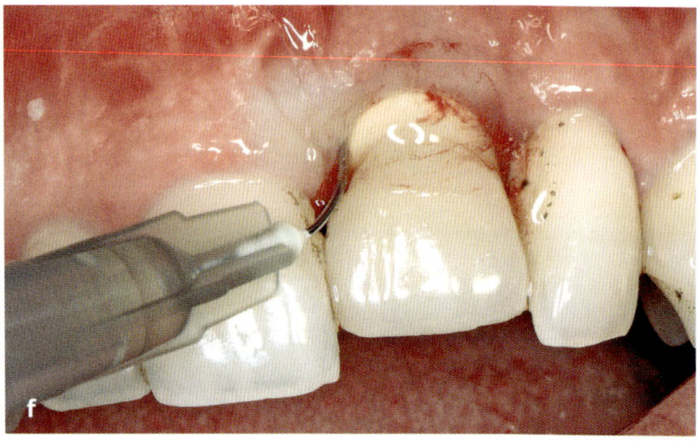

Figs 9-6d–f (d) Cross-sectional views of the CBCT scan revealed the severity of bone destruction. **(e)** Air debriding decontamination with PERIOFLOW and erythritol spray after disclosure of biofilm, oral hygiene instructions, and AIRFLOW. **(f)** 1% chlorhexidine gel was irrigated submucosally. The same gel was prescribed to the patient for use at home three to four times daily for 4 weeks.

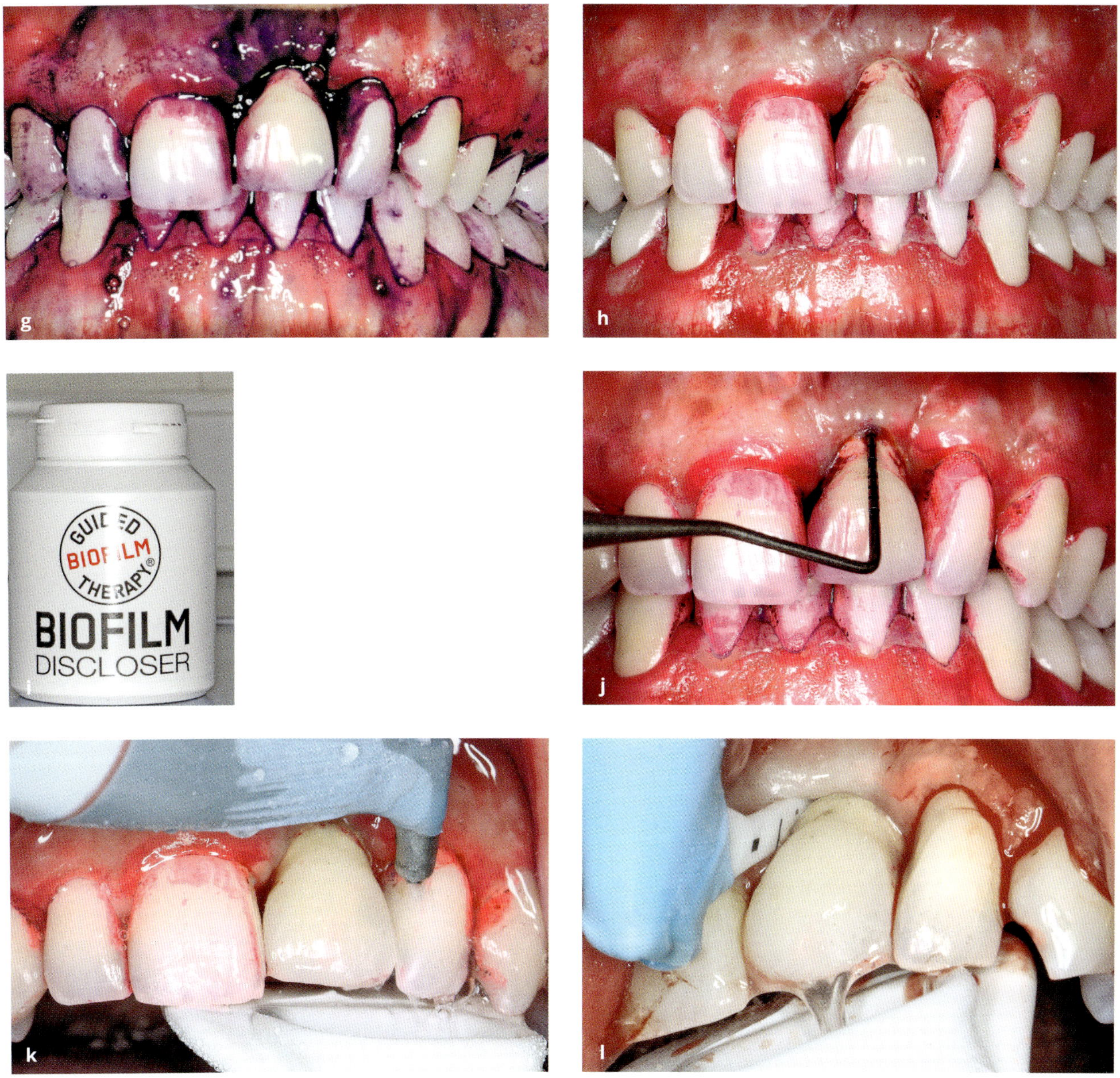

Figs 9-6g–l **(g)** Four weeks later, reevaluation was performed. The use of a disclosing agent revealed abundant biofilm at the interproximal areas. **(h)** After water irrigation, large deposits of biofilm could be seen. Once again, detailed oral hygiene instructions were given to the patient. **(i)** Package of disclosing pellets. **(j)** Despite the remaining dental biofilm, a significant reduction in inflammation (less bleeding) and depth of the peri-implant pockets at 6 mm was noted. **(k)** The GBT protocol was repeated thoroughly. The inclination of the handpiece can be observed during the use of AIR-FLOW. **(l)** The nozzle of the PERIOFLOW handpiece can be seen.

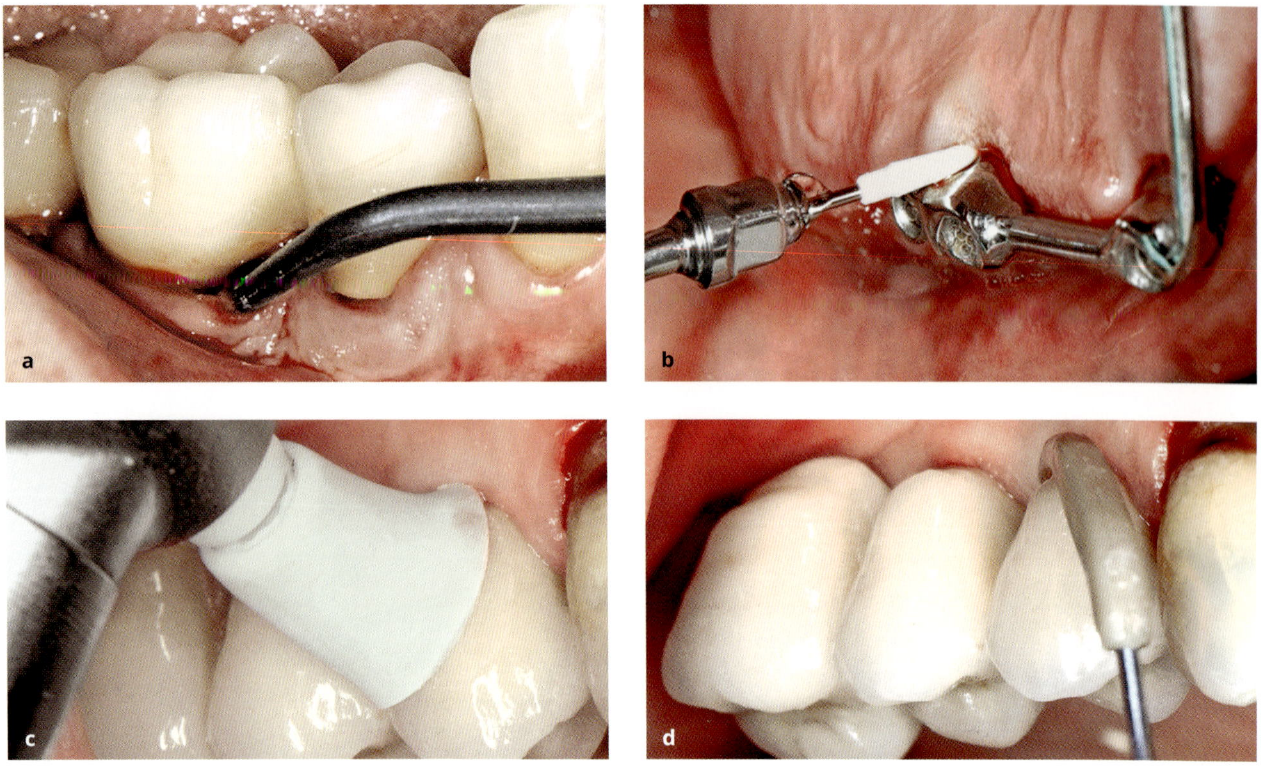

Figs 9-7a–d **(a)** Application of a carbon fiber curette. **(b)** Ultrasonic tip made of polyetheretherketone **(PI)**. **(c)** Rubber cup and polishing paste. **(d)** An ultrasonic tip made of synthetic material (NSK, Tokyo, Japan) is only one of the instruments used for the management of peri-implant inflammation.

The reasons for the replacement of the mechanical debridement guideline with the GBT application guideline are:[24]

- GBT does not damage the titanium surfaces and restoration materials;
- greater removal of biofilms is achieved, even in deep peri-implant pockets;
- it less time-consuming compared to other methods;
- it is better accepted by the patient compared to other procedures, as it is nearly painless.

For the mechanical debridement of deposits, a variety of instruments and devices have been employed (Figs 9-7a–d and 9-8a–d).[20,25–29] Using devices and instruments to remove soft and hard deposits can cause damage to the implant surfaces and restoration materials (Figs 9-9a, b and 9-10a–d).[30–33]

First, the mechanical effect may lead to the removal of the protective oxide layer from titanium surfaces. It has been claimed, although not substantiated, that, in some cases, the recreation of the oxide layer may not be reestablished entirely. The result of the use of various devices or instruments for titanium surfaces, which typically depends on the material and its roughness, are shown in Figs 9-11a–f, 9-12a–f, and 9-13a–f.

Scratches on the titanium surface, and detachment of titanium particles and restoration materials, constitute unwanted situations that are blamed for greater biofilm accumulation, mechanical irritation, or even possible foreign-body reactions (Figs 9-14a, b, 9-15, 9-16a–e, 9-17, and 9-18a–d).[33,34]

The application of stainless steel or other metallic hand or ultrasonic instruments is not recommended during cause-related therapy of peri-implant mucositis.[11,12,34] On the other hand, in cases of peri-implantitis, implant surface modification has often been advocated, that is, implantoplasty. However, before the introduction of a special nozzle for air debriding decontamination using PERIOFLOW, the only device that was able enter peri-implant pockets to remove deposits was a thin metallic ultrasonic tip (Figs 9-19 and 9-20).[35]

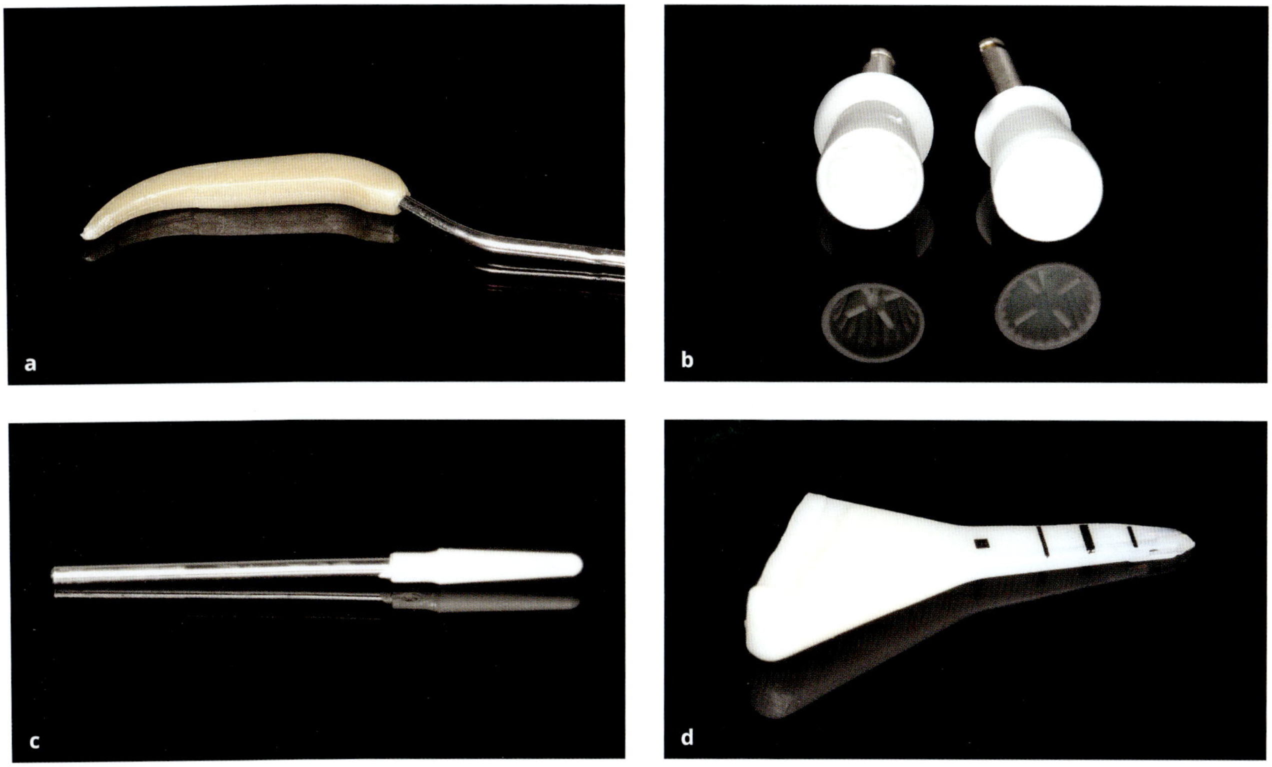

Figs 9-8a–d (a) Ultrasonic tip made of synthetic material (NSK). **(b)** Rubber cups for polishing, used in combination with polishing pastes. **(c)** Ultrasonic tips made of polyetheretherketone. **(d)** Single-use nozzle with three points for irrigation, for subgingival air debriding decontamination, which was adapted to the PERIOFLOW handpiece.

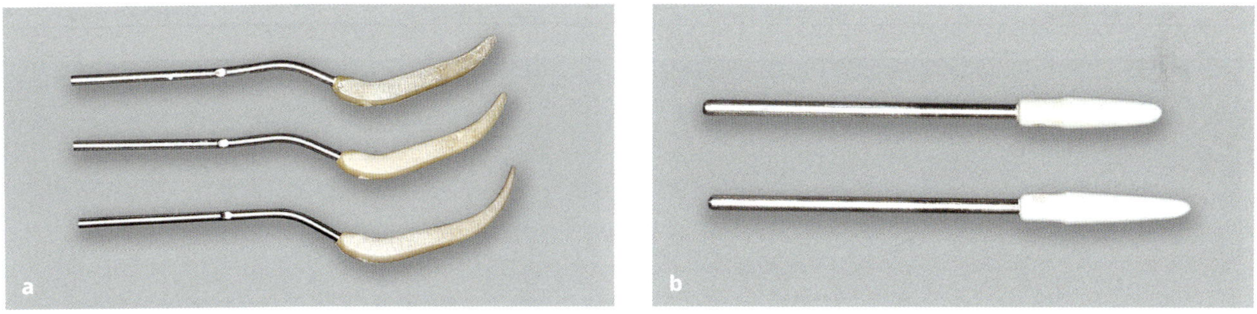

Figs 9-9a, b Gradual wear of a new plastic tip. The material that is slowly abraded may be retained on the implant surface, with unknown consequences for the course of the therapeutic outcome.

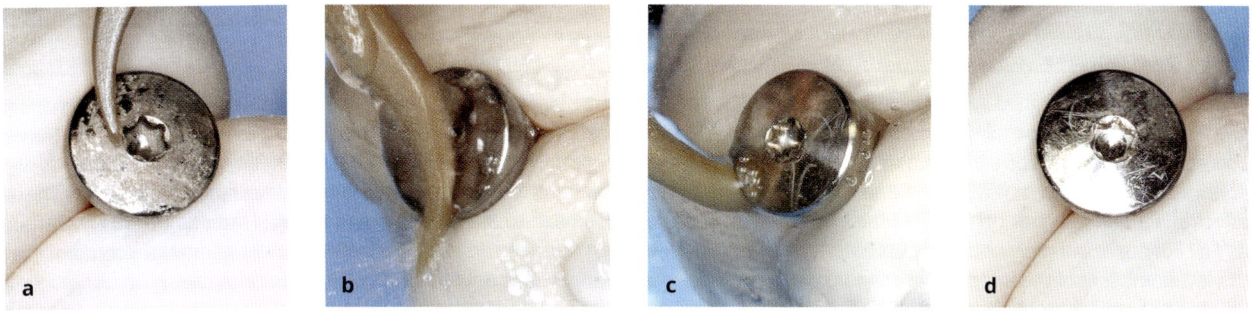

Figs 9-10a–d Removal of biofilm from the healing abutment, which remained in the mouth for 6 weeks. Evidently, the use of instruments made of synthetic materials may cause damage to the titanium surface.

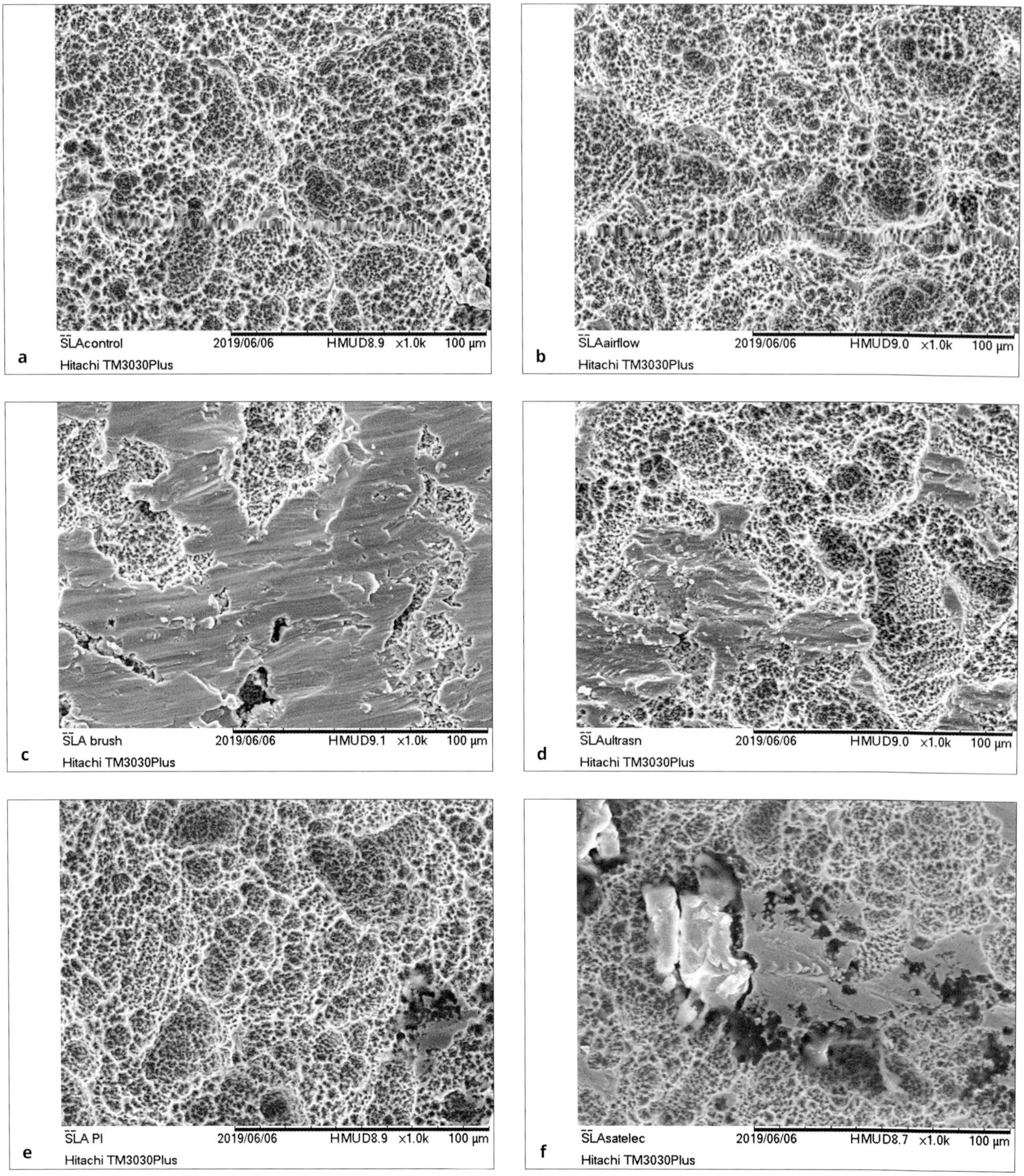

Figs 9-13a–f Comparative evaluation of different tools used to remove biofilms from implant surfaces. The images are micrographs taken with a scanning electron microscope at ×1,000 magnification. **(a)** Sandblasted and acid-etched (SLA) titanium surface, which served as the control surface. **(b)** Effect of AIRFLOW application with erythritol on a titanium surface. No alteration of the titanium surface can be observed. **(c)** Effect of the application of a titanium brush on the SLA titanium surface. The surface is almost completely damaged. **(d)** Effect of a metallic ultrasonic tip (SATELEC) on the SLA surface. At this magnification, the damage caused is substantial. **(e)** The effect of the application of an ultrasonic tip made of polyetheretherketone on the SLA surface can be seen. A small, abraded piece of polyetheretherketone is visible on the lower right side of the image; the surface of the titanium is slightly altered. **(f)** Effect of the application of an ultrasonic tip made of synthetic material on the SLA surface. Significant damage of the titanium surface and abraded pieces of synthetic material are obvious.

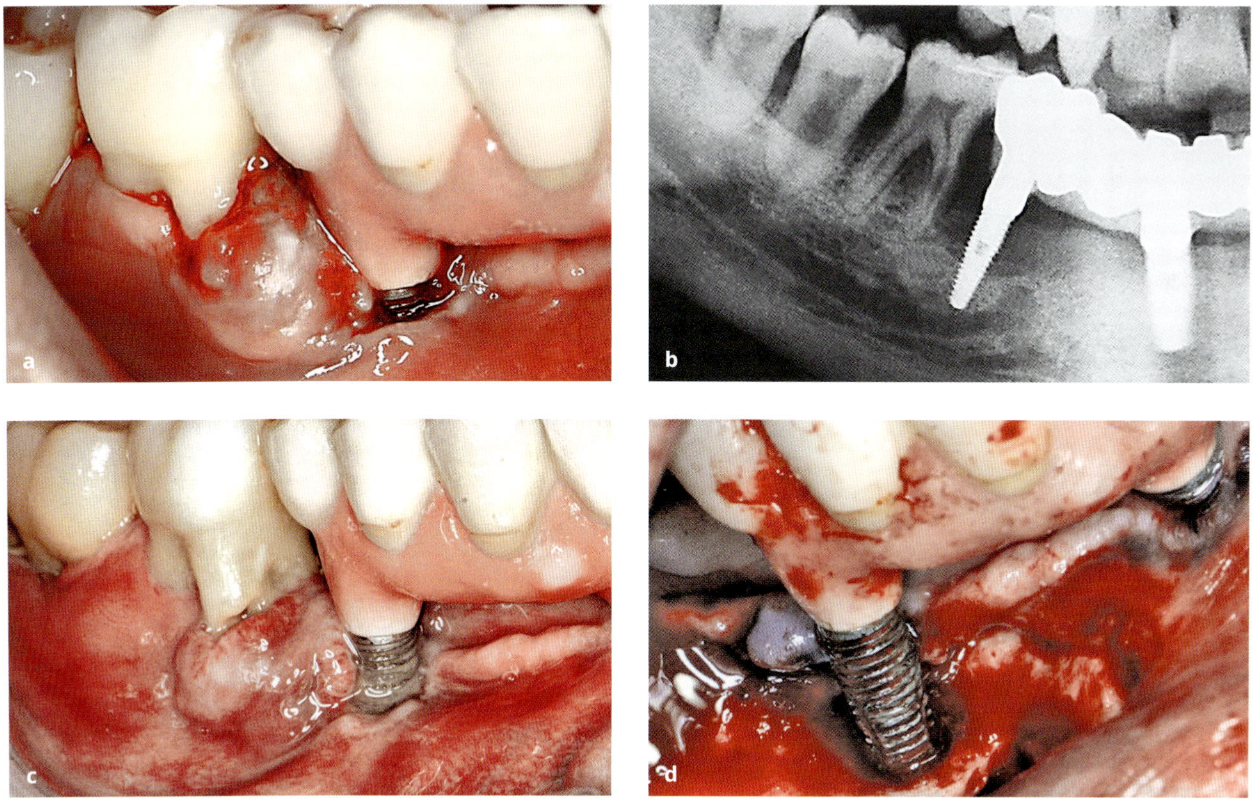

Figs 9-14a–d **(a and b)** Clinical and radiographic images of a tumor at the distal aspect of implant no. 45, with bleeding and a fragile surface. The lesion is clearly correlated to the implant surface. Radiographically, it seems to be associated with resorption of the root of no. 46. The patient had the implants for 4 years. The radiographs and clinical image taken after the surgical procedures are shown in Fig 4-7. **(c)** After cause-related therapy, the tissues shrank but the tumor did not. **(d)** The tumor was removed, a biopsy specimen was taken, and the sample was sent for histologic examination. Severe bone destruction and thread exposure can be seen (surgical images courtesy of Dr George Vilos).

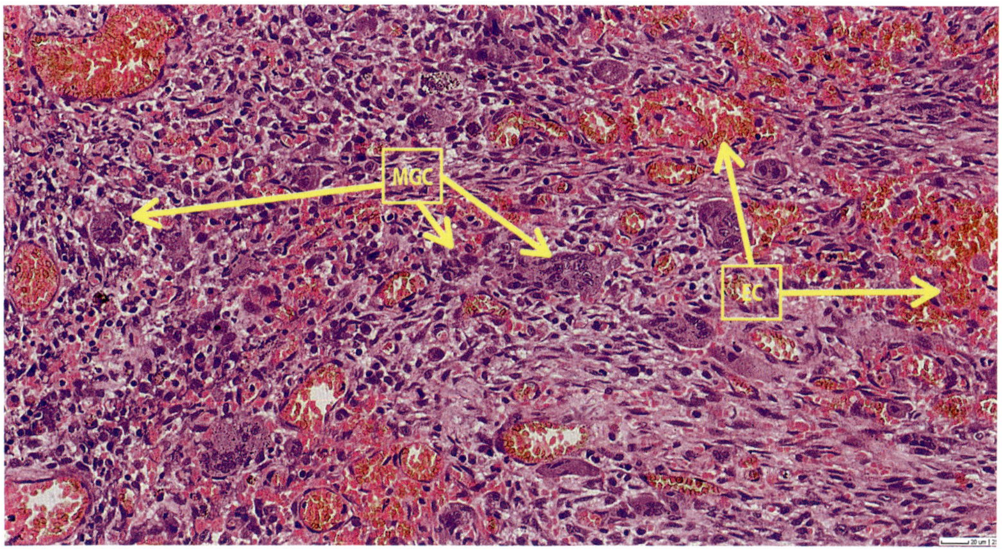

Fig 9-15 Histologic image from the tumor biopsy diagnosed a peripheral giant cell granuloma. Multinuclear giant cells (MGCs) and erythrocytes (ECs) are shown. The tissue has many macrophages (the cells with round purple nuclei), as well as fibroblasts, which are similar to macrophages but smaller in size and with slightly more angular nuclei (courtesy of Professor N. Nikitakis).

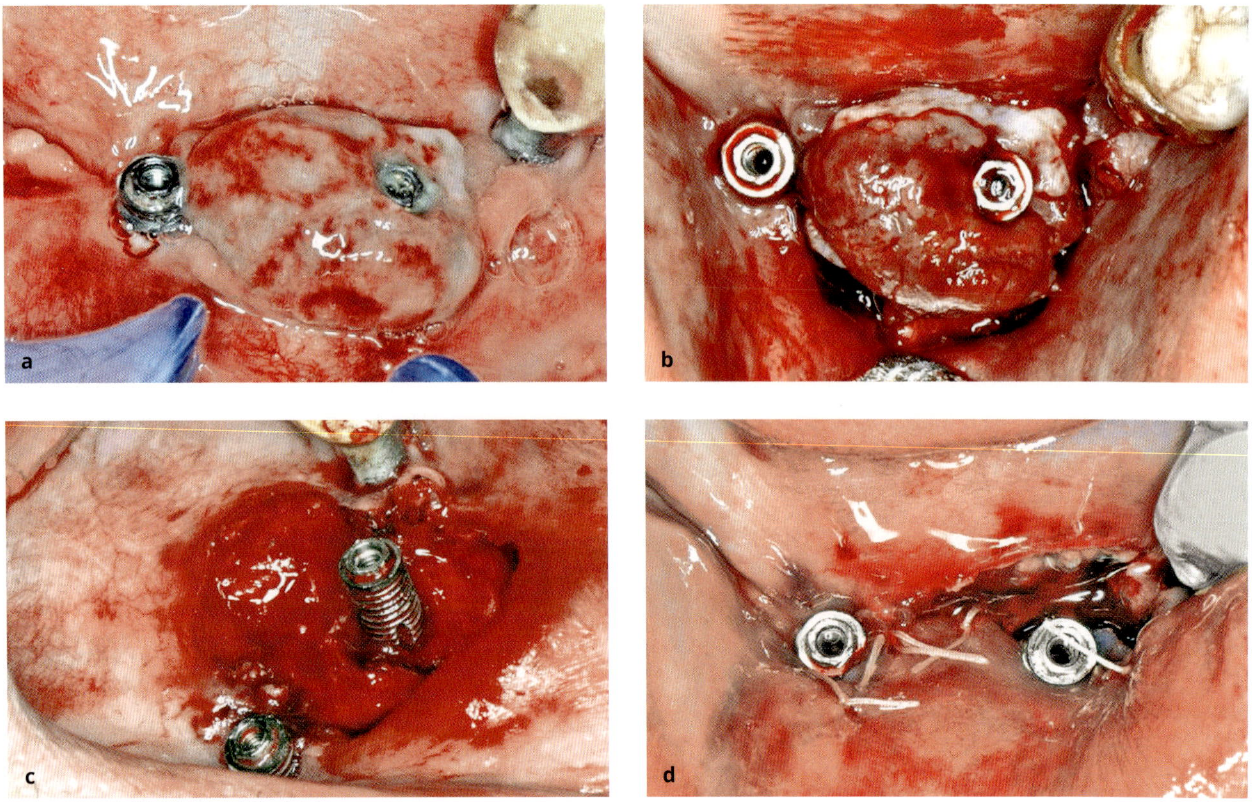

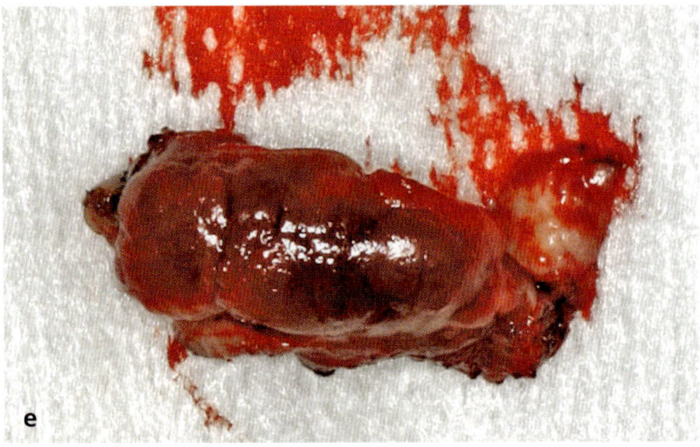

Figs 9-16a–e (a) Two years later, an exophytic mass with similar clinical features rapidly developed in the anterior mandible; it was related to the two implants. **(b)** The mass was surgically prepared for an excision biopsy specimen to be taken. **(c and d)** After tumor excision and suturing. **(e)** The large, removed tumor was sent for histologic examination (surgical images courtesy of Dr George Vilos).

Fig 9-17 Histologic image from the tumor biopsy, which diagnosed a peripheral giant cell granuloma. Multinuclear giant cells (MGCs) and erythrocytes (ECs) are shown, while the black spots are hemosiderin granules; collagen fibers can also be seen. Many macrophages (the cells with round purple nuclei), as well as fibroblasts, which are similar to macrophages but a little smaller in size and with slightly more angular nuclei, can be seen (courtesy of Dr D. Vlahodimitropoulos).

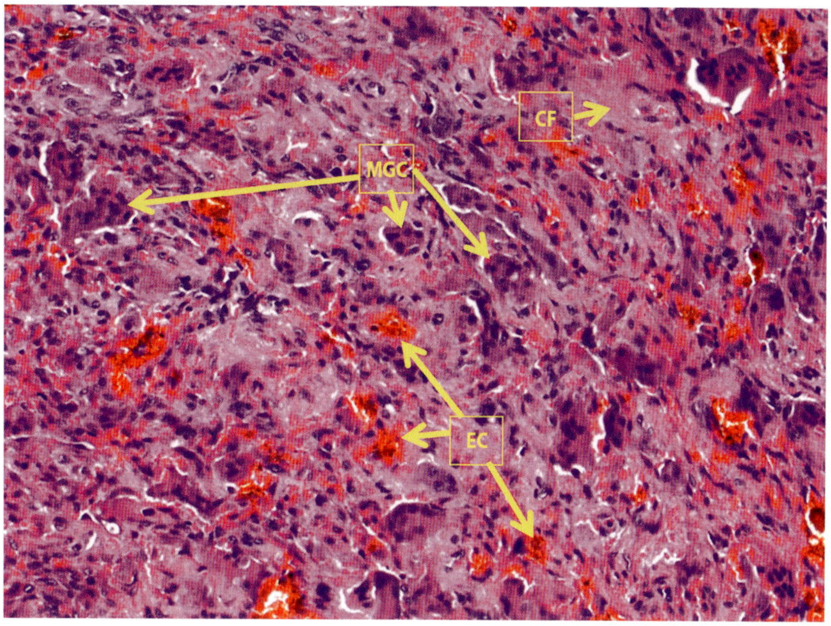

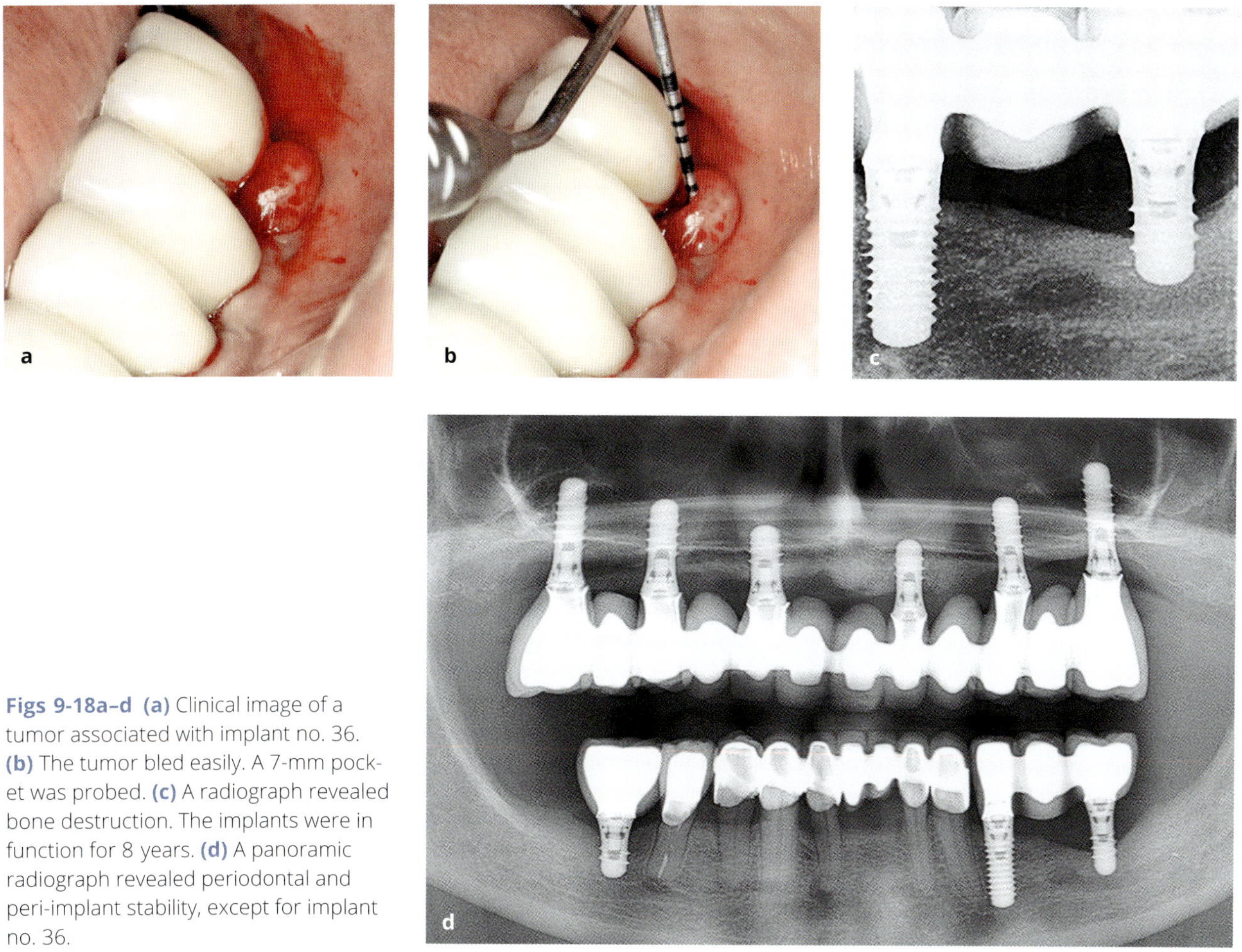

Figs 9-18a–d **(a)** Clinical image of a tumor associated with implant no. 36. **(b)** The tumor bled easily. A 7-mm pocket was probed. **(c)** A radiograph revealed bone destruction. The implants were in function for 8 years. **(d)** A panoramic radiograph revealed periodontal and peri-implant stability, except for implant no. 36.

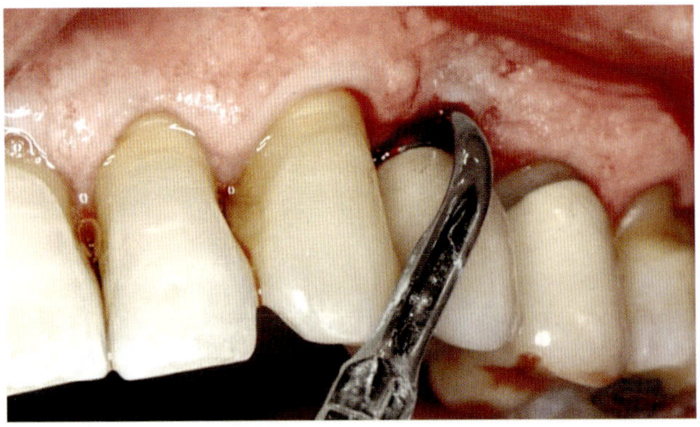

Fig 9-19 Metallic ultrasonic tip placed into the peri-implant pocket. In the past, because of the lack of other tools for mechanical debridement of peri-implant pockets, such approaches were chosen.

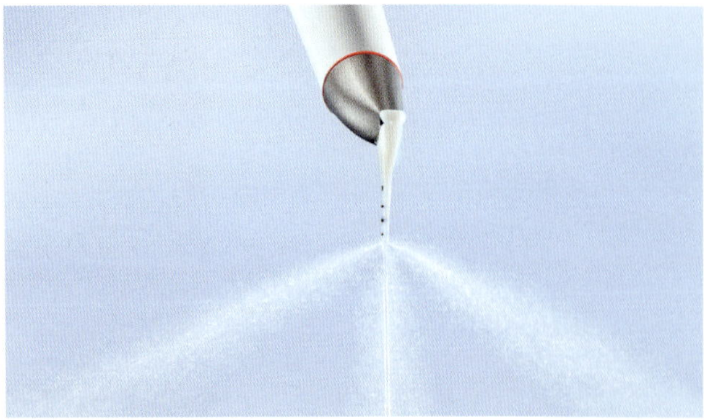

Fig 9-20 Three-point spraying nozzle used for decontamination by means of air polishing up to 9 mm subgingivally.

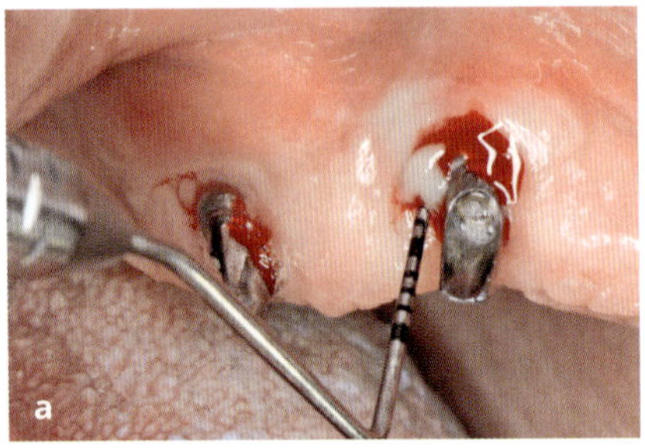

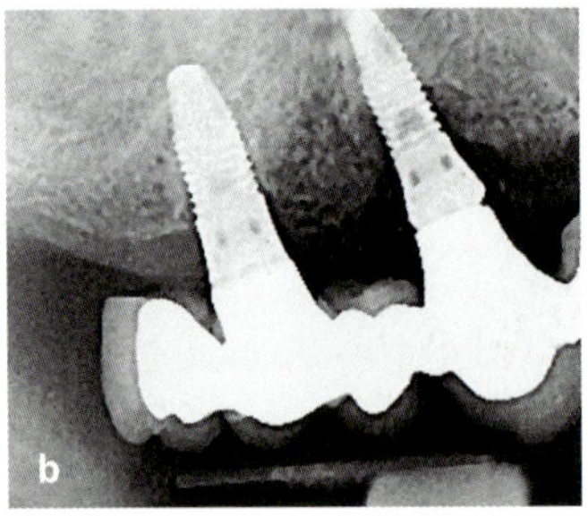

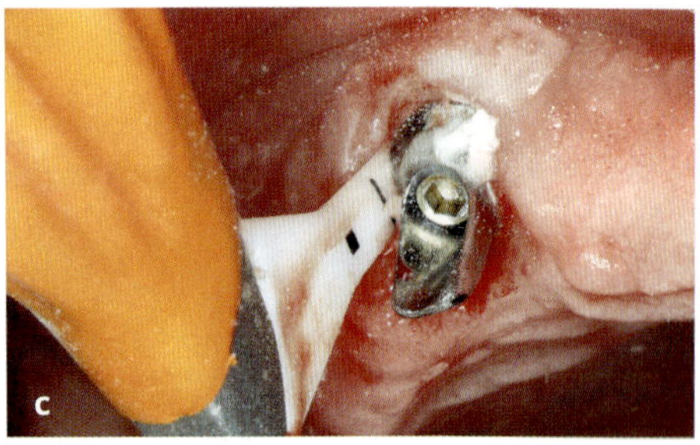

Figs 9-21a–c (a and b) Clinical and radiographic images of peri-implantitis. Pocket formation and bleeding on probing were substantial, while the radiograph revealed bone destruction. (c) Prior to the corrective phase of therapy, steps A and B of the CIST protocol were applied. The elastic nozzle and agglutination of the erythritol powder can be seen.

Nevertheless, the inability to remove deposits from grooves between implant threads was the most significant reason why cause-related therapy of peri-implantitis was unsuccessful in eliminating inflammation. Even if everything mentioned in the list was performed, followed by surgical flap reflection to access the grooves between implant threads, removal of microbial biofilms and elimination of inflammation was difficult. This is indirectly supported by the high percentages of recurrence of peri-implantitis. New methods and technologies, such as the GBT protocol and photodynamic therapy,[35–38] appear to be promising (Figs 9-21a–c).

The second addition to the CIST protocol concerns laser applications during treatment of peri-implant mucositis and peri-implantitis. Lasers may be used for the decontamination of the implant surface[39] and removal of granulation tissue (Fig 9-22).[22]

Limited data regarding the utility of lasers in the context of initial therapy for the treatment of peri-implantitis[40–42] support that there is a short-term difference in both clinical and biologic parameters (Figs 9-23a–h).[43–45]; however, this implies the need for specialized training in and knowledge of laser applications, expensive equipment, and a disciplined maintenance care program. Moreover, the clinician should realize that laser applications may need to be repeated frequently. A more detailed discussion of laser applications in peri-implant therapy is provided in Chapter 16 (Figs 9-24a–f).

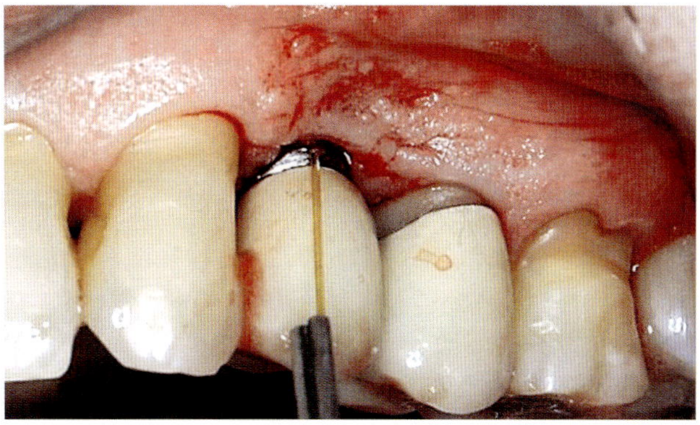

Fig 9-22 A 300-µm optical fiber was used for laser irradiation of the peri-implant pocket. Optical fibers were used with Nd:YAG and diode lasers.

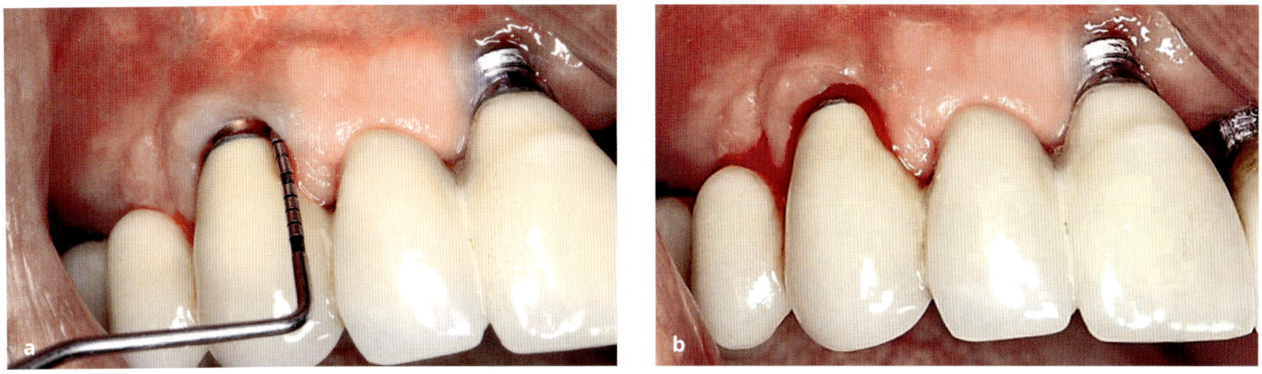

Figs 9-23a, b Clinical images of peri-implantitis. A 7-mm pocket and intense BOP are obvious.

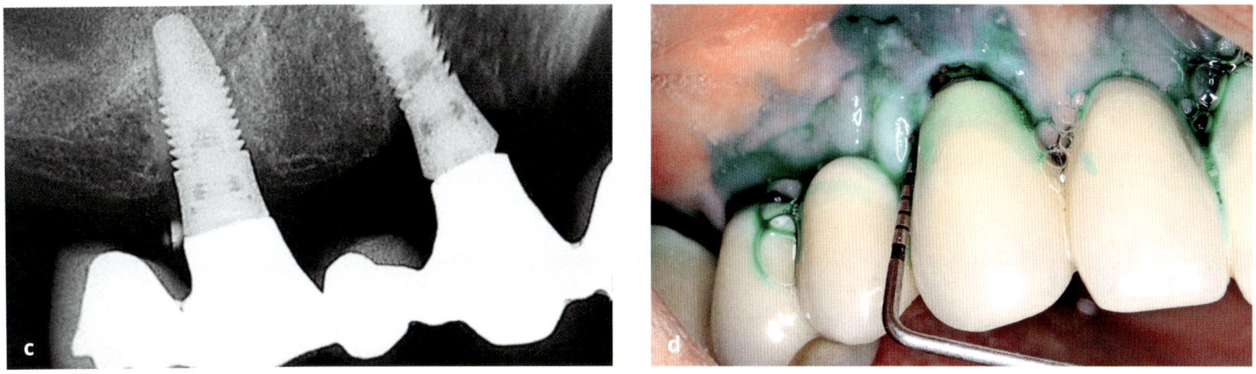

Figs 9-23c, d **(c)** The radiograph revealed bone destruction. **(d)** EmunDo photothermal therapy (A.R.C Laser, Nuremberg, Germany) was used. The indocyanine green photosensitizer can be seen, as well as the pocket depth at the distal site of implant no. 13.

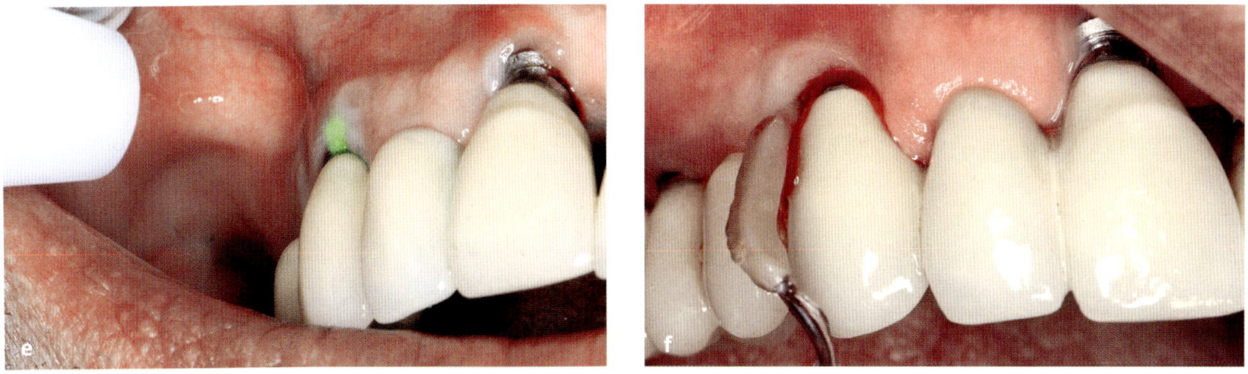

Figs 9-23e, f **(e)** Irradiation of the pockets through the peri-implant mucosa (only the first of the three optical fibers used is shown). **(f)** Removal of deposits with a plastic NSK tip.

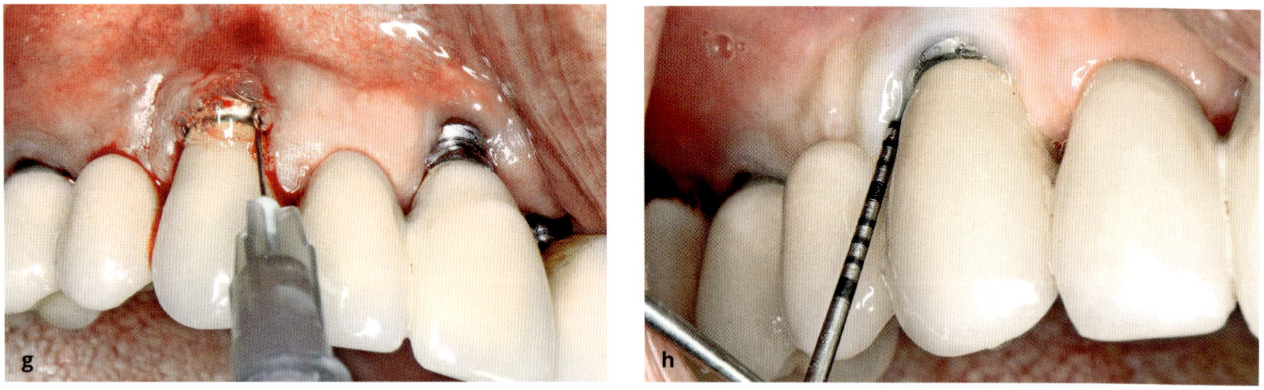

Figs 9-23 g, h **(g)** Irrigation with chlorhexidine gel. Chlorhexidine would also be applied by the patient at home, according to the CIST protocol. **(h)** Six weeks after the second application of EmunDo, the reduction of pocket depth and elimination of inflammation can be seen.

9.1 Patient motivation using dental biofilm disclosure

The effectiveness of any therapy depends on whether or not the patient complies with the oral hygiene guidelines and instructions. The use of a disclosing agent for biofilms is significant because both the patient and clinician can see the surfaces where bacteria remain. Furthermore, the technique, means, and time needed to effectively remove all the disclosed biofilm are assessed and estimated.[46]

9.2 Establishment of successful communication

The proper approach for patient motivation contributes to the establishment of a relationship of trust between the patient and the clinician. It is clear that a positive treatment outcome is the product of mutual efforts from both parties. For this approach, clinicians should possess good communication skills, knowledge of psychology, and the ability to manage human behavior.[47,48]

People communicate with each other and develop typical, neutral, friendly, close, bad, or good relationships. The establishment of a sufficient level of communication and, therefore, collaboration with patients presenting with different profiles is indeed challenging.

Three models of communication between the patient and dental practitioner have been described[11,12]:

1. The leading model, which constitutes the traditional way of communicating with the patient. This is an approach whereby the clinician imposes their opinion on the patient. In other words, it involves "one-way" communication from the individual in a position of authority to the other, who does not possess knowledge on the subject. It may be an effective method if a trusting relationship already exists between the patient and practitioner or if an acute and urgent problem must be handled. The information to be given should be valid, apt, and individualized.
2. The condescending model, where the clinician dedicates a lot of time not only to listening to the patient, but also to understanding the anxiety, disappointment, or externalization of thoughts and emotions that are often quite irrelevant to the initial reason for the patient to be in the clinic. This model aims to provide the patient with encouragement and support. However, it should be applied with caution, without crossing boundaries in the patient–doctor relationship.
3. The guiding model, where the practitioner directs patients through inductive discussion to motivate them to change their beliefs or behaviors. This is a "two-way" communication model and is useful to help patients change their smoking habits, for example.

Apart from these communication models, the dental practitioner must also know that each individual

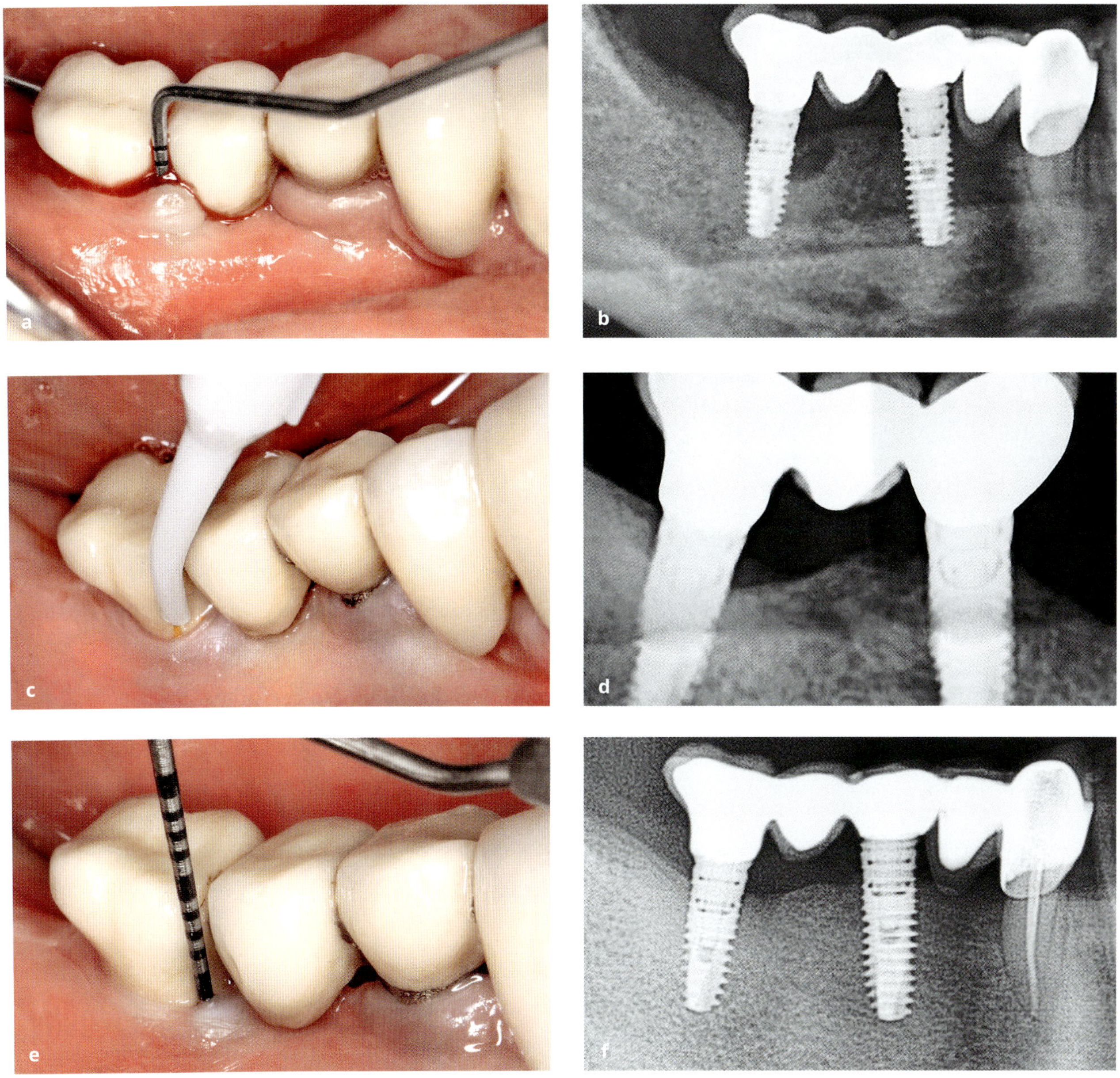

Figs 9-24a–f (a and b) Clinical and radiographic images of a patient with peri-implantitis. The initial plan was to perform surgery, possibly using guided bone regeneration. (c) Steps A and B of the CIST protocol preceded, with complementary application of a 980-nm laser for bactericidal effect. (d) The improvement of clinical parameters was such that surgery was avoided. Control of inflammation, combined with the patient being consistent in the application of the maintenance care program and daily oral hygiene, led to this improvement. The radiograph was taken 3 years after the initial phase of treatment. Partial filling of the intraosseous defect can be observed. (e) Six years after the initial phase of therapy, the pockets were eliminated. (f) The radiograph 6 years after therapy revealed the filling of the intraosseous defect with bone.

may respond better to a visual, auditory, or mixed comprehension approach, depending on how they understand new information. Usually, the clinician cannot distinguish what type of learner the patient represents. Therefore, they should inform patients of the situation in the oral cavity and support this with a discussion and simultaneous visualization. For this reason, biofilm disclosure may be helpful.

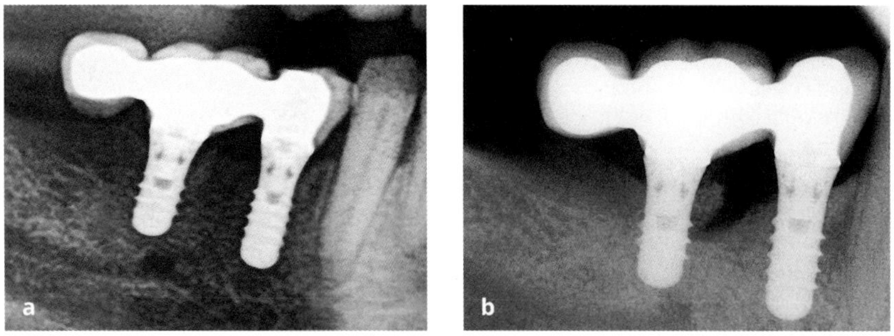

Figs 9-25a, b **(a)** Radiograph after placement of the implant restoration and **(b)** 2.5 years later. Unilateral bone destruction may be observed due to the presence of a foreign body **(b)** (case treated at the Postgraduate Clinic of Periodontology, Dental School, National and Kapodistrian University of Athens, Athens, Greece).

9.3 Methods of oral hygiene

Oral hygiene refers to mechanical procedures only.[49] There is no alternative way to apply daily and effective oral hygiene other than by using a toothbrush and interdental cleaning devices. Chemical agents may be applied for a specific time period only. Methods for administering oral hygiene are individualized, depending on the anatomy of the peri-implant tissues, the type and design of the restorations, and the patient's skills. The optimal toothbrush is one that can be used by the patient effectively. According to a recent study, electric ultrasonic toothbrushes (for example Philips Sonicare, Amsterdam, The Netherlands) may have an advantage in being slightly more effective in biofilm control.[50] In case of inefficient biofilm removal, changing toothbrush may motivate the patient to perform better oral hygiene. In any case, effective biofilm removal is associated with the time devoted to brushing. This is clear to patients once they try to remove the disclosed biofilm with a toothbrush. They will also realize how much time is required to use interdental cleaning devices effectively. The latter comprise dental floss and especially mini flossers, SuperFloss, and interdental brushes. All interdental cleaning devices are efficient as long as they are used correctly.[11,12] The selection of devices depends on the types of restoration, access, and the width of the interdental spaces. Where interdental brushes are selected, those with very large metallic elements should be avoided.[11,12]

Chemical agents do not replace mechanical biofilm removal. However, they may be included during treatment for peri-implant mucositis because several clinical studies have shown that they improve the therapeutic outcome, reducing BOP.[51]

Should the implant restoration obstruct access for effective oral hygiene, it should be corrected or replaced. Insufficient oral hygiene not only causes peri-implant mucositis, but is also the most crucial risk factor for peri-implantitis.[1–3,5] Peri-implant mucositis occurs more frequently in patients with cemented compared to screw-retained restorations.[52] When cemented restorations are selected, care should be taken to remove excess cement. Cement remnants facilitate biofilm accumulation and soft tissue inflammation, and may lead to bone destruction.[53,54] The peri-implant sulcus should also be examined and cleaned after impression taking. If impression material remains in the sulcus, this will lead to peri-implant mucositis and, if not treated early, to iatrogenic peri-implantitis (Figs 9-25a, b and 9-26a–f).[55]

9.4 Early information on and regular reminder of the value of a maintenance care program

The clinician must inform the patient diagnosed with peri-implant mucositis about the importance of consistent compliance with the maintenance care therapy at the very first appointment.[23] After treatment of peri-implant mucositis, inadequate attendance of maintenance care appointments will lead to a high incidence of peri-implantitis. A study found that within 5 years after an initial diagnosis of mucositis, peri-implantitis reached 44%, whereas the incidence of peri-implantitis in patients treated for peri-implant mucositis and who were fully compliant with the maintenance care program reached only 18%.[56]

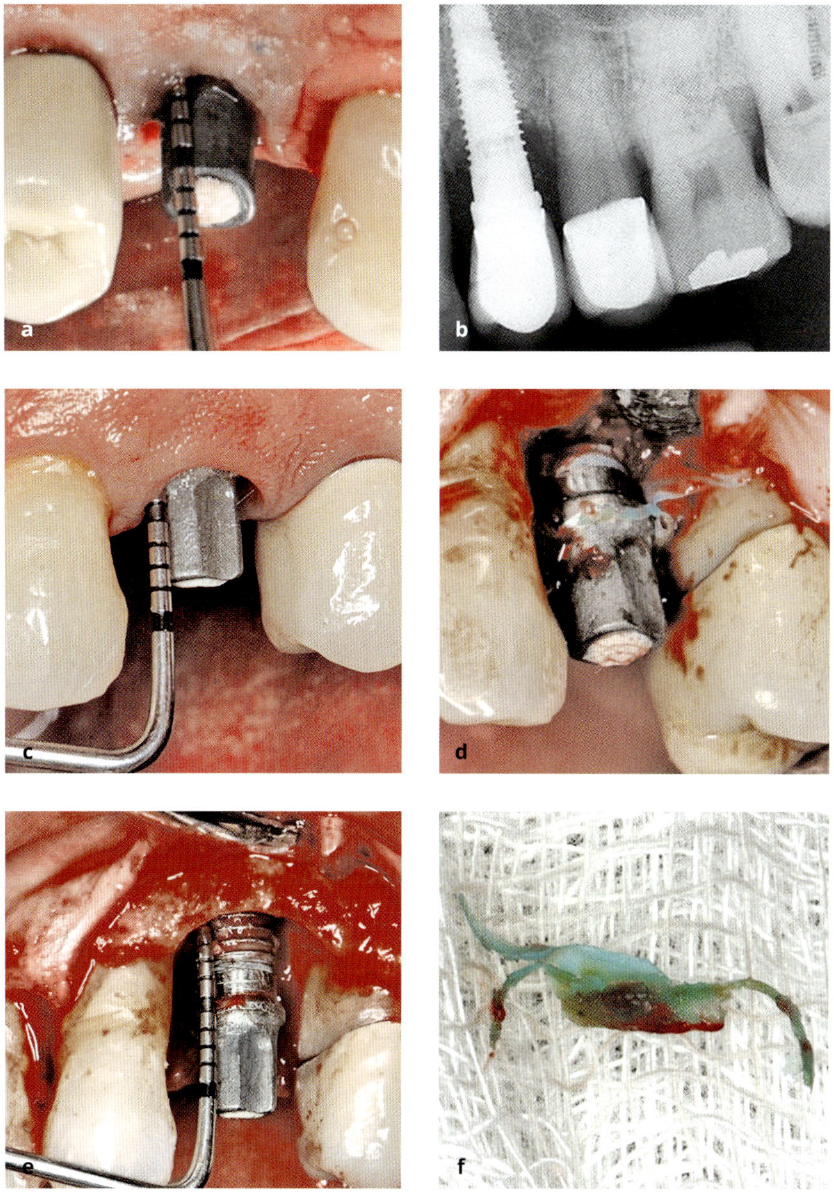

Figs 9-26a–f (a) Ten days after placement of the restoration, the patient reported pain. Clinical examination revealed deep pockets at implant no. 24. **(b)** The radiograph revealed severe bone destruction. **(c)** A probing pocket depth of 9 mm mesial of no. 24 was diagnosed. **(d)** Immediately after reflection of a mucoperiosteal flap, a piece of impression material was found. This resulted in iatrogenic peri-implantitis. **(e)** After removal of the granulation tissue, the extent and severity of bone destruction were clear. **(f)** The impression material was trapped in the peri-implant sulcus (case treated at the Postgraduate Clinic of Periodontology, Dental School, National and Kapodistrian University of Athens, Athens, Greece).

References

1. Theofanatos GD, Parashis AO. Etiology and treatment of peri-implant inflammation during supportive implant therapy. Per Anal 2008;19:173–214.
2. Schwarz F, Becker J. Peri-Implant Infection. Etiology, Diagnosis, Treatment. London: Quintessence, 2009.
3. Froum SJ. Dental Implant Complications: Etiology, Prevention and Treatment. Hoboken, NJ: John Wiley & Sons, 2015.
4. Gupta S, Kaushik M. Peri-implantitis management from periodontal perspective. Saarbrücken: LAP LAMBERT Academic Publishing, 2016.
5. Heitz-Mayfield LJA. Peri-implant diseases: diagnosis and risk indicators. J Clin Periodontol 2008;35:292–304.
6. Renvert S, Roos-Jansåker A-M, Claffey N. Non-surgical treatment of peri-implant mucositis and peri-implantitis: a literature review. J Clin Periodontol 2008;35:305–315.
7. Lopez MA, Passarelli PC, Marra M, et al. Antimicrobial efficacy of photodynamic therapy (PDT) in periodontitis and peri-implantitis: a systematic review. J Biol Regul Homeost Agents 2020;34:59–65.
8. Esposito M, Grusovin MG, Worthington HV. Treatment of peri-implantitis: what interventions are effective? A Cochrane systematic review. Eur J Oral Implantol 2012;5(suppl):S21–S41.

9. Karoussis IK, Kotsovilis S, Feloutzis A, Fourmousis I. Diagnosis and treatment of peri-implantitis. Odontostomatologica Progress 2009;63:168–195.
10. Karoussis IK, Gkogkos A, Prevezanos I, Vrotsos I. Biological complications. Diagnosis and treatment of peri-implantitis. Odontostomatologica Progress 2012;66:384–411.
11. Vrotsos IA, Karoussis IK. Periodontology-Implantology. Athens: BETA Publications, 2016.
12. Lang NP, Lindhe J. Clinical Periodontology and Implant Dentistry, vol. 2. Hoboken, NJ: John Wiley & Sons, 2015.
13. Coli P, Sennerby L. Is peri-implant probing causing over-diagnosis and over-treatment of dental implants? J Clin Med 2019;8:1123.
14. Lang NP, Wilson TG, Corbet EF. Biological complications with dental implants: their prevention, diagnosis and treatment. Clin Oral Implants Res 2000;11:146–155.
15. Araujo MG, Lindhe J. Peri-implant health. J Periodontol 2018;89(suppl 1):S249–S256.
16. Mombelli A, Lang NP. The diagnosis and treatment of peri-implantitis. Periodontol 2000 1998;17:63–76.
17. Dhir S, Mahesh L, Kurtzman GM, Vandana KL. Peri-implant and periodontal tissues: a review of differences and similarities. Compend Continuing Educ Dent 2013;34:e69–e75.
18. Belser U, Martin W, Zung R, et al. Implant Therapy in the Esthetic Zone. Single-Tooth Replacement. ITI Treatment Guide. Berlin: Quintessence Publishing, 2007.
19. Kotsovilis S, Karoussis IK, Trianti M, Fourmousis I. Therapy of peri-implantitis: a systematic review. J Clin Periodontol 2008;35:621–629.
20. Sahm N, Becker J, Santel T, Schwarz F. Non-surgical treatment of peri-implantitis using an air-abrasive device or mechanical debridement and local application of chlorhexidine: a prospective, randomized, controlled clinical study. J Clin Periodontol 2011;38:872–878.
21. Renvert S, Lindahl C, Roos Jansåker A-M, Persson GR. Treatment of peri-implantitis using an Er:YAG laser or an air-abrasive device: a randomized clinical trial. J Clin Periodontol 2011;38:65–73.
22. Schwarz F, Sculean A, Rothamel D, Schwenzer K, Georg T, Becker J. Clinical evaluation of an Er:YAG laser for nonsurgical treatment of peri-implantitis: a pilot study. Clin Oral Implants Res 2005;16:44–52.
23. Wilson TG. A typical implant maintenance visit. In: Wilson T Jr, Harrel S (eds). Dental Implant Failure. Cham: Springer, 2019:83–92.
24. Shrivastava D, Natoli V, Srivastava KC, et al. Novel approach to dental biofilm management through guided biofilm therapy (GBT): a review. Microorganisms 2021;9:1966.
25. Sculean A, Bastendorf K-D, Becker C, et al. A paradigm shift in mechanical biofilm management? Subgingival air polishing: a new way to improve mechanical biofilm management in the dental practice. Quintessence Int 2013;44:475–477.
26. Schwarz F, Bieling K, Bonsmann M, Latz T, Becker J. Nonsurgical treatment of moderate and advanced peri-implantitis lesions: a controlled clinical study. Clin Oral Investig 2006;10:279–288.
27. Sanz M, Bäumer A, Buduneli N, et al. Effect of professional mechanical plaque removal on secondary prevention of periodontitis and the complications of gingival and periodontal preventive measures: consensus report of group 4 of the 11th European Workshop on Periodontology on effective prevention of periodontal and peri-implant diseases. J Clin Periodontol 2015;42(suppl 16):S214–S220.
28. Renvert S, Samuelsson E, Lindahl C, Persson GR. Mechanical non-surgical treatment of peri-implantitis: a double-blind randomized longitudinal clinical study. I: clinical results. J Clin Periodontol 2009;36:604–609.
29. Rühling A, Kocher T, Kreusch J, Plagmann HC. Treatment of subgingival implant surface with Teflon-coated sonic and ultrasonic scaler tips and various implant curettes. An in vitro study. Clin Oral Implants Res 1994;5:19–29.
30. Tribst JPM, Dal Piva AMO, de Lima DR, Borges ALS, Bottino MA. Simulated damage of two implant debridement methods: nonsurgical approach with Teflon and stainless steel hand scalers. J Indian Soc Periodontol 2018;22:340–344.
31. Sahrmann P, Winkler S, Gubler A, Attin T. Assessment of implant surface and instrument insert changes due to instrumentation with different tips for ultrasonic-driven debridement. BMC Oral Health 2021;21:25.
32. Valderrama P, Blansett JA, Gonzalez MG, Cantu MG, Wilson TG. Detoxification of implant surfaces affected by peri-implant disease: an overview of non-surgical methods. Open Dent J 2014;8:77–84.
33. Xin W, Yu L, Yuan F, Haode C, Dehua L. Macrophage polarization in aseptic bone resorption around dental implants induced by Ti particles in a murine model. J Periodontal Res 2019;54:329–338.
34. Wilson TG Jr. Bone loss around implants—is it metallosis? J Periodontol 2021;92:181–185.
35. Riben-Grundstrom C, Norderyd O, André U, Renvert S. Treatment of peri-implant mucositis using a glycine powder air-polishing or ultrasonic device: a randomized clinical trial. J Clin Periodontol 2015;42:462–469.
36. Lerario F, Roncati M, Gariffo A, et al. Non-surgical periodontal treatment of peri-implant diseases with the adjunctive use of diode laser: preliminary clinical study. Lasers Med Sci 2016;31:1–6.
37. Roncati M, Lucchese A, Carinci F. Non-surgical treatment of peri-implantitis with the adjunctive use of an 810-nm diode laser. J Indian Soc Periodontol 2013;17:812–815.
38. Sculean A, Deppe H, Miron R, Schwarz F, Romanos G, Cosgarea R. Effectiveness of photodynamic therapy in the treatment of periodontal and peri-implant diseases. Monogr Oral Sci 2021;29:133–143.
39. Nejem Wakim R, Namour M, Nguyen HV, et al. Decontamination of dental implant surfaces by the Er:YAG laser beam: a comparative in vitro study of various protocols. Dent J 2018;6:66.
40. Kreisler M, Götz H, Duschner H. Effect of Nd:YAG, Ho:YAG, Er:YAG, CO_2, and GaAlAs laser irradiation on surface properties of endosseous dental implants. Int J Oral Maxillofac Implants 2002;17:202–211.

41. Romanos G, Ko H-H, Froum S, Tarnow D. The use of CO2 laser in the treatment of peri-implantitis. Photomed Laser Surg 2009;27:381–386.
42. Romanos GE, Gupta B, Yunker M, Romanos EB, Malmstrom H. Lasers use in dental implantology. Implant Dent 2013;22:282–288.
43. Schwarz F, Bieling K, Nuesry E, Sculean A, Becker J. Clinical and histological healing pattern of peri-implantitis lesions following non-surgical treatment with an Er:YAG laser. Lasers Surg Med 2006;38:663–671.
44. Schwarz F, Sculean A, Rothamel D, Schwenzer K, Georg T, Becker J. Clinical evaluation of an Er:YAG laser for nonsurgical treatment of peri-implantitis: a pilot study. Clin Oral Implants Res 2005;16:44–52.
45. Ashnagar S, Nowzari H, Nokhbatolfoghahaei H, Yaghoub Zadeh B, Chiniforush N, Choukhachi Zadeh N. Laser treatment of peri-implantitis: a literature review. J Lasers Med Sci 2014;5:153–162.
46. Fasoulas A, Pavlidou E, Petridis D, Mantzorou M, Seroglou K, Giaginis C. Detection of dental plaque with disclosing agents in the context of preventive oral hygiene training programs. Heliyon 2019;5:e02064.
47. Waylen A, Makoul G, Albeyatti Y. Patient–clinician communication in a dental setting: a pilot study. Br Dent J 2015;218:585–588.
48. Misra S, Daly B, Dunne S, Millar B, Packer M, Asimakopoulou K. Dentist–patient communication: what do patients and dentists remember following a consultation? Implications for patient compliance. Patient Prefer Adherence 2013;7:543–549.
49. Silverstein LH, Kurtzman GM. Oral hygiene and maintenance of dental implants. Dent Today 2006;25:70–75.
50. Digel I, Kern I, Geenen EM, Akimbekov N. Dental plaque removal by ultrasonic toothbrushes. Dent J 2020;8:28.
51. Liu S, Li M, Yu J. Does chlorhexidine improve outcomes in non-surgical management of peri-implant mucositis or peri-implantitis? A systematic review and meta-analysis. Med Oral Patol Oral Cir Bucal 2020;25:e608–e615.
52. Dalago HR, Schuldt Filho G, Rodrigues MAP, Renvert S, Bianchini MA. Risk indicators for peri-implantitis. A cross-sectional study with 916 implants. Clin Oral Implants Res 2017;28:144–150.
53. Linkevicius T, Puisys A, Vindasiute E, Linkeviciene L, Apse P. Does residual cement around implant-supported restorations cause peri-implant disease? A retrospective case analysis. Clin Oral Implants Res 2013;24:1179–1184.
54. Staubli N, Walter C, Schmidt JC, Weiger R, Zitzmann NU. Excess cement and the risk of peri-implant disease—a systematic review. Clin Oral Implants Res 2017;28:1278–1290.
55. Hashim D, Cionca N. A comprehensive review of peri-implantitis risk factors. Curr Oral Health Rep 2020;7:262–273.
56. Costa FO, Takenaka-Martinez S, Cota LOM, Ferreira SD, Silva GLM, Costa JE. Peri-implant disease in subjects with and without preventive maintenance: a 5-year follow up. J Clin Periodontol 2012;39:173–181.

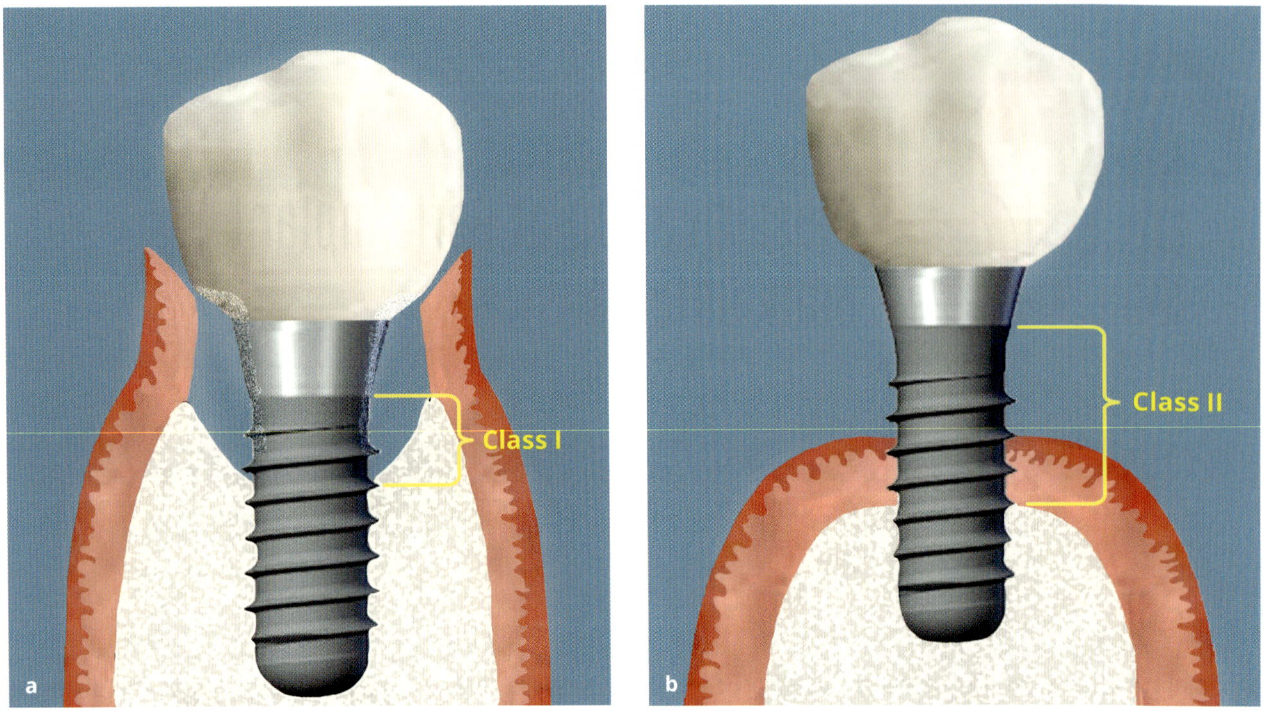

Figs 10-1a, b Schematic representation of **(a)** an intraosseous and **(b)** a supra-alveolar peri-implant bony defect.

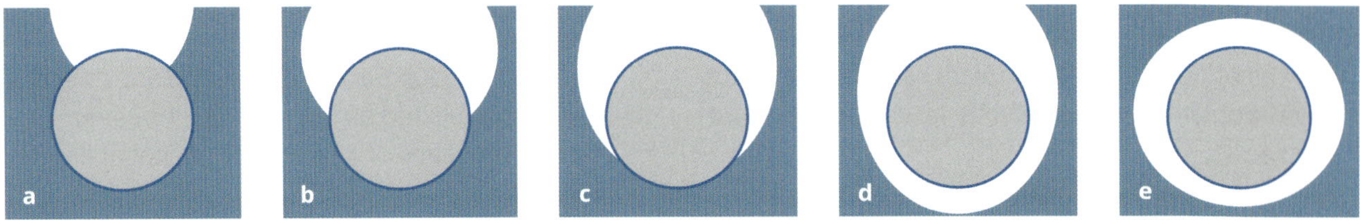

Figs 10-2a–e Schematic representation of the morphology of peri-implant bony defects. The alveolar ridge is depicted in blue in cross-section, the implant in gray, and the horizontal morphology of the bony defect in white (modified after Schwarz and Becker).[10]

as the linear distance between the bony walls and the body of the implant. This classification is complex and provides information only for some categories of intraosseous defects.

In most cases, without flap elevation, information on the morphology of a defect is inadequate. However, the intraoperative picture of an implant with peri-implantitis may vary according to several factors. These factors include the morphology of the alveolar ridge, the distance between adjacent implants or an implant and the neighboring tooth, and the severity of disease.

In 2004, Vanden Bogaerde[7] proposed a classification of peri-implant bony defects, highlighting the importance of having intact bony walls around the intraosseous defect for successful therapy:

- Closed defects: these are characterized by the preservation of intact bony walls.
- Open defects: these are characterized by the lack of one or more bony walls.

This classification presented the advantage that it may correctly guide the choice of regenerative procedure for the closed defect type. On the other hand, it classified all other cases, in which one or more walls were missing, in the same category. However, the morphology of a peri-implant bony defect may vary from the most commonly observed, namely circumferential bony defects, to the rarest, horizontal bone loss.

A simple classification that classifies intraosseous defects into five categories to facilitate the choice of

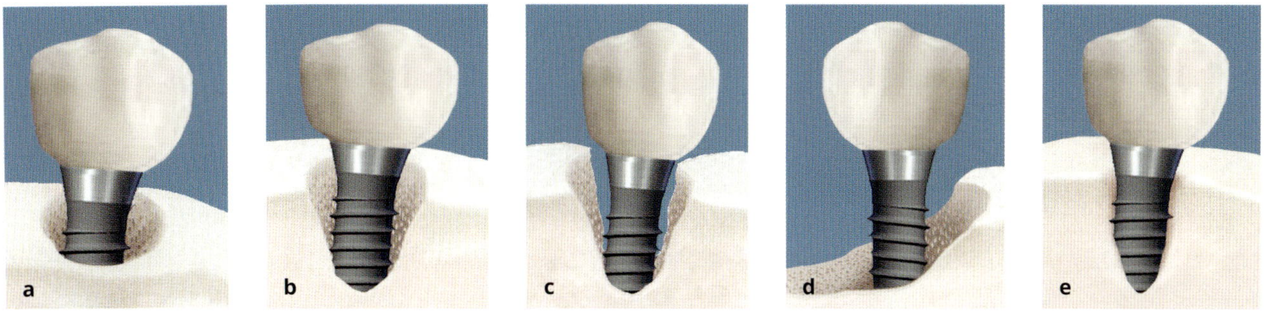

Figs 10-3a–e Schematic representation of the morphology of peri-implant bony defects: **(a)** four-wall, **(b)** three-wall, **(c)** two-wall, and **(d)** one-wall defect, and **(e)** dehiscence.

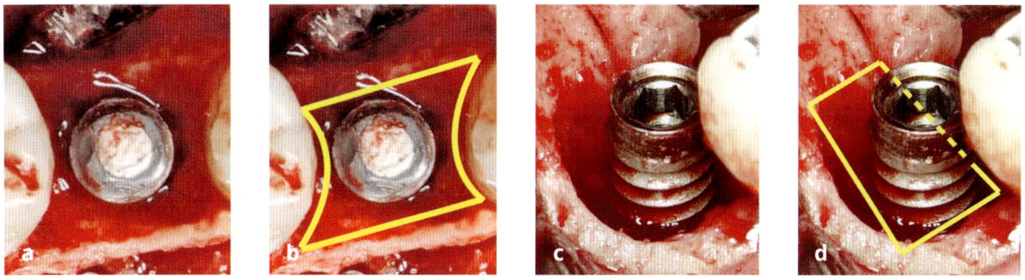

Figs 10-4a–d Four-wall bony defects.

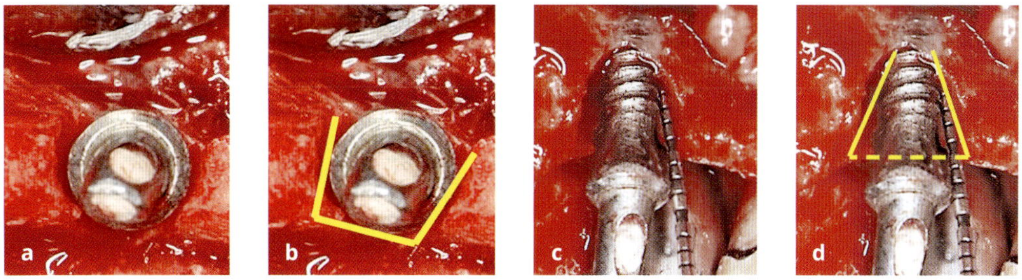

Figs 10-5a–d Three-wall bony defects.

surgical approach was proposed by Renvert and Giovannoli.[8]

Peri-implant bony defects are classified as follows according to the number of remaining bony walls (Figs 10-3a–e):[9–11]

- circumferential, crater-like, four-wall defects;
- three-wall defects;
- two-wall defects;
- one-wall defects;
- dehiscence.

In a circumferential, crater-like, four-wall bony defect, bone walls surround the implant in a 360-degree manner (Figs 10-4a–d). In the absence of the buccal, or lingual or palatal, bony plate, the lesion is considered a three-wall defect (Figs 10-5a–d). If only two of the bony walls surrounding the implant remain, then it is considered a two-wall defect. Loss of the buccal, and lingual or palatal, bony plate is usually observed (Figs 10-6a–d). If only one bony wall remains, the peri-implant bony defect is considered a one-wall defect (Figs 10-7a–d). Finally, exposure of implant threads on one side of the implant, while no bone is lost on the other sides, is called a dehiscence (Figs 10-8a, b). This is most often located on the buccal surface of the implant and is usually caused by the placement of a large-diameter implant in a narrow alveolar ridge or a buccally misplaced implant. This is common in cases where bone regeneration should have been performed but was avoided (iatrogenic defect).

The same classification applies in the case of adjacent implants having been placed at a minimal

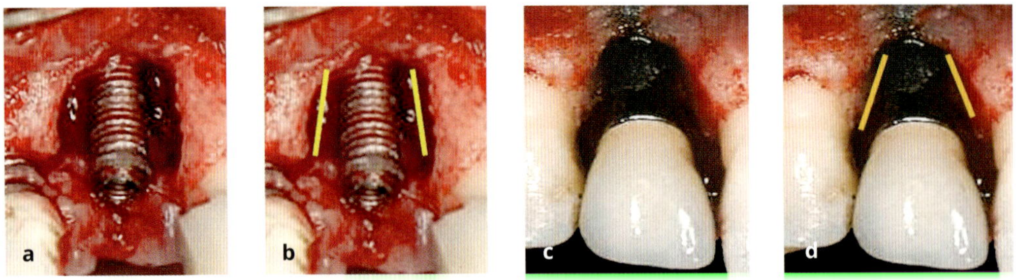

Figs 10-6a–d Two-wall bony defects.

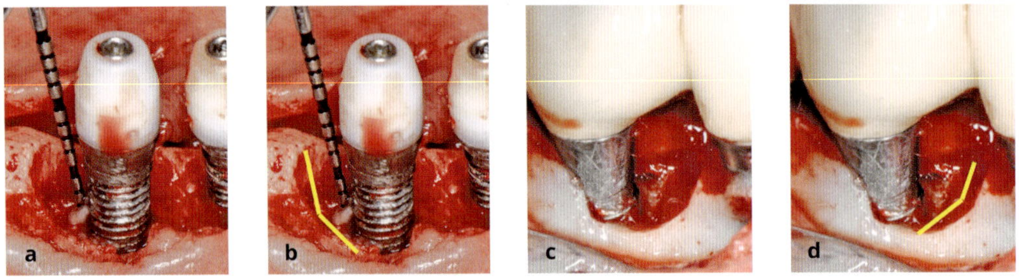

Figs 10-7a–d One-wall bony defects. **(a)** and **(b)** are the same and so are **(c)** and **(d)**, but with the course of the bony wall marked in yellow in **(b)** and **(d)**.

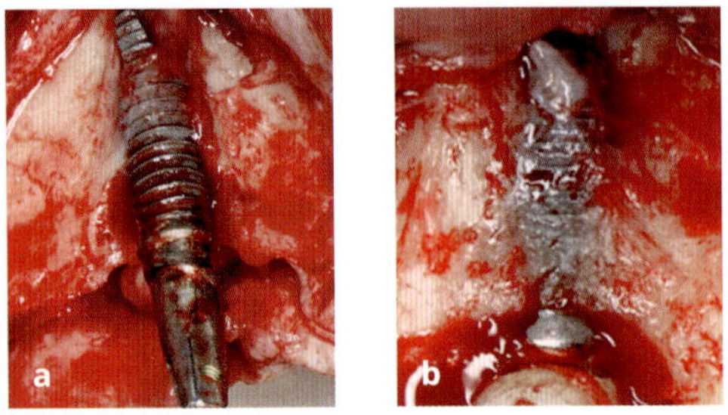

Figs 10-8a, b Dehiscence defects.

distance from each other, resulting in bone loss between them. In the event of complete loss of the four bony walls of each implant, bone loss is considered as horizontal.[12] In addition, combinations of the categories of intraosseous defects are often observed. In fact, more walls are usually located at the apical part of the defect and fewer at the coronal part.

The most important factor that will determine the choice of surgical technique is the morphology of the peri-implant bony defect.[1–3,10] With a one- or two-wall defect, an access flap will be selected for debridement of the implant surface, or a resective technique with an "apically" positioned flap with or without bone surgery.[13] In contrast, the application of a regenerative technique, mainly guided bone regeneration, is chosen in cases of three- or four-wall bony defects or dehiscence (Fig 10-9).[14,15]

In regenerative surgery, it is advisable to remove the implant-supported restoration wherever possible, to use a coronally repositioned flap, and to cover the affected implants. Although the results on the potential benefits of submucosal healing in the outcome of a regenerative technique over transmucosal healing are conflicting,[16] clinical experience suggests that the results with submerged healing are particularly favorable.

The choice of regeneration is preferable compared to access flaps and implant surface disinfection in terms of the degree of bone filling of the defect.[17]

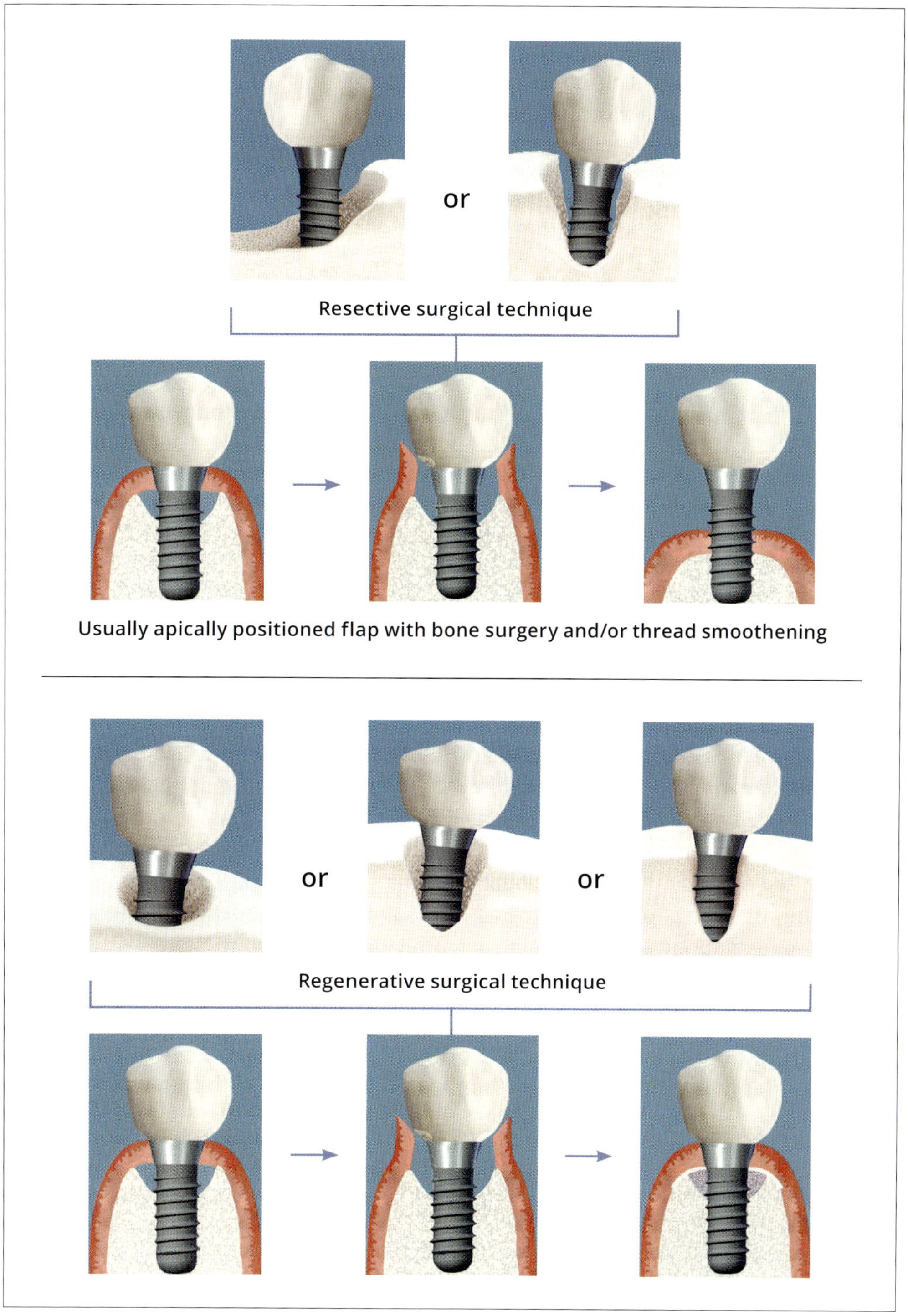

Fig 10-9 Schematic representation of surgical technique selection depending on the morphology of the peri-implant bony defect. In one- or two-wall defects, resective surgical techniques are applied. Guided bone regeneration is applied to three- or four-wall bony defects and dehiscence.

10.2 Radiographic criteria

Radiographs are used to diagnose bone loss around teeth and implants.[18] If clinical signs of inflammation are found (bleeding on probing or suppuration), a radiograph is needed to determine possible bone loss. The information provided by the radiograph should be evaluated in conjunction with clinical measurements to identify the morphology of the peri-implant bony defect.[4,19] Periapical radiographs do not provide information on bony defects located

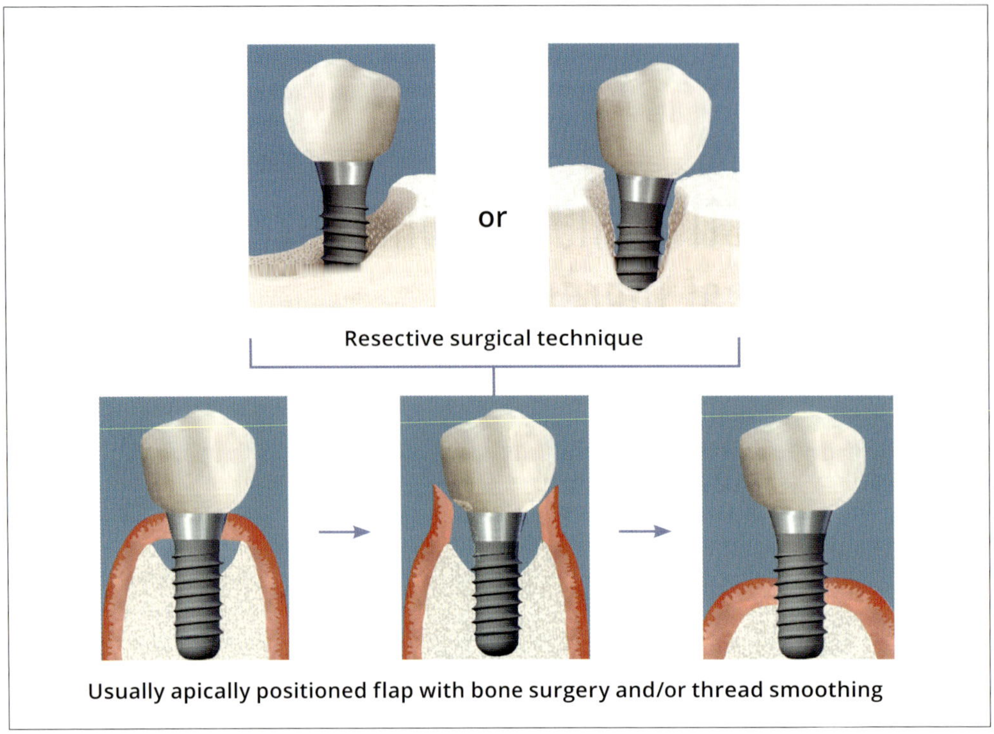

Fig 11-1 In cases of one- or two-wall bony defects, a full-thickness flap is elevated, biofilm is removed, bone surgery for pocket elimination or reduction is performed, an exposed thread may be smoothed when necessary, and the flap is sutured apically to achieve pocket elimination or reduction.

When the morphology of peri-implantitis lesions[28] allows the application of guided bone regeneration, better outcomes may be obtained than by simply applying an access flap and disinfecting the implant surface.[29]

Experimental studies that histologically examined the results of different techniques concluded that the use of membranes with or without bone grafts led to higher rates of re-osseontintegration[30,31] compared to open flap debridement of the implant surface alone.[32]

As mentioned in Chapter 10, the morphology of peri-implant lesions is one of the important factors that determine the choice of surgical technique.[28] If the peri-implant intraosseous defect consists of one or two bony walls or if there is horizontal bone loss, usually an access flap will be selected (open flap debridement) including resective surgery (apically repositioned flap combined with bone surgery) (Fig 11-1).[33] In intraosseous defects consisting of three or four bony walls, application of a regenerative technique may be selected (Fig 11-2).

The most commonly used regenerative technique is guided bone regeneration. However, there are interesting reports on the positive effect of recombinant human bone morphogenetic protein-2[34] or plasma rich in growth factors combined with autologous bone graft,[35] on bone regeneration and re-osseointegration compared to only a graft or open flap debridement. However, the use of bone morphogenetic proteins or commercial growth factors is almost prohibitive because of the extremely high cost. On the other hand, the use of plasma rich in growth factors, despite being substantially advertised, has not been researched adequately in the treatment of peri-implantitis.[36]

Complete control of inflammation in the case of peri-implantitis is usually achieved by performing additional surgery. The reason for this is that biofilm removal from the implant surface is more effective when carried out after flap elevation, compared to a flapless approach. Surgery to treat peri-implantitis may lead to an improvement in inflammatory markers, regardless of the technique used.[37]

Many studies have confirmed that the roughness of the implant surface promotes osseointegration.[38,39] A rough surface induces the migration of mesenchymal cells, thereby accelerating new bone formation. On the other hand, roughness is a disadvantage if peri-implantitis affects that surface. The rough surface is exposed to microbial colonization, and microbial retention is greater compared to a smooth surface. Furthermore, it is more difficult to

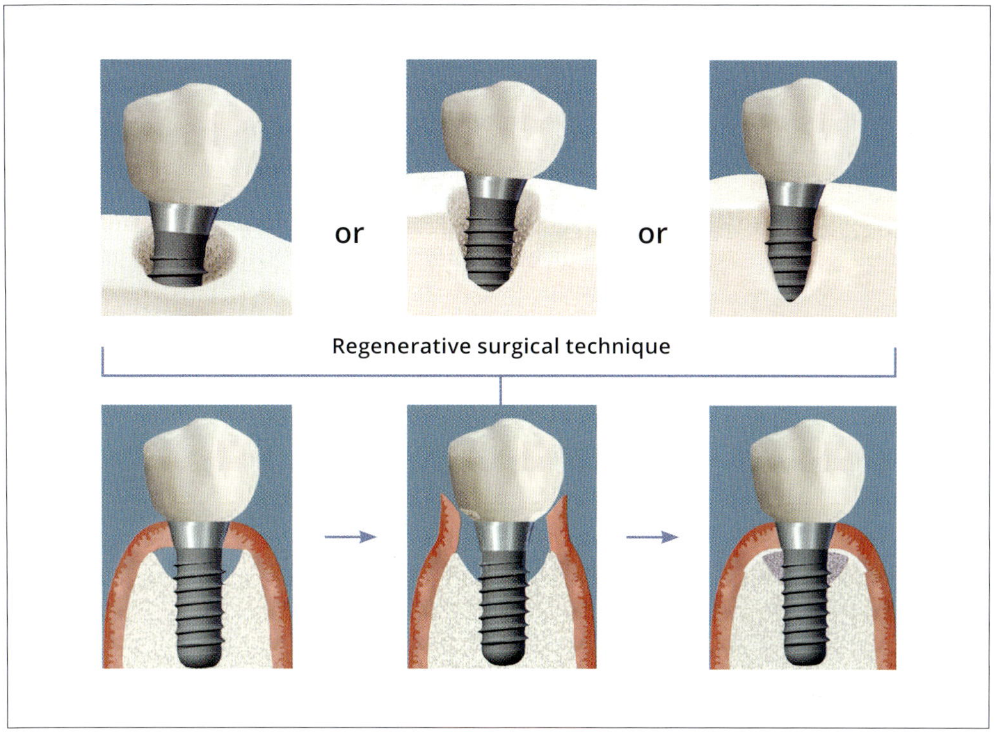

Fig 11-2 In intraosseous defects involving three or four bony walls and in bone dehiscence, a full-thickness flap is elevated. After this, debridement, smoothing of the exposed threads when necessary, and placement of bone graft and membrane are performed. The membrane may need to be fixed with titanium pins or sutures. Surgery is completed with flap suturing to achieve bone regeneration.

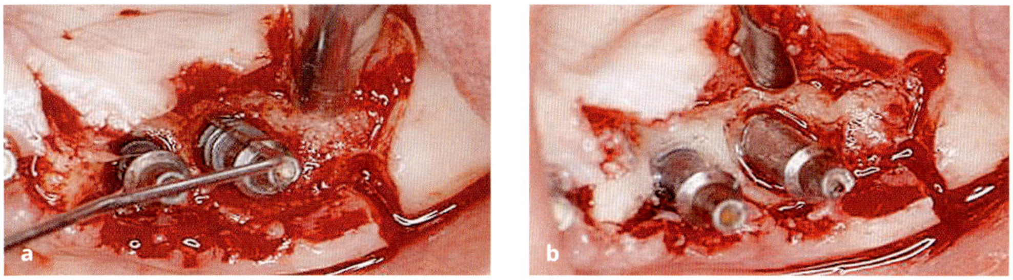

Figs 11-3a, b Intraoperative photographs **(a)** before and **(b)** after after completion of the smoothing of the exposed implant threads.

remove biofilms from a rough surface.[40] Thus, progression of bone loss may be faster. Under no circumstances should the clinician think that implants with a rough surface are more likely to present with peri-implantitis. Exposure of a rough surface to the pocket environment is the result and not the cause of bone loss.

On the other hand, the surface of the implant influences the outcome of bone regeneration during surgical treatment of peri-implantitis. Animal studies have shown that the regenerative potential and likelihood of re-osseointegration increases when implants have a rough surface.[2] However, when a non-regenerative surgical technique is selected, an attempt to remove the threads from the implant surface has been advocated. This procedure is known as implantoplasty and aims to more easily remove biofilms during maintenance care (Figs 11-3a, b).

Limited scientific evidence supports the notion that laser treatment, in addition to other therapies, improves treatment outcomes.[41,42] In a study by Bach et al,[43] patients with peri-implantitis received cause-related therapy as in stages A and B of the cumulative interceptive supportive therapy (CIST) protocol, followed by surgery (resective or regenerative). Finally, all patients attended maintenance care appiintments every 6 months. At each appointment, clinical, radiologic, and microbiologic examination were performed. In one group of patients, additional diode laser disinfection of the implant surface was performed during resective or regenerative surgery, and in each recall session. After the second year of the posttreatment follow-up, patients receiving additional laser disinfection showed better results.

Correspondingly, microbiologic studies have shown a beneficial bactericidal effect achieved by using additional laser radiation. This concerns the most important periodontal pathogens, such as *Aggregatibacter actinomycetemcomitans*, *Porphyromonas gingivalis,* and *Prevotella intermedia* during treatment of peri-implantitis.[44,45]

Some studies[9] have reported a short-term beneficial effect on presumptive pathogenic microorganism reduction in the peri-implant pockets. After 6 months, the microbiome was similar in non-laser-treated peri-implantitis sites.

11.1 Surgical techniques

Several techniques used in the surgical treatment of peri-implantitis have been modified from those used in periodontics.[1] The fact that many of these techniques have been used since the beginning of the last century has provided periodontists with the experience and familiarity needed to deal with peri-implantitis.

11.1.1 Biofilm removal or open flap debridement with repositioned full-thickness flaps

This is a technique in which biofilms are removed and the surface of the implant is disinfected after a full-thickness flap is elevated. When designing the flap, care is taken to preserve all the soft peri-implant tissues (ie, to avoid removing soft tissues during the incision). The flap is then repositioned and sutured at its original position.

It is imperative to combine this surgical technique with papillary preservation. The latter was introduced in 1985 by Takei et al[46] and was later modified by Cortellini et al.[47] Its aim is to maintain the integrity of the interdental or "interimplant" papilla, the smallest possible amount of tissue loss, and the best possible postoperative esthetic result. This flap design is also chosen in regenerative surgery to protect regenerative materials from exposure.

With regard to the interdental papillary preservation technique, the initial incision and elevation of the flap are performed first palatally or lingually; then the papilla are carefully detached so that they are part of the flap that will be elevated into a buccal position. Modification of the technique consists of a diagonal incision of the interdental papilla, for example, from the adjacent buccal interdental space of one tooth or implant to the corresponding adjacent palatal or lingual interdental space of the adjacent tooth or implant, so that half of the interdental papilla remains in the buccal flap and the other half in the palatal or lingual flap. Varying the technique is advantageous in the case of narrow interdental spaces.

Open flap debridement cannot be used to eliminate deep peri-implant bony defects. To achieve effective inflammation control, especially when there are deep pockets, flap elevation is required to give access for the removal of biofilms and disinfection of the implant surface. This is otherwise unlikely, especially in the spaces between the infected threads (Figs 11-4a–l). Indications for this type of surgery are:

- areas of inflammation after the application of stages A and B of the CIST protocol;
- when the morphology of the intraosseous lesion does not allow bone surgery for peri-implant pocket elimination, nor bone regeneration;
- as cause-related therapy, when regeneration has been decided on, but when after stages A and B of the CIST protocol, the pockets continue to exudate pus;
- when soft tissues should not be sacrificed or apically repositioned for esthetic reasons;
- in the case of horizontal bone destruction and an absence of deep intraosseous pockets.

Contraindications for this type of surgery are:

- intraosseous pockets whose morphology requires the choice of another technique;
- presence of pseudo-pockets when no bone damage is documented.

The advantages of the technique are:

- it leads to the elimination of inflammation;
- it causes little discomfort to the patient;
- it is relatively simple to implement.

The disadvantage of this technique is that it does not eliminate or fill intraosseous defects. The preoperative phase involves:

- application of stages A and B of the CIST protocol (oral hygiene instructions, AIRFLOW and PERIO-FLOW [EMS Dental, Nyon, Switzerland], mechanical calculus removal);
- verification of the effectiveness of oral hygiene;
- removal of the implant-supported restoration when this is feasible.

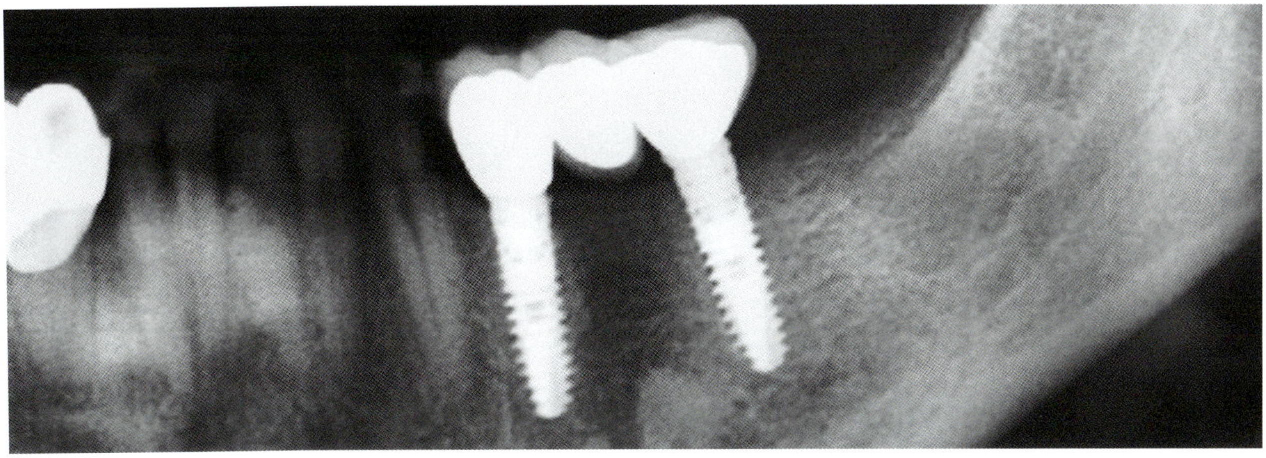

Fig 11-4a Initial radiograph of a patient after functional loading of implants.

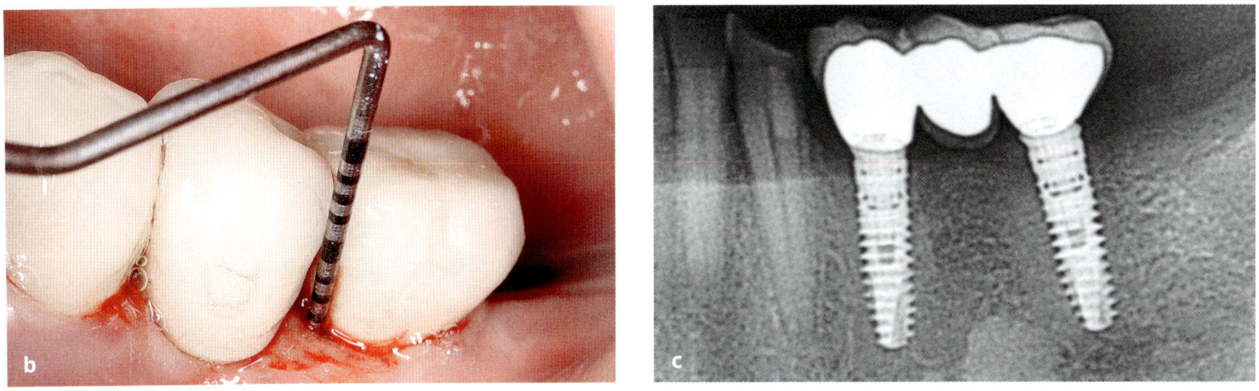

Figs 11-4b, c Clinical and radiographic images of the patient 5 years after implant placement. For the previous 4 years, the patient had abandoned the individualized maintenance care program. Pockets and signs of bone destruction without crater formation are visible.

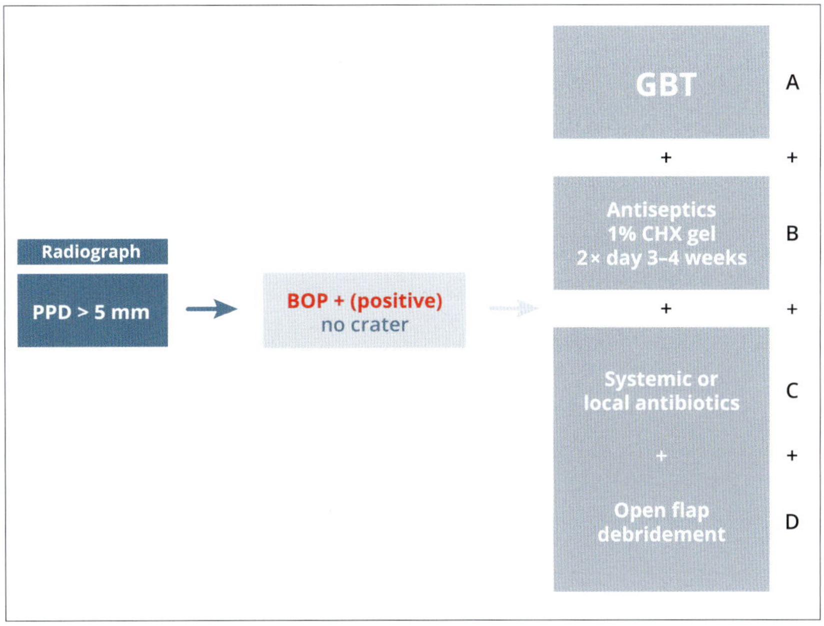

Fig 11-4d Proposed approach to corresponding cases according to the current data. CHX, chlorhexidine; GBT, guided biofilm therapy; PPD, periodontal probing depth.

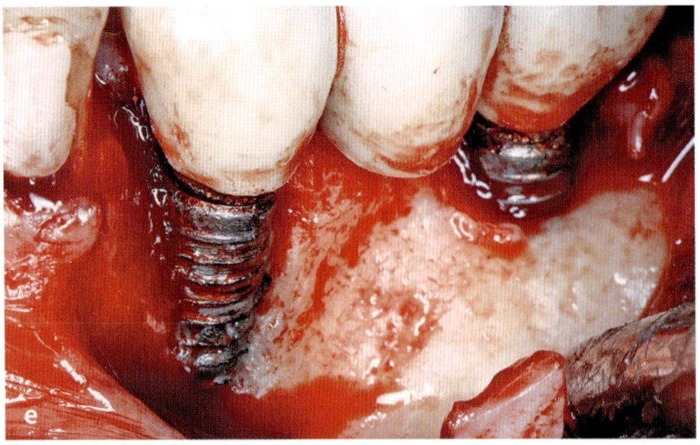

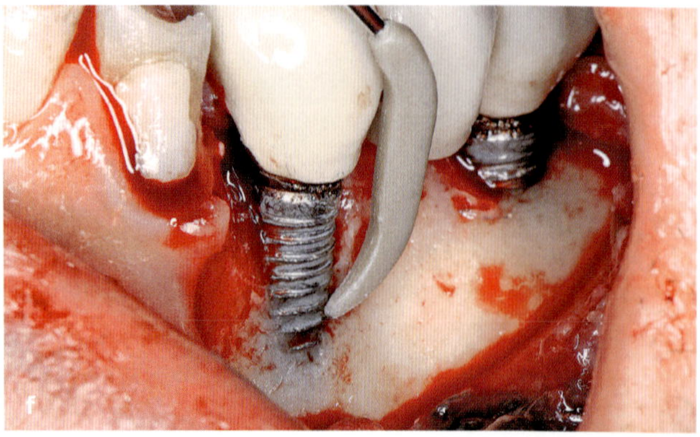

Figs 11-4e, f (e) After the inflammation control phase (stages A and B) under perioperative antibiotics (stage C), surgery was performed with a full-thickness flap to access the surfaces of the implants (stage D). **(f)** Removal of deposits using a plastic ultrasonic tip (NSK, Tokyo, Japan).

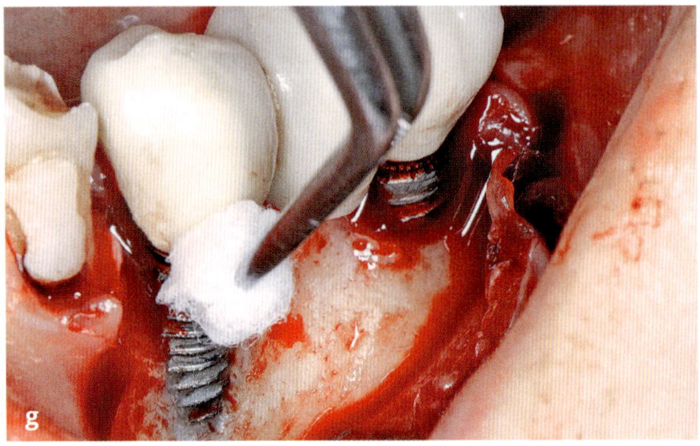

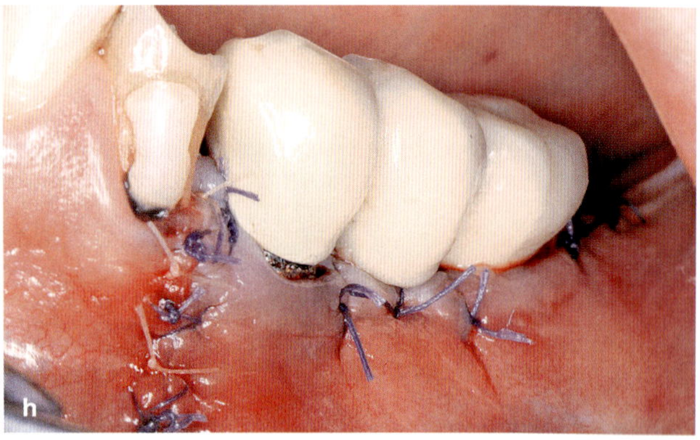

Figs 11-4 g, h (g) Subsequently, repeated cleansing (abrasive) movements were performed with gauze or cotton swabs soaked in saline. **(h)** Suturing followed. Suturing under the partial restoration was done with a horizontal mattress suture with a Laurel loop.

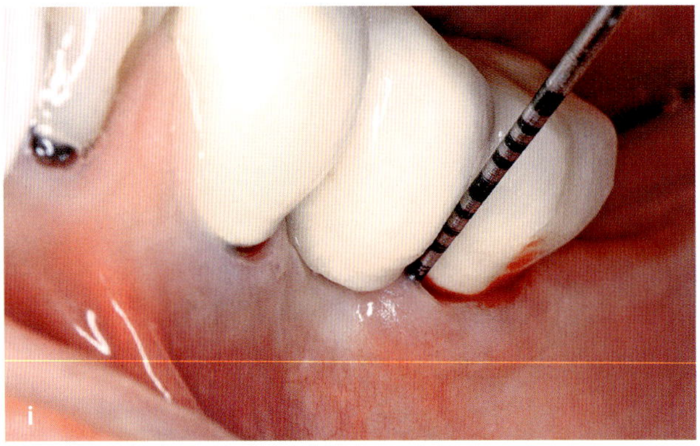

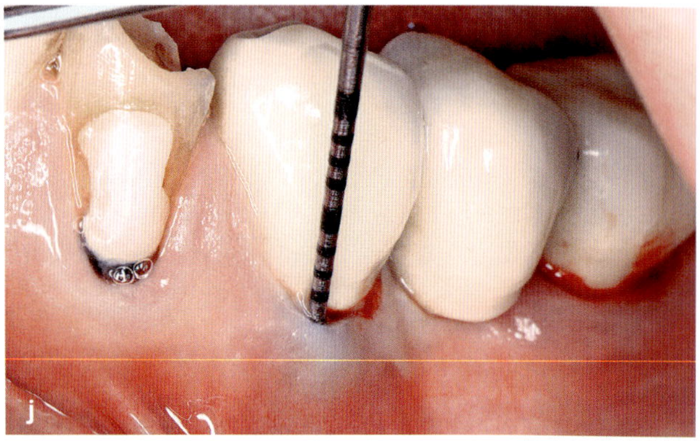

Fig 11-4i, j One year after surgery, BOP was observed, but the peri-implant soft tissue attachment was maintained. Stages A and B of the CIST protocol were implemented and the patient attended an individualized maintenance care program every 3 months.

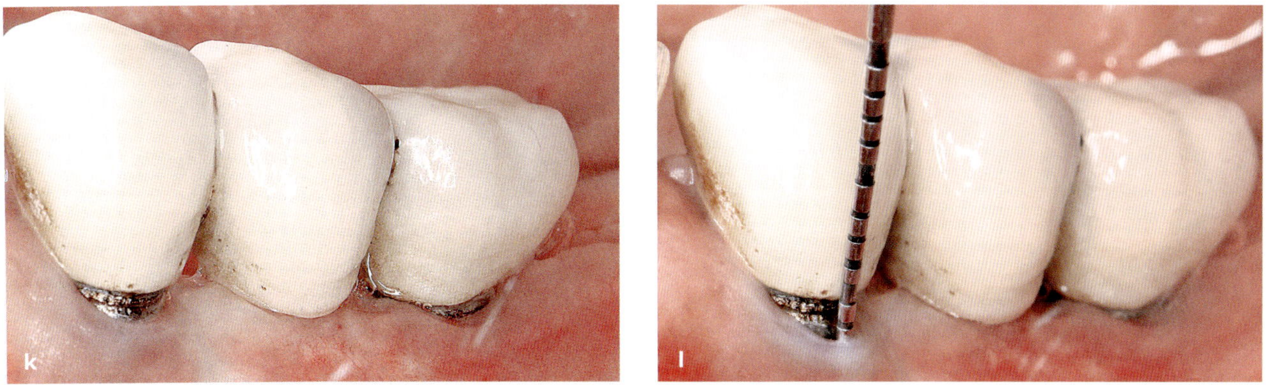

Figs 11-4k, l Five years after the operation. The patient complied consistently with the strict maintenance care program, but also with daily application of effective oral hygiene. Peri-implant health was preserved.

The surgical phase involves:

- anesthesia with vasoconstrictors;
- incision with a no. 15 or 15c scalpel or an ophthalmic blade depending on the dimensions of the necks of the adjacent teeth and the distances between adjacent implants. The incision does not extend around the perimeter of the implants. A basic condition is that the connective tissue between the buccal and palatal or lingual flap has been sufficiently separated in the interproximal (interdental) areas;
- buccal flap elevation with a Prichard no. 3 or Glickman P24G elevator, just below the margin of the alveolar bone (1 to 2 mm), but not beyond the mucogingival junction. In the maxilla, elevation beyond the mucogingival junction may lead to apical repositioning of the flap because of muscle traction;
- elevation of the palatal or lingual flap;
- removal of granulation tissue. Once the incision has been made carefully, no soft tissue remains, neither as a "collar" nor as parts of the interdental papilla in contact with the bone or the adjacent surfaces of the implants. Usually, granulation tissue is easily detached from the tension of the periosteal elevator and follows the flap on which it adheres;
- treatment of the implant surfaces with AIR-FLOW,[8,9] plastic or metallic ultrasonic instruments,[48,49] and titanium brushes.[50] The restriction on the contact of metal instruments on the titanium surface is removed because its threads have already come into contact with the pocket environment. Interestingly, rubbing the implant surface with gauze or cotton swabs soaked in saline has been done successfully to remove biofilms (Figs 11-5a–e, 11-6a, b, and 11-7a, b);
- smoothing of the implant threads.[51] This practice leads to greater accessibility during the maintenance care phase and facilitates the patient's efforts in administering daily oral hygiene (Figs 11-8a–e). However, it is not possible in implants with a small diameter if there is a risk of perforation of the inner shaft or implant fracture. Because of the reduction in mechanical strength, implantoplasty should be avoided;
- if thread smoothing is not possible, Er:YAG (2,940 nm), CO_2 (10,600 nm), diode lasers (980 or 810 nm), or photodynamic therapy may be used for disinfection of the implant surfaces[6,7,41–44];
- rinsing with saline;
- flap repositioning;
- suturing with continuous or single interrupted sutures using 4-0 or 5-0 sutures with a 16-mm-long nontraumatic needle.
- avoidance of periodontal dressings.

Er:YAG lasers are a completely safe choice for disinfection of the implant surface, do not damage the titanium surface, and do not increase the temperature of the surrounding tissues.[7,44]

CO_2 lasers have a small depth of penetration into soft tissues (0.2 mm). However, high power during their use may cause a significant increase in temperature with catastrophic consequences for the osseointegration of the apical part of the implant. Although it can be used in the treatment of peri-implantitis, it is not the first choice for clinicians because it is difficult to handle.[52–54]

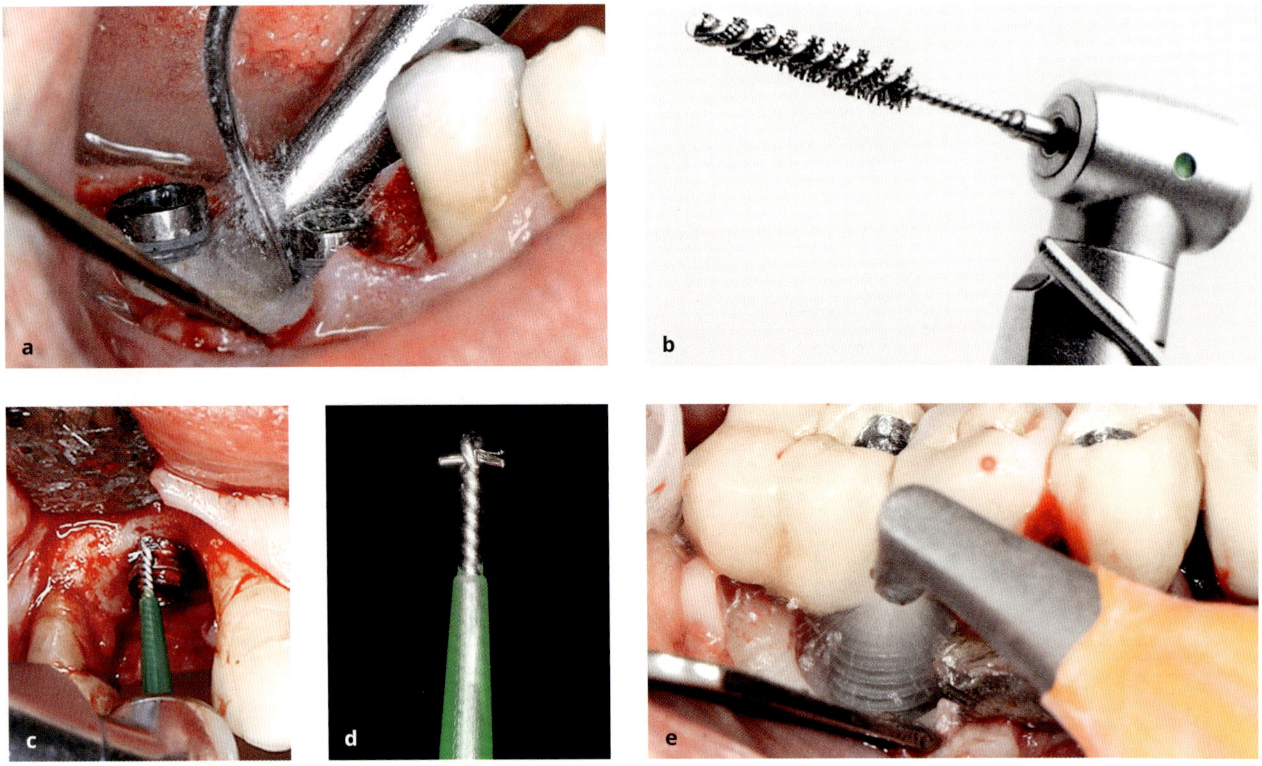

Figs 11-5a–e Instruments and devices used to remove deposits from the implant surface. **(a)** Metallic ultrasonic tip. **(b to d)** Disposable titanium brushes adapted to a handpiece with a surgical motor. **(e)** AIRFLOW. During its application, the spray must not be directed toward the area between the flap and the bone to avoid development of emphysema.

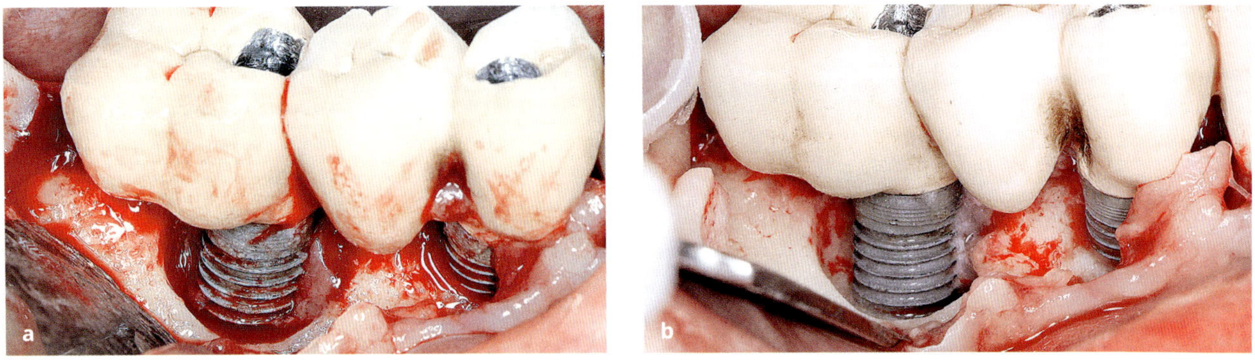

Figs 11-6a, b Exposed titanium surfaces **(a)** before and **(b)** after AIRFLOW application, showing the cleanliness of the implant surfaces.

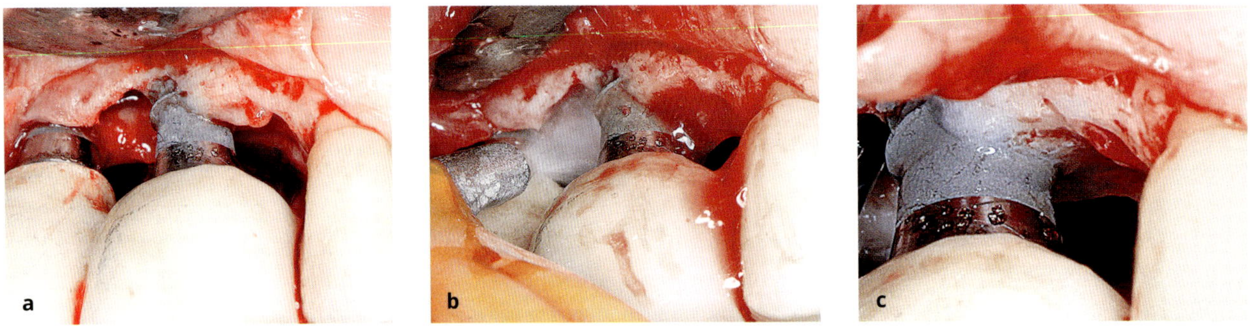

Figs 11-7a–c **(a)** The implant surface was exposed to the pocket environment before open flap debridement. **(b)** Application of AIRFLOW with erythritol. **(c)** The cleanliness of the surface can be seen immediately after the application of AIRFLOW.

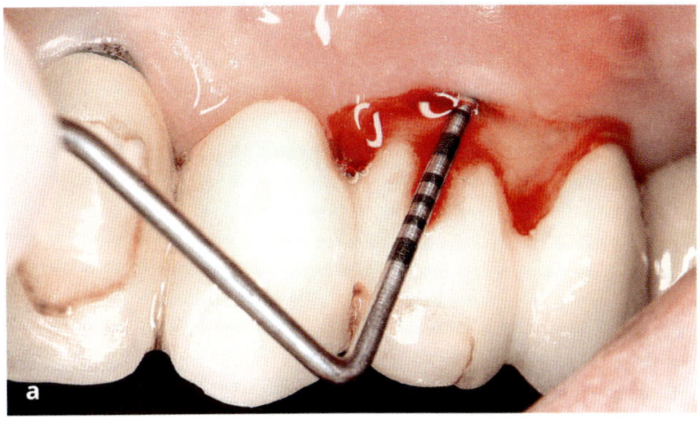

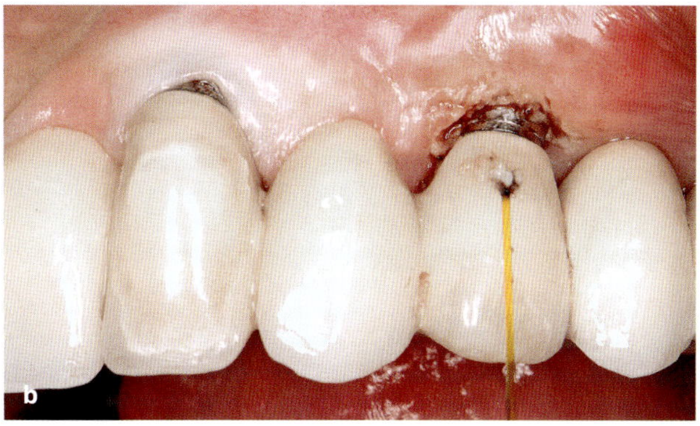

Figs 11-8a, b (a) Three years after placement of a connective tissue graft to increase the thickness of the keratinized peri-implant mucosa at no. 24, the patient presented with edema and pain inthe area. Probing revealed a bleeding pocket and pus formation. **(b)** After debridement (not presented), a 980-nm (1 W) diode laser was used for bactericidal effect and concomitant de-epithelialization.

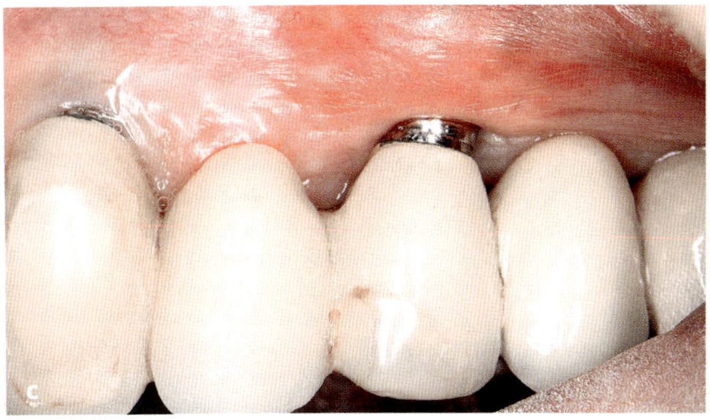

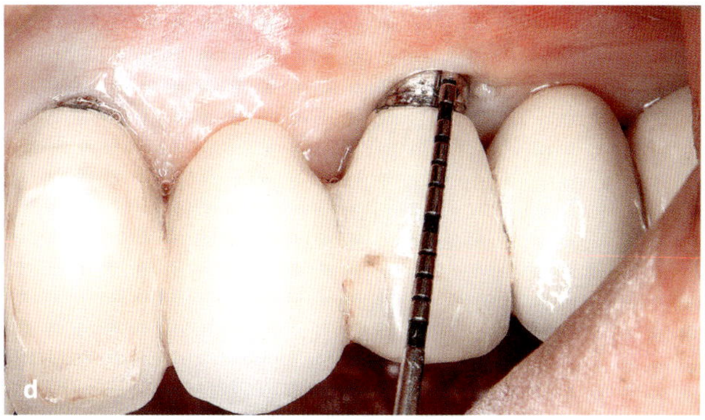

Figs 11-8c, d One year after the procedure, peri-implant health can be seen and no pocket is found.

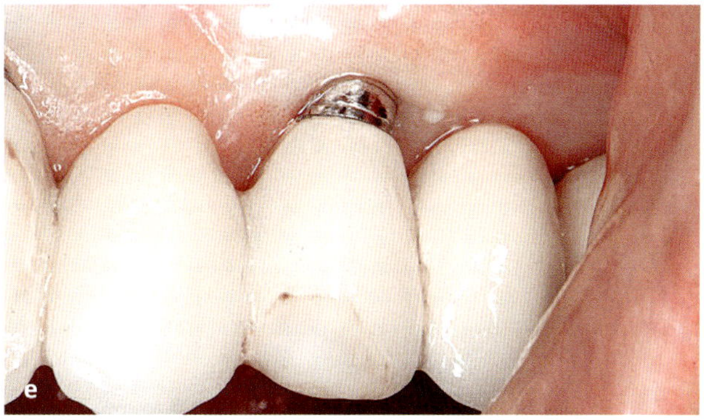

Fig 11-8e Two years after treatment, the stability of the result can be seen. The width and thickness of the keratinized mucosa is maintained (the grafting procedure is shown in Figs 13-10a–d).

Regarding diode lasers,[6,41] the results of in vitro studies have shown that they do not cause damage to the titanium surface as with Nd:YAG lasers. However, high power or long application time may cause a significant rise in temperature, with negative consequences for the osseointegration of the apical part.

Because of the increase in temperature caused by lasers, the clinician should keep the following in mind:

- The critical temperature for osseointegration damage is 47°C.
- This temperature may be produced when using diodes for 9 seconds at 2.5 W, 12.5 seconds at 2 W, 18 seconds at 1.5 W, or 30.5 seconds at 1.0 W.
- When used to disinfect implant surfaces, diode lasers should be employed for a short time (< 25 seconds) and at low power (≤ 1 W) to avoid damage to the bone.

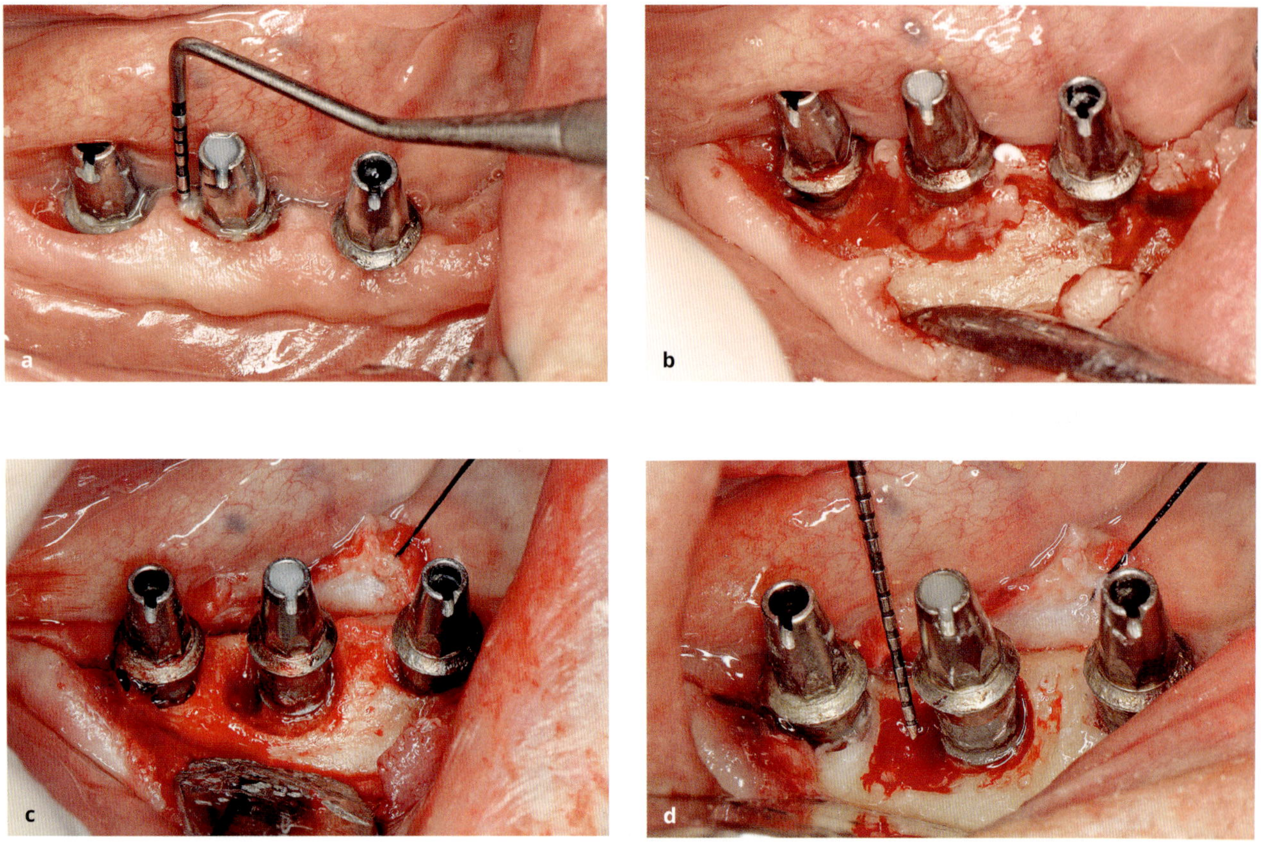

Figs 11-9a–d **(a)** Probing revealed a pocket depth of 7 mm and BOP. **(b)** An intrasulcular incision was made; a flap was elevated to continue as a partial-thickness flap, in case the defect was suitable for bone regeneration. **(c)** After removal of the granulation tissue, the depth of the intraosseous defects and the number of bony walls were examined. **(d)** Once it was confirmed that the defect was not suitable for regeneration but for resective surgery, osteoplasty was carried out to eliminate the depth of the intraosseous defects.

Limited data suggest that the EmunDo protocol may have an advantageous bactericidal effect. Indocyanine green highly absorbs photons with a 810-nm wavelength. As indocyanine green selectively binds with microbial cell membranes, radiation absorption leads to a large increase in temperature only in the microbial cells that are destroyed.[55,56] This is because very little power is used (200 to 500 mW), and cannot induce damage to the surrounding area.

As shown in a recent systematic review, Er:YAG and CO_2 lasers and photodynamic therapy are effective in controlling inflammation (Figs 11-8a–e).[57]

11.1.2 Resective surgery

Resective techniques describe the apical repositioning of full or partial-thickness flaps, peri-implant bone surgery, resection of the peri-implant mucosa (the term gingivectomy does not apply because gingiva are dependent on the presence of teeth) and modification (smoothing) of the implant surface (implantoplasty).[18]

Resective surgery aims to eliminate or significantly reduce the depth of the peri-implant pockets by removing soft tissue or placing the margin of its mucosal walls apically. To achieve this, surgery is often also required in the bone peripheral to the implant. Placement of the peri-implant mucosal margin at a more apical level is done either through flap elevation, which will be performed apically, or by removing part of the soft tissues. Excision of part of the soft tissues is done using mucosectomy or by designing a flap so that the incision is not made in intrasulcular fashion, but at some distance from the margin of the free mucosa. This flap is called a partially resective repositioned flap (Figs 11-9a–j). It is ideal for removing the portion of the peri-implant mucosa after all the other stages of surgery have been completed and just before suturing. This, of course, requires special surgical skills. There are specific indications

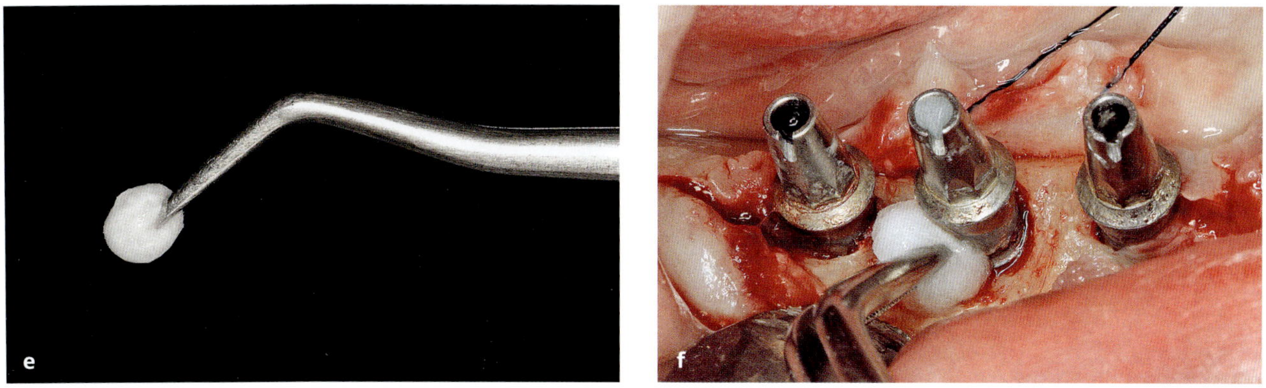

Figs 11-9e, f **(e)** Fuse immersed in saline. **(f)** Use of a cotton pellet at the implant site.

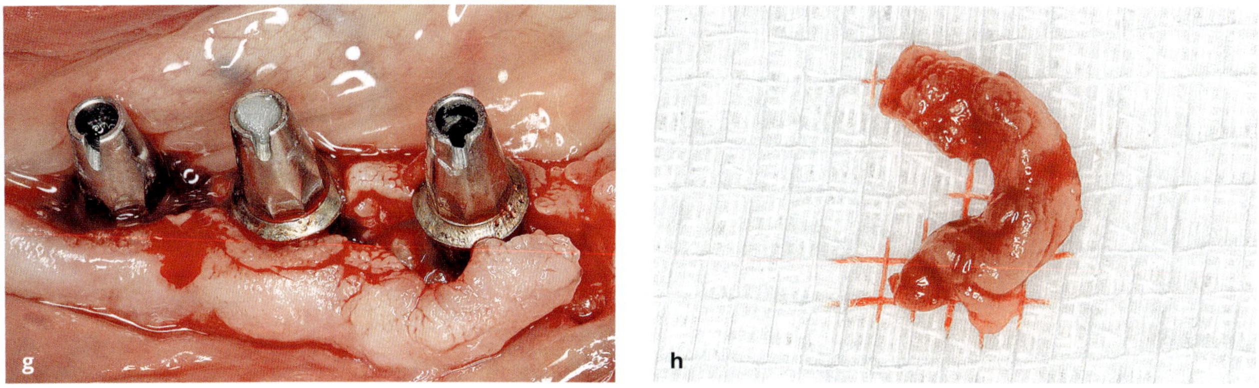

Figs 11-9g, h **(g)** If the thickness and width of the keratinized tissues allow it, careful thinning of the flaps may be performed using a scalloped incision to achieve a reduction in pocket depth during healing. **(h)** The part of the soft tissues that was removed from the buccal flap.

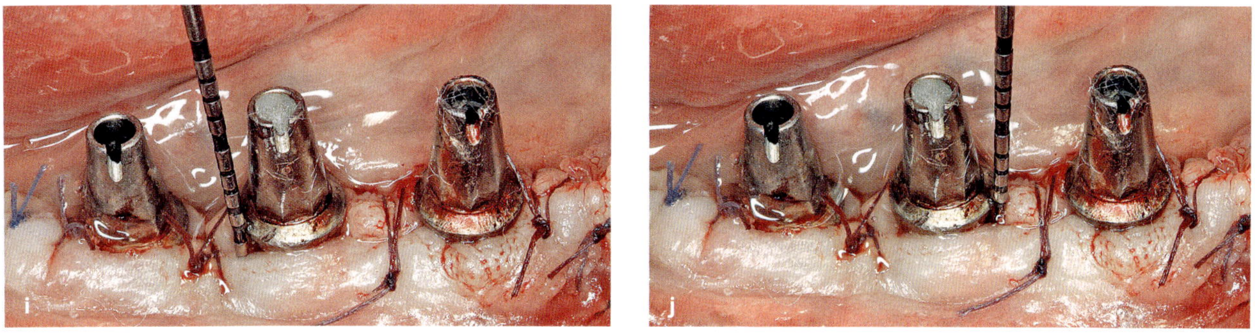

Figs 11-9i, j As can be seen with the periodontal probe, the distance from the peri-implant mucosal margin to the alveolar bone does not exceed 4 mm.

and conditions for each technique. The main objectives of these techniques are:

- to acquire an optical field for effective removal of biofilms and disinfection of the surface of the affected implants;
- to establish a peri-implant mucosa and bone architecture that allows the patient to apply effective oral hygiene and the dental practitioner to effectively apply the therapeutic preventive measures required during the maintenance care phase. To achieve this goal, implant thread smoothing, when feasible, is advocated;
- to ensure long-term maintenance of the attachment level;
- to establish a peri-implant sulcus with the smallest possible depth so that it is accessible for administration of oral hygiene products and easily manageable during the maintenance phase.

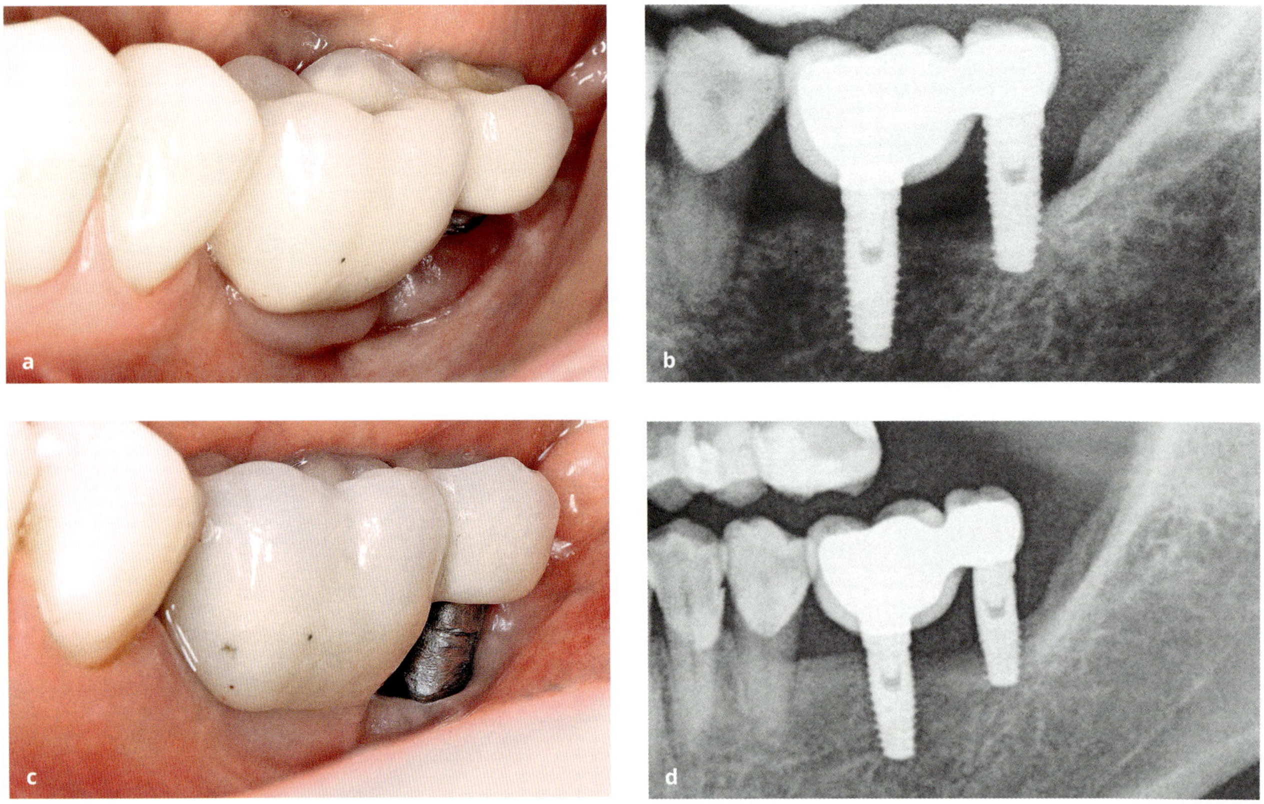

Figs 11-10a–d (a and b) Clinical and radiographic images of peri-implantitis in implant no. 37. The anatomy of the area makes the apical displacement of the soft peri-implant tissues a particularly demanding process. **(c and d)** Clinical and radiographic images 3 years after surgery. Extensive apical displacement was achieved and the stability of the peri-implant tissues is evident (this is the treatment of the case shown in Figs 3-12a–d).

11.1.3 Apically repositioned flaps

Apically repositioned flaps may have full thickness, partial thickness, or a combination of the two. A full-thickness flap is usually preferred when surgery is performed in the maxilla; a combination of full- and partial-thickness flaps is usually preferred when the mandible is concerned. A partial-thickness flap is prepared with a scalpel, which cuts the soft tissues parallel to the surface of the alveolar ridge. This results in a mucosal flap, while the periosteum, together with parts of the connective tissue, are left attached to the bone. Apically repositioned flaps aim to eliminate the depth of the peri-implant pockets (Figs 11-10a–d).[58]

11.1.4 Apically repositioned full-thickness flaps

This is the technique in which the entire zone of keratinized tissue together with the periosteum is detached and repositioned more apically (at the level of the crest of the alveolar ridge) to eliminate the existing peri-implant pockets. Because of the bone loss caused by peri-implantitis, part of or the entire zone of keratinized mucosa is no longer "attached" to the underlying bone. It forms the soft tissue wall of the peri-implant pocket. Removal of the soft tissues by mucosectomy, a procedure similar to gingivectomy, would lead to pocket elimination if bone loss is horizontal. However, the main issue in most cases where the zone of keratinized mucosa is narrow is the risk of causing a mucogingival problem. A lack of keratinized tissues is a risk factor for peri-implant diseases. For this reason, an apically repositioned flap is usually chosen, where all the soft peri-implant tissues are included in a full-thickness flap, displaced and sutured more apically.

Indications for this type of surgery are:

- presence of peri-implant pockets that involve implants in areas that will not be esthetically compromised if part of the implants is showing;

- when it is not feasible to apply regenerative techniques because of the morphology of the lesions or due to heavy smoking;
- a narrow zone of keratinized mucosa, which does not allow mucosectomy with an external bevel excision even if bone loss is not combined with intraosseous defects (horizontal loss);
- bone defects involving one or two bony walls that require ostectomy or osteoplasty.

Contraindications for this type of surgery are:
- when the smile reveals the peri-implant mucosa. When there is excessive gingival display, a major esthetic problem may be created not only because "black triangles" are revealed in the position of the interdental papilla, but also because part of the implants will be displayed;
- treatment of peri-implantitis in the mandible, where the elevation of a full-thickness flap beyond the mucogingival junction leads to a coronal movement of the flap due to forces exercised. In this case, vertical incisions may have to be chosen.

Advantages of the technique are as follows:
- It can be used to eliminate or greatly reduce the depth of the peri-implant pockets.
- It facilitates the preservation of the existing keratinized mucosa and the determination of the postoperative position of the margin of the free peri-implant mucosa.
- It offers the option of bone surgery (ostectomy and osteoplasty).
- It offers access for debridement by means of air-polishing or ultrasonic instruments.
- It facilitates the repositioning of the flap at a level chosen by the clinician.

Disadvantages of the technique are as follows:
- It requires special care when detaching the peri-implant mucosa in patients with a thin phenotype. As mentioned, no scalpel incision is required around the implant because the peri-implant mucosa does not contain Sharpey fibers. In implants, connective tissue fibers generally run parallel to the long axis of the implant or around it. It is important to separate the connective tissue in the cross-sectional direction of the buccal and palatal or lingual flap. If the correct dissection is not made, applying force to a fine soft tissue phenotype may lead to flap tearing that complicates the technique and increases morbidity.
- Apical soft tissue displacement may cause esthetic or phonetic problems. It is not uncommon for a fixed prosthesis to be replaced with a denture to address these problems (Figs 11-11a–t). Another potential issue arises in teeth adjacent to implants that show bony defects involving one or two bone walls. If the supporting bone needs to be removed from an adjacent tooth to reduce the depth of the intraosseous defect of the peri-implant pocket, this will inevitably result in attachment loss.

The preoperative phase involves the following:
- the application of stages A and B of the CIST protocol (oral hygiene instructions, AIRFLOW and PERIOFLOW, mechanical debridement) or the application of laser to control microorganisms in sessions before these procedures take place. The latter should be performed at least 2 weeks before the day of surgery, so that tissues have been given time to heal from cause-related treatment;
- checking of the effectiveness of oral hygiene;
- removal of the implant-supported restoration if feasible.

Anesthesia for this type of surgery involves:
- administration of local anesthesia (with the addition of vasoconstrictors) in the maxilla, whereas in the mandible, a combination of inferior alveolar nerve block anesthesia with terminal anesthesia is usually selected. Achieving depth of anesthesia, as well as hemostasis, facilitates surgical manipulation;
- detection of the underlying crest of the alveolar ridge with a metallic periodontal probe with the surgical field anesthetized. Thus, a clear picture of both the depth and orientation of the pockets is revealed.

The technique for this surgery involves making an incision in the adjacent areas with a no. 15, 12, 12b, or an ophthalmic blade. Subsequently, using an Orban knife (Hu-Friedy, Chicago, IL, USA), an attempt is made to cut the attached soft tissue that may not have been accessed using a scalpel, at the bottom of the adjacent peri-implant pockets. As with any periodontal surgery, the incision is started at the distal point of the area and is directed toward the mesial aspect. Thus, surgical suction follows the scalpel and Orban knife so that throughout the procedure, the field of

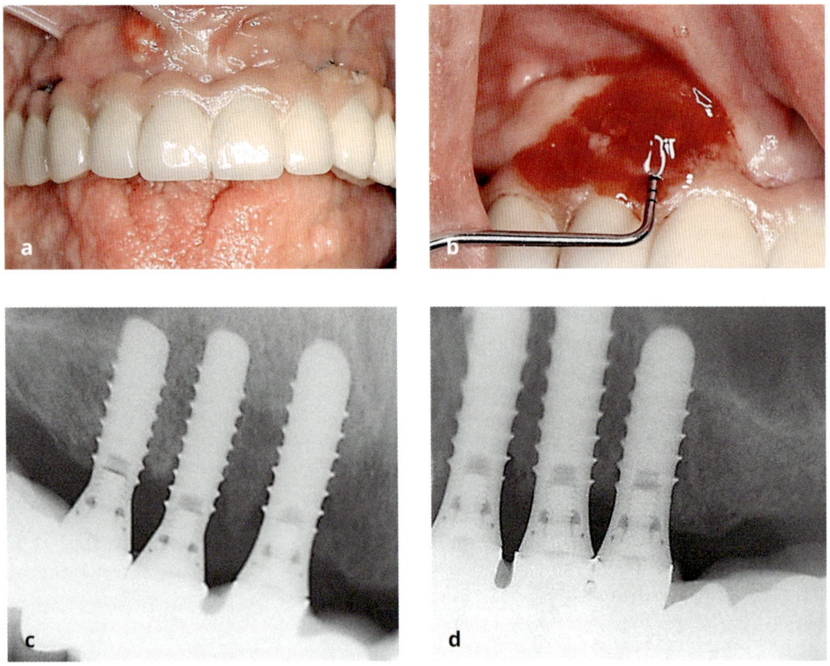

Figs 11-11a–d (a and b) Clinical images of a patient who did not respond to the therapeutic maintenance care program, 6 years after implant placement. Drainage of the abscess in site no. 12 led to an outflow of pus and blood and resulted in pain relief. **(c and d)** Bone loss is visible on the radiographs.

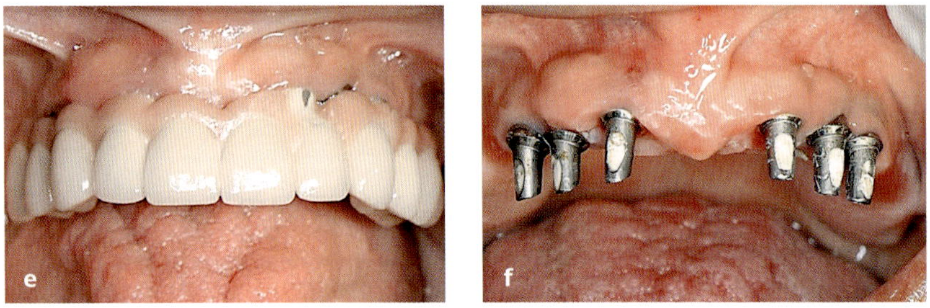

Figs 11-11e, f After the inflammation control phase (stages A and B), which was performed according to the classic CIST protocol, a significant clinical improvement was observed. The fistula remained in site no. 12. To apply stages A and B, ideally the fixed restoration should be removed to facilitate access. If a cement-retained fixed prosthesis is inserted, the porcelain may break.

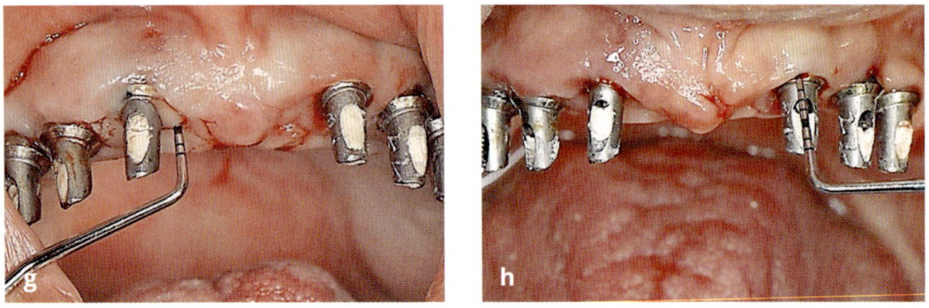

Figs 11-11 g, h Increased pocket depth and pus formation were observed.

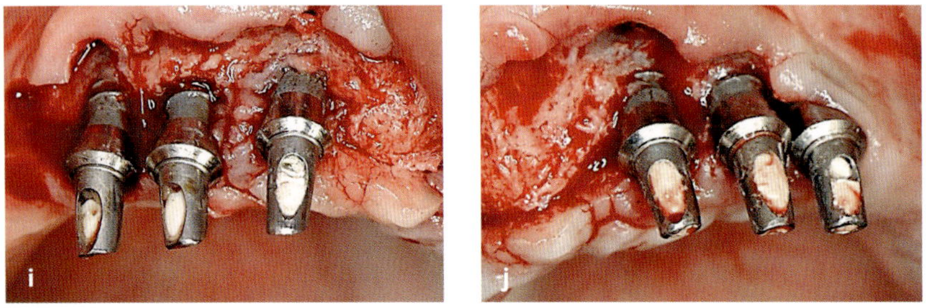

Figs 11-11i, j After flap elevation, the exposed implant surfaces can be seen.

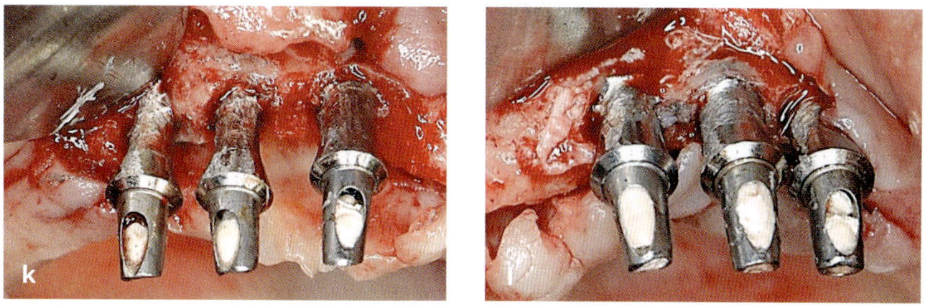

Figs 11-11k, l The surface of the implants was disinfected. Removal of the granulation tissue, thread smoothing, and thinning of the flaps for better adaptation during suturing were performed.

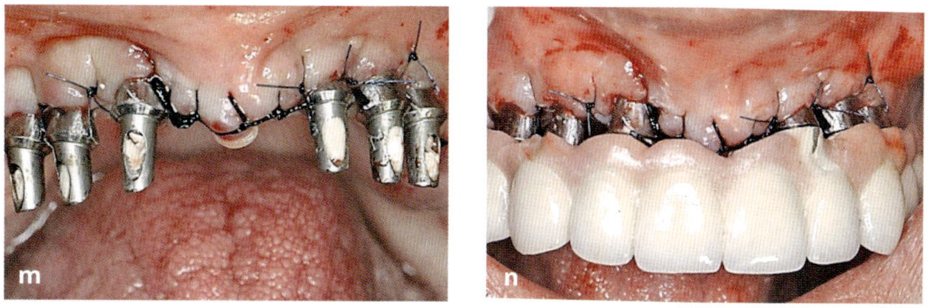

Figs 11-11m, n (m) Apical flap repositioning achieved a reduction of pocket depth. **(n)** The esthetic result was suboptimal.

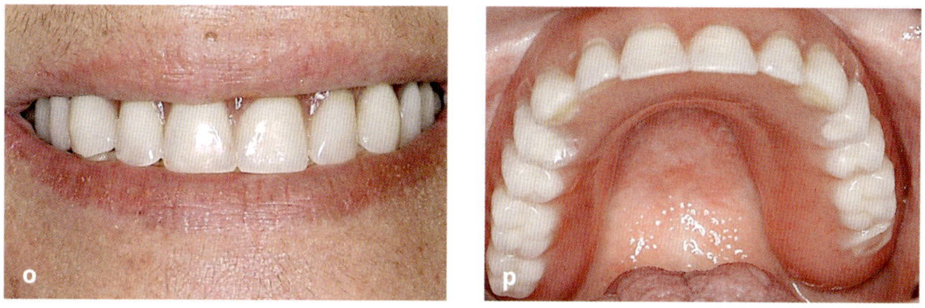

Figs 11-11o, p To meet the esthetic needs, replacement of the fixed prosthetic restoration with a removable prosthesis was necessary.

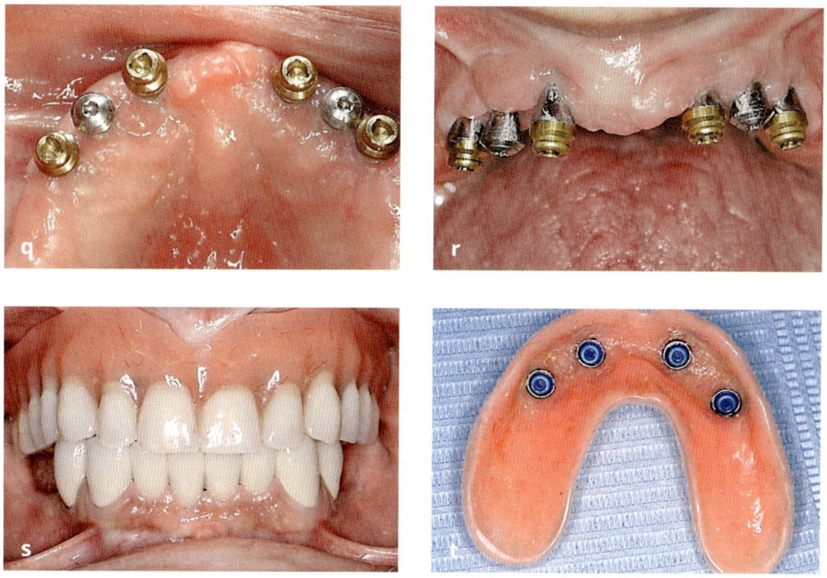

Figs 11-11q–t Clinical images of the patient 1 year after surgery. Maintenance of peri-implant tissue health can be seen. Of the six implants, only four were used for the prosthesis.

view is relatively dry. If the flap is designed without vertical incisions but as an envelope flap, it must extend sufficiently to ensure adequate vision and comfort of handling, while at the same time avoiding tension at the edges of the flap. Unlike apically repositioned flaps around teeth, no simultaneous thinning of the flap is sought at the implant sites. If needed, it may be postponed until completion of the bone surgery. Thus, postoperative exposure of the alveolar bone should be avoided.

If vertical releasing incisions are needed, they are always made on the buccal surface to avoid injury of the lingual nerve or major palatine arteries. The vertical incision is made at a tooth or implant site beyond the last element to be treated. The vertical incision should be beveled to ensure better adaptation of the flap during suturing, and to encourage faster healing (placement of the blade at an angle of about 45 degrees to the surface of the soft tissue). The incision should be initiated at a location 1 mm apical to the mucogingival junction and be drawn in a coronal direction, ending at the proximal or distal line angle of the tooth or implant. The incision should end at the base of the interdental papilla and never split its tip.

A Prichard no. 3 periosteal elevator is used for flap elevation in a thick mucosal phenotype, or a Glickman P24G if it is applied to an area with a thin mucosal phenotype. The elevator is inserted into the incision at an angle of about 30 degrees and its movement is always controlled and semicircular along the surgical field. It should never be moved only in a perpendicular direction. Slippage of the elevator and subsequent perforation of the flap is a possible complication, resulting in healing delays, pain, and patient discomfort.

If, at some point, the elevator encounters resistance, it should be withdrawn and the procedure should be continued with a scalpel.

After the buccal flap is treated with a sterile gauze soaked in saline, the elevation process is repeated on the lingual side.

After elevation of the palatal or lingual flap, removal of the granulation tissue begins by using a Crane-Kaplan sickle CK-6, a Younger-Good 7/8 scaler (Hu-Friedy), with custom-designed cutting burs (Fig 11-12). It is convenient to use an ultrasonic device with a thin and long instrument to remove soft tissue remnants. Once removal of granulation tissue is completed, bleeding is dramatically reduced, then any biofilms are removed using AIRFLOW.

Whenever feasible, after disinfecting the implant surface with AIRFLOW, the implant threads may be smoothed. The technique is described later in this chapter.

Bone surgery may be performed to reduce the depth of the intraosseous defects or eliminate them completely, with round diamond burs of various diameters, or grooved tungsten carbide burs especially designed for this purpose (Figs 11-13 to 11-15).

Leveling the walls of an adjacent crater, once it has been decided that no regenerative technique is going to be employed, is done by using a diamond bur smaller than the proximal–distal dimensions of the lesion wall so that its base can form the future bony crest between the implant and the adjacent tooth. Bur movement must always be in an apicocoronal direction so as not to affect the apical part of the implants.

Suturing is done with resorbable sutures, polyglycolic acid (PGA) or Vicryl 4-0 or 5-0 (Ethicon, Raritan, NJ, USA); 12-mm or 16-mm atraumatic needles are recommended. Vertical mattress sutures are normally used to better control placement of the edge of the peri-implant mucosa, mainly in the region of the interdental papilla. They may be performed so that the initial insertion of the needle is made at a more apical point than the level from which the tissues have been elevated to achieve better apical flap adaptation by pressing the knot to rest on the most apical buccal insertion point (periosteal or subperiosteal suture). This technique helps to position the flap exactly at the level chosen by the clinician; at the same time, it provides a satisfactory flap adaptation for the alveolar ridge (Figs 11-16a, b).

Postoperative care consists of the following:

- application of pressure to the flaps immediately after suturing, using a gauze soaked in saline for 3 to 4 minutes to prevent a hematoma;
- daily rinsing with 0.1% to 0.2% chlorohexidine for 1 month; no periodontal dressing needs to be used;
- removal of sutures after 10 to 12 days;
- administration of perioperative antibiotics, documented by and at the discretion of the clinician. Amoxicillin should be administered with a loading dose of 2 g 1 hour before surgery and then 1 g every 8 hours for 4 to 7 days. In patients who are allergic to penicillin, broad-spectrum alternatives are preferred, ideally clindamycin. The loading dose is 600 mg 1 hour before surgery and then 300 mg every 6 hours for 4 to 7 days;

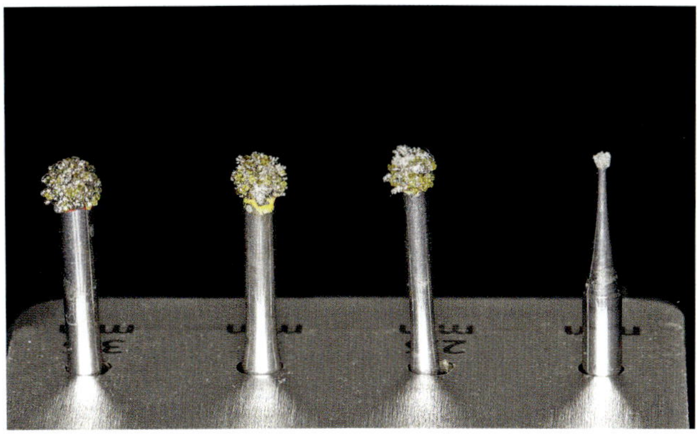

Fig 11-12 Special cutting burs of various diameters for the removal of granular tissue from intraosseous defects.

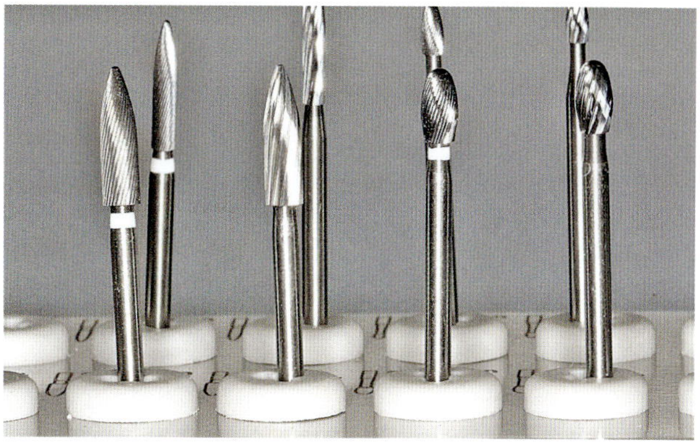

Fig 11-13 Specially designed tungsten carbide burs for thread smoothing. The ones with the white band are used for final smoothing.

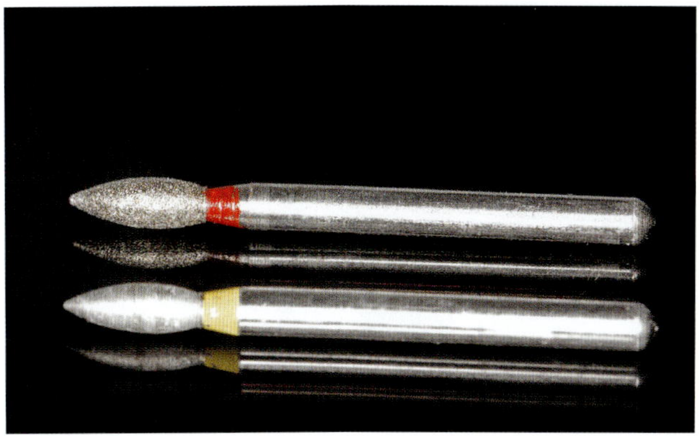

Fig 11-14 Diamond burs of different roughnesses for composite resin smoothing, which can also be used for final smoothing.

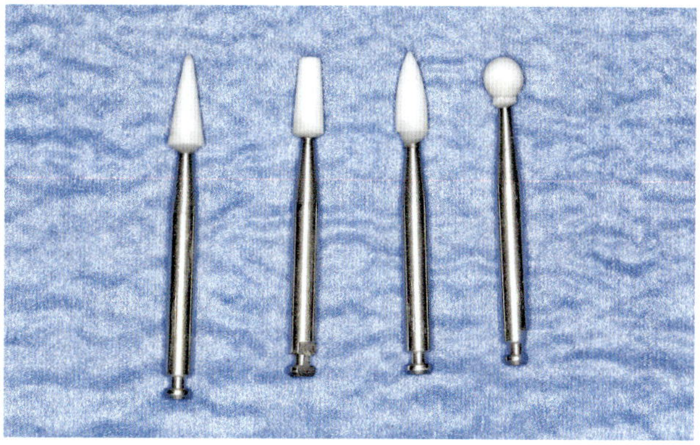

Fig 11-15 Smoothing Arkansas burs used after diamond burs.

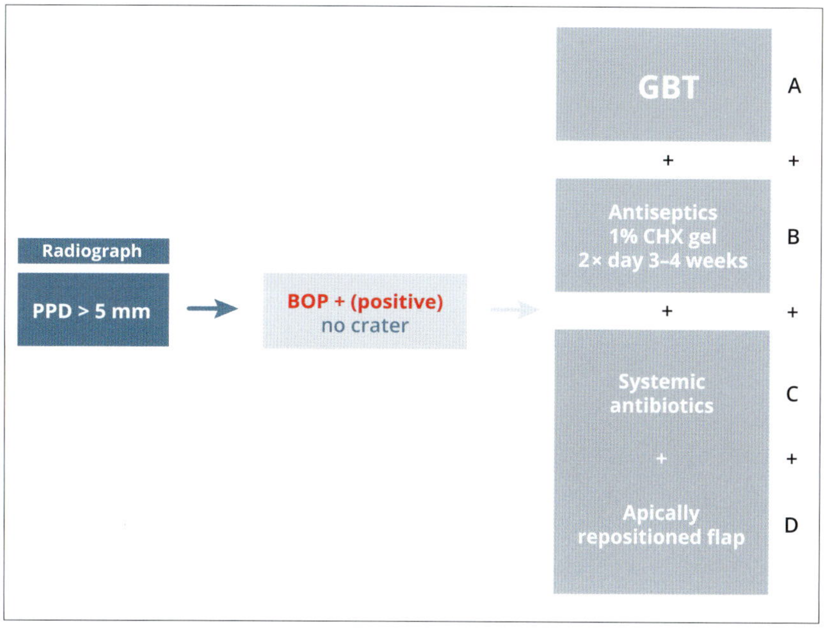

Fig 11-16a Proposed approach, according to modern data, for cases where an apically repositioned flap is indicated. CHX, chlorhexidine; GBT, guided biofilm therapy; PPD, periodontal probing depth.

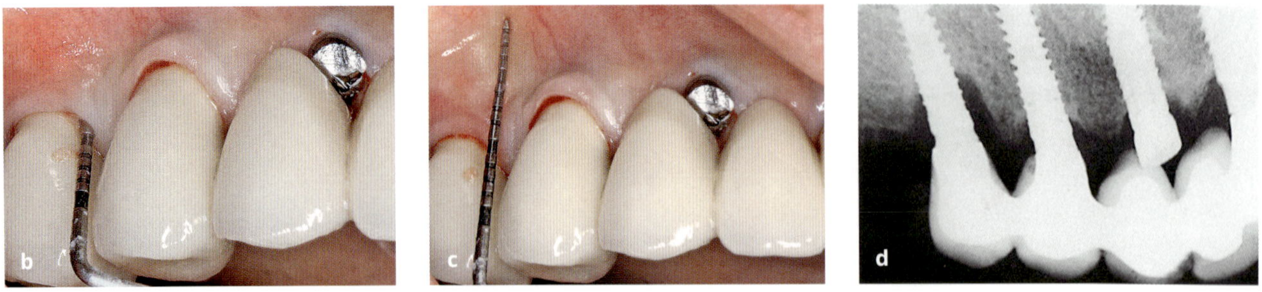

Figs 11-16b–d (b and c) During the clinical examination, a pocket depth of 9 mm was detected. **(d)** Radiograph showing bone loss due to peri-implantitis in implant no. 15 in a patient whose implants were placed 10 years previously.

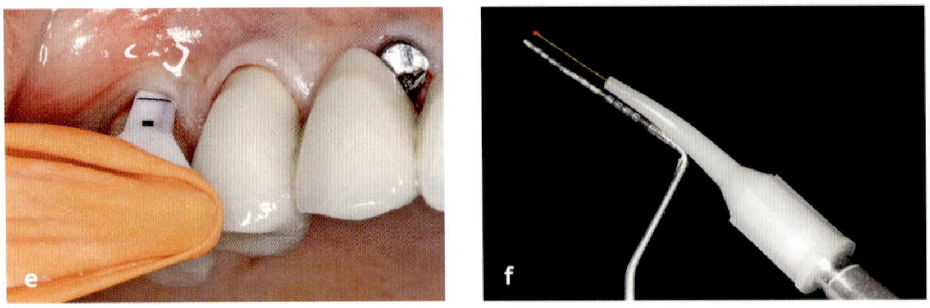

Figs 11-16e, f (e) Guided biofilm therapy. The image shows the application of PERIOFLOW where the tip reaches 9 mm inside the peri-implant pocket. **(f)** Adjusting the optical fiber (300 μm) of a 980-nm diode laser so that it enters the desired depth. Irradiation is intended for bactericidal effect and is carried out continuously with a power of 1 W.

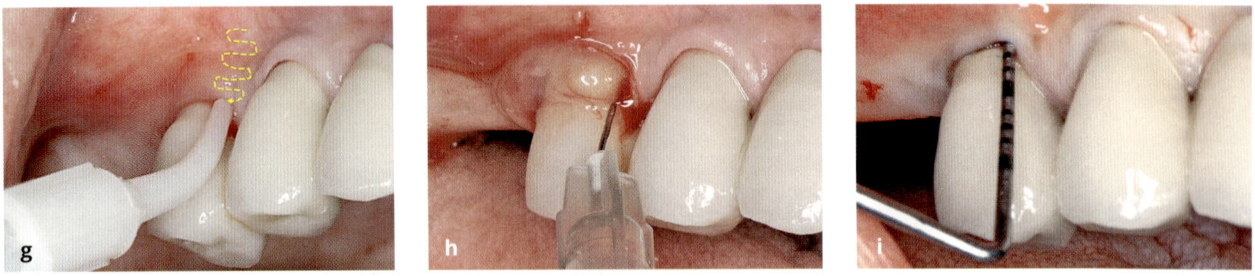

Figs 11-16 g–i (g) The optical fiber has entered the depth of the pocket; with serpentine movements, irradiation is carried out. The optical fiber comes out gradually, covering a vertical distance of about 1 mm every 2 seconds. **(h)** 1% chlorhexidine gel was injected and the same formulation was prescribed to the patient for home use. **(i)** Five weeks after the implementation of stages A and B of the CIST protocol. There is a decrease in the measured depth of the peri-implant pocket and shrinkage of the soft tissues.

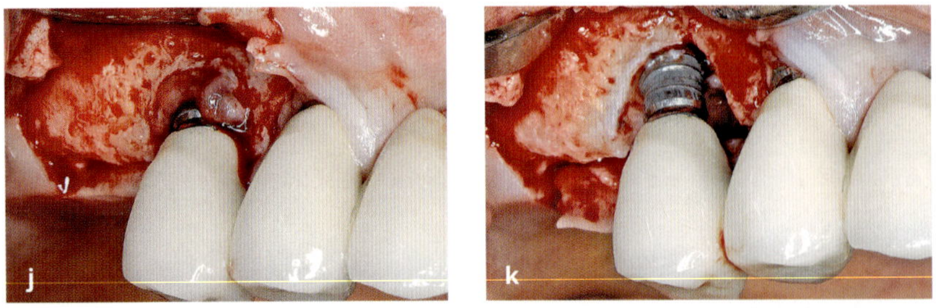

Figs 11-16j, k (j) After full thickness flap elevation. **(k)** After removal of the granulation tissue from the intraosseous peri-implant defect. A two-wall bony defect was noted.

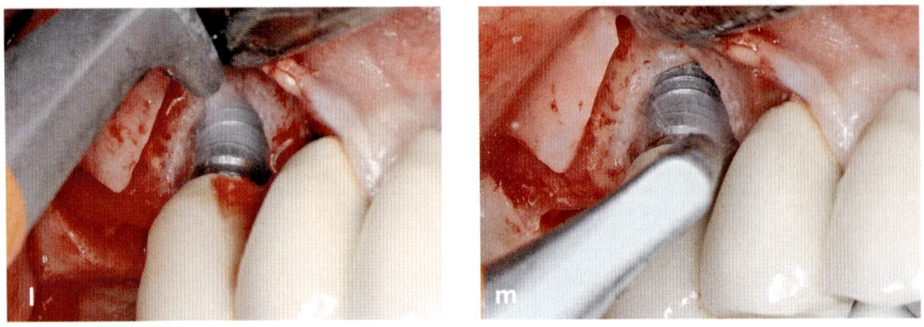

Figs 11-16l, m AIRFLOW application first to the neck and then to the bone–implant contact area. The erythritol spray beam was not directed between the flap and the bone to avoid emphysema.

Figs 11-16n, o **(n)** The clarity of the implant surface can be observed after rinsing with saline. **(o)** The process of thread smoothing began with special tungsten carbide burs of various shapes, initially to remove roughness.

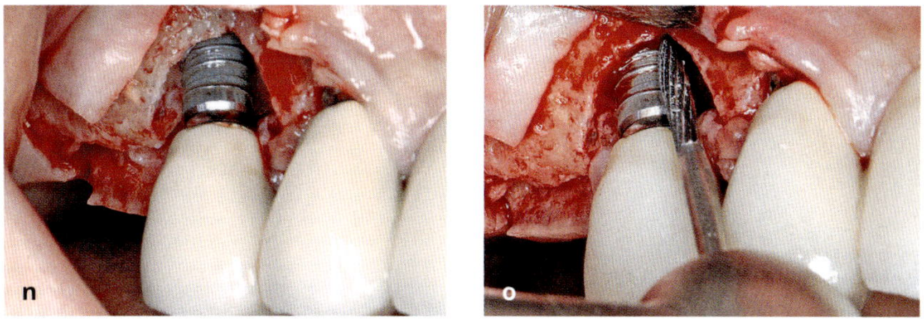

Figs 11-16p, q Then, diamond burs were used to further smooth the surface.

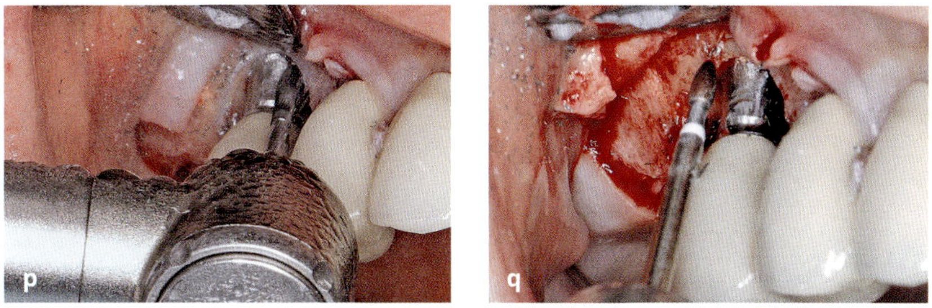

Figs 11-16r, s **(r)** This is followed by osteoplasty to reduce the size of the intraosseous component. **(s)** Slimming of the palatal flap for better adaptation but also to remove titanium particles that have escaped from the measures taken to limit them.

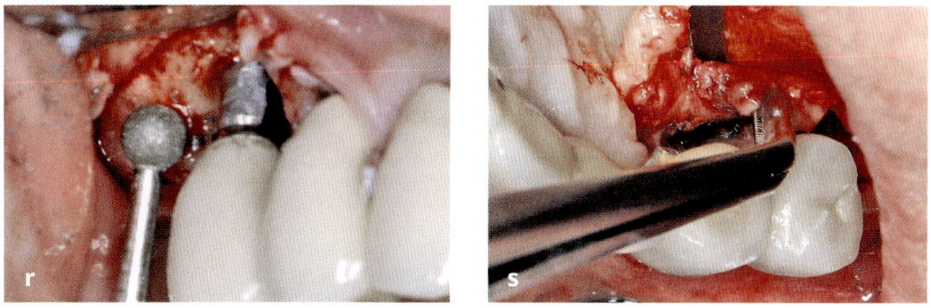

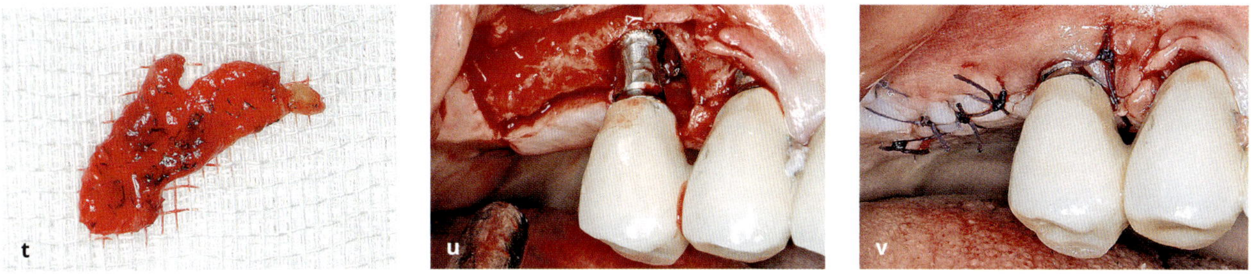

Figs 11-16t–v **(t)** Despite the use of strong surgical suction and placement of gauze pieces, escape of titanium particles on the lingual or palatal side is usually unavoidable. **(u)** After completion of the procedure, the distal intraosseous defect had been eliminated and conditions that would favor biofilm removal during the maintenance care phase were achieved. It was decided to leave the proximal wall of the lesion without bone surgery. **(v)** After flap suturing.

Figs 11-16w, x Images **(w)** before and **(x)** immediately after suture removal. Good healing and absence of inflammation are evident.

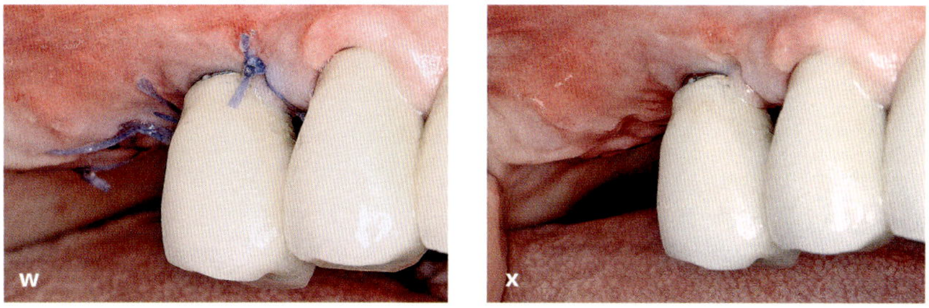

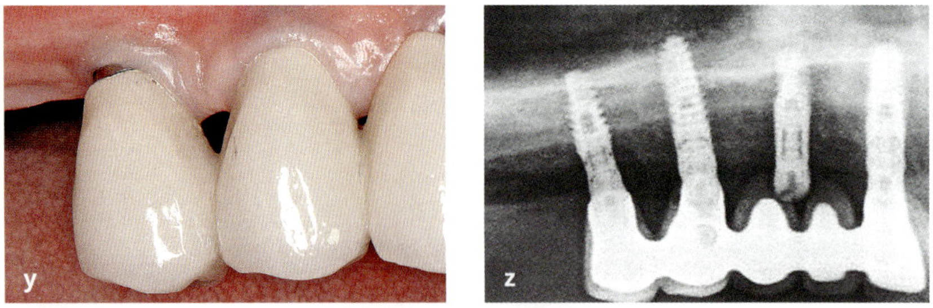

Figs 11-16y, z **(y)** Clinical image 2 years after surgery. **(z)** Part of the panoramic radiography showing the improvement of the peri-implant bone in implant no. 15: elimination of the intraosseous defect distally, reduction of the intraosseous pocket depth mesially, and thread smoothing 2 years after treatment completion.

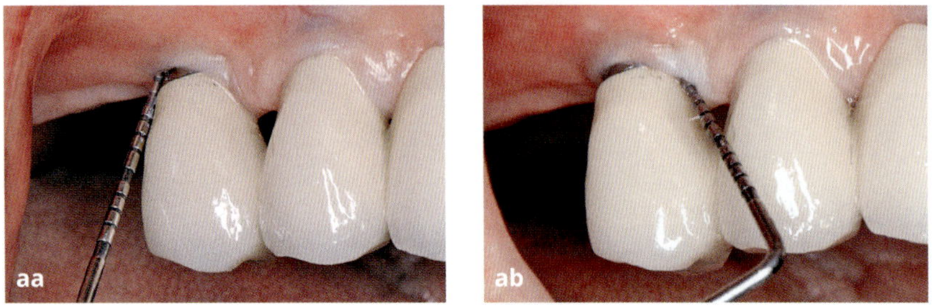

Figs 11-16aa, ab A 3-mm distal and 4-mm mesial peri-implant sulcus of implant no. 15 was detected.

- use of painkillers recommended on the first day and then at the patient's discretion;
- administration of anti-inflammatory analgesic; this provides significant help, preventing the onset of severe swelling or pain. However, caution is needed when there is a history of high blood pressure to avoid a hypertensive crisis.

11.1.5 Apically repositioned partial-thickness flaps

In this technique, the flaps are not elevated completely but are prepared with a 15 or 15c scalpel that runs parallel to the surface of the alveolar ridge. The flap consists of epithelium and part of the connective tissue of the peri-implant mucosa, while the rest of the connective tissue remains attached together with the periosteum to the underlying bone. If bone surgery is necessary, the flap is initially raised as a full-thickness flap. As soon as it is elevated below the alveolar ridge crest, it is split into a partial-thickness flap. This enables better flap adaptation and displacement (Figs 11-17a–f).

Indications for this type of surgery are:

- when there are peri-implant pockets around implants, usually in the mandible;
- when it is not feasible to apply regenerative techniques because of the morphology of the defects or due to heavy smoking;
- when there is a narrow zone of keratinized mucosa that does not allow mucosectomy with external bevel resection even when bone loss is not combined with intraosseous defects (horizontal loss).
- presence of one- or two-wall bony defects, the treatment of which requires ostectomy or osteoplasty.

A contraindication for this type of surgery is when smiling displays the peri-implant mucosa of maxillary anterior implants.

The advantages of the technique are as follows:

- It offers the option of eliminating or greatly reducing peri-implant pocket depth.
- It makes it possible to suture the flap to the periosteum and stabilize it at the desired height. This is beneficial for surgery in the mandible, where a full-thickness flap would result in coronal movement.

The disadvantages of the technique are as follows:

- It requires special attention and skills during preparation. A specially trained dental nurse may be needed to provide support in the operating room.
- Healing is by secondary intention when contact between the buccal and lingual or palatal flaps is not achieved in interdental areas.

The processes for preoperative care and anesthesia are identical to those for the apically repositioned full-thickness flap.

The technique consists of two vertical (releasing) incisions made with a 15 or 15c scalpel, or ophthalmic

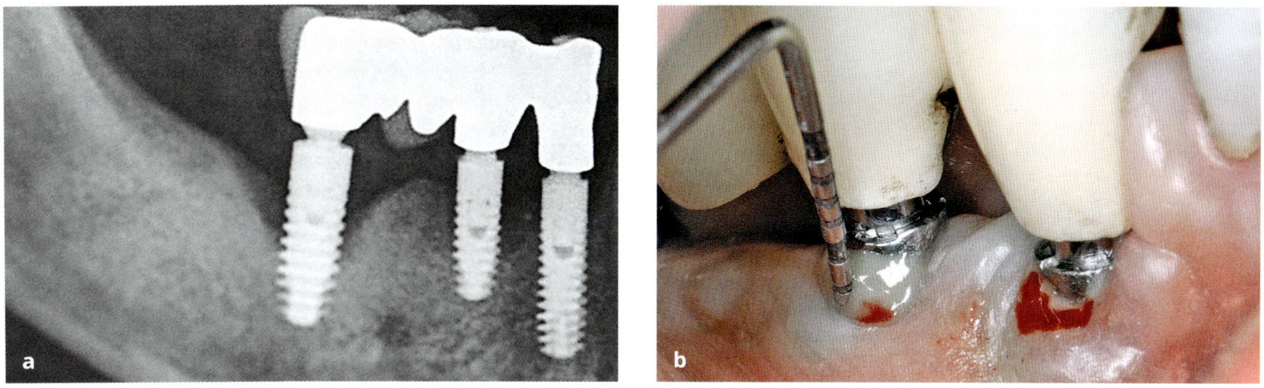

Figs 11-17a, b (a) Radiographic image of a patient with peri-implantitis, in whom osteoplasty and thread smoothing were undertaken. Osteoplasty aimed to eliminate or reduce the depth of the pockets; thread smoothing aimed to reduce the retention of biofilm and improve the ability to remove the microbial load during maintenance care sessions. **(b)** The clinical picture shows the presence of pockets as well as bleeding and pus formation on probing.

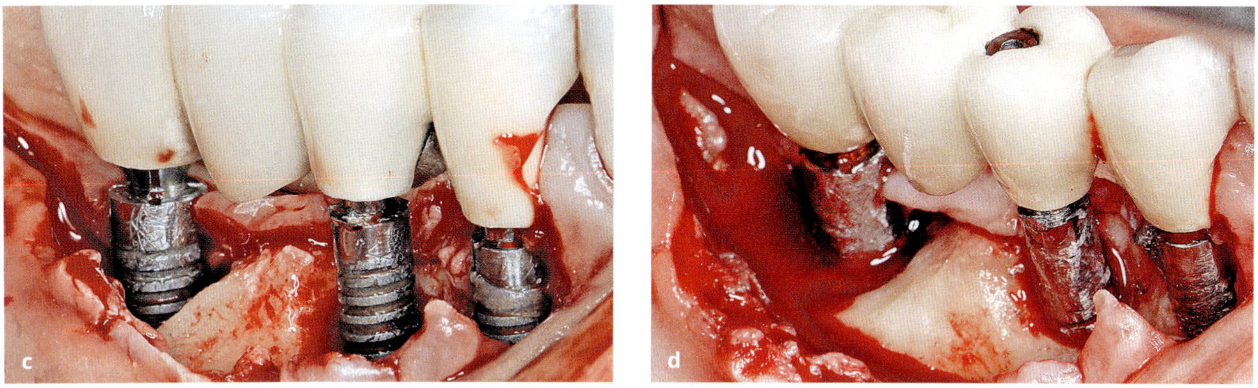

Figs 11-17c, d (c) Intraoperative image showing the resorbed bone crest and implant thread exposure. **(d)** After thread smoothing and polishing and during bone surgery, for apical repositioning of the soft tissues and reduction of peri-implant pocket depth.

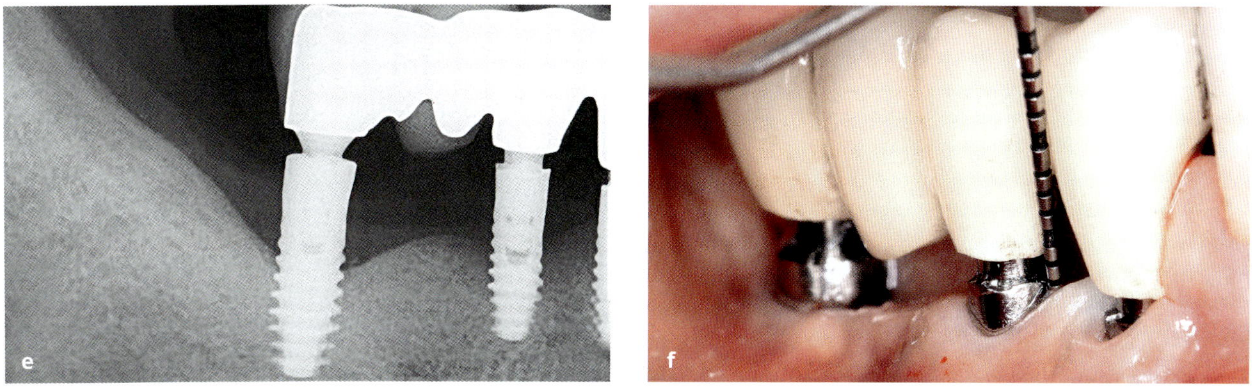

Figs 11-17e, f (e) The radiograph shows the same area 6 years after surgery. **(f)** The clinical picture confirmed the achievement of the goal of bone surgery and thread smoothing and polishing; the therapeutic effect was maintained for 6 years.

blades that extend from the mucogingival junction to the free peri-implant mucosa and define the vertical sides of the flap. The vertical incisions are made, as for any flap, from an apical to a coronal direction to avoid complications. They are joined by a horizontal incision, which is prepared at the margin of the peri-implant mucosa. This incision reaches the bone crest, just as described for the full-thickness flap.

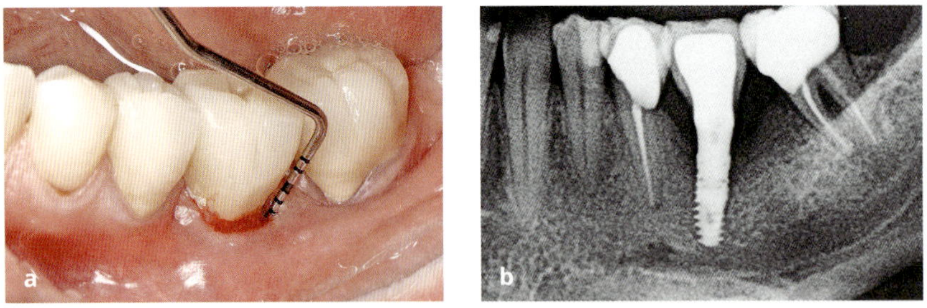

Figs 11-18a, b (a) Clinical image of peri-implantitis showing attachment loss of the peri-implant tissues, a pocket, and inflammation detected by the secretion of blood and pus on probing. **(b)** Radiograph showing angular bony defects around the implant.

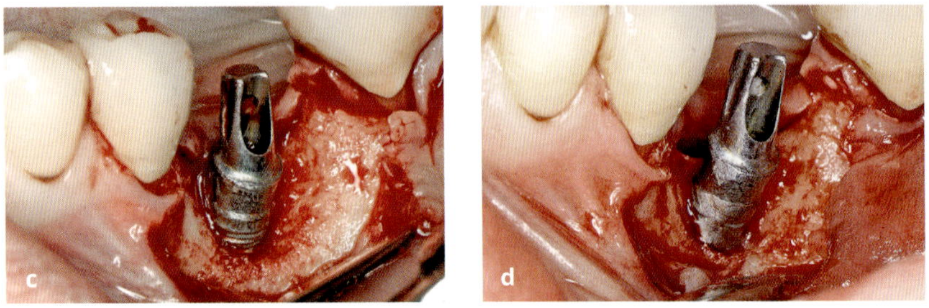

Figs 11-18c, d (c) After elevation of a full-thickness flap, the two-wall bony defect and exposed threads are visible. **(d)** After thread smoothing and polishing to achieve better access to remove the microbial load during the maintenance care program.

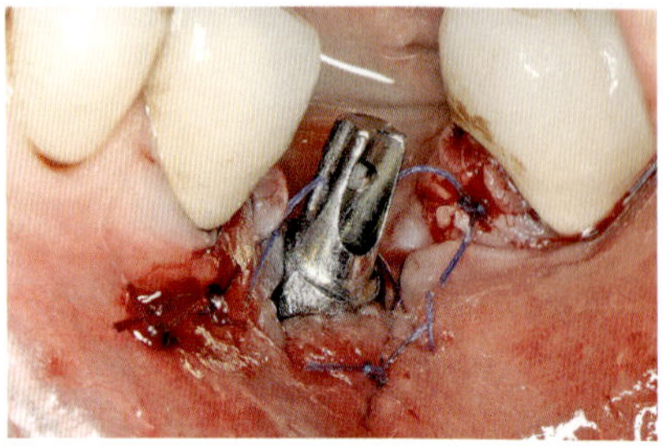

Fig 11-18e Periosteal suturing to achieve tissue healing in an apical position, with the aim of eliminating the pocket.

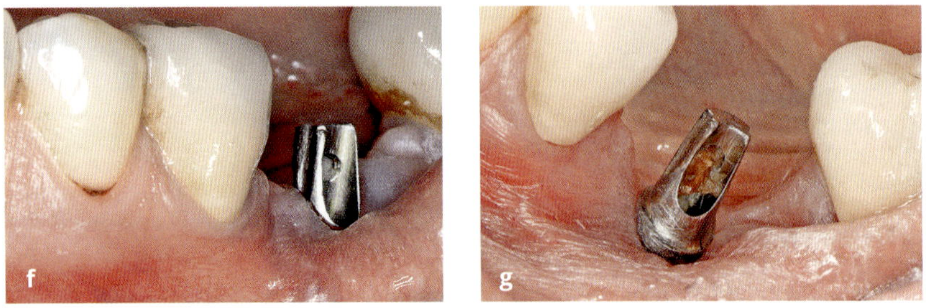

Figs 11-18f, g (f) Before performing apical repositioning of the flap. **(g)** One year after surgery. Significant apical displacement of the peri-implant tissue, which resulted in pocket depth reduction, is evident.

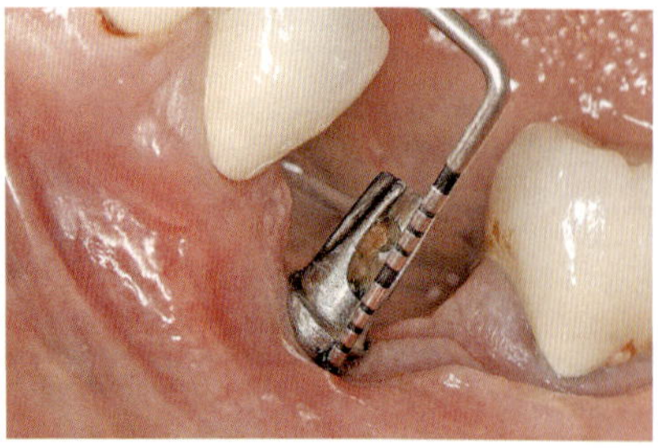

Fig 11-18h Two years after surgery, the crown was removed. A 4-mm peri-implant sulcus was detected. To improve the prognosis, the patient was advised to have a free gingival graft to increase the keratinized mucosa.

When preparing vertical incisions, the tip of the scalpel does not rest on the bone, thus keeping part of the periosteum intact and providing a partial-thickness flap.

Starting from the proximal vertical incision and keeping the blade parallel to the bone, moving from the tip to the margin of the peri-implant mucosa, separation of the flap from the periosteum is begun with the help of surgical forceps. Preparation of a partial-thickness flap is only performed at the buccal site. At the lingual or palatal site, the flap is always prepared as a full-thickness flap. Apical displacement is achieved by removing part of the coronal mucosa after all other procedures are completed and before suturing (Figs 11-18a–h, 11-19a–j, and 11-20a–h).

After all the necessary procedures have been performed as described for an apically repositioned full-thickness flap, a periosteal suture with 5-0 resorbable sutures (PGA or Vicryl) with a P-3 atraumatic needle will stabilize the flap in the desired position.

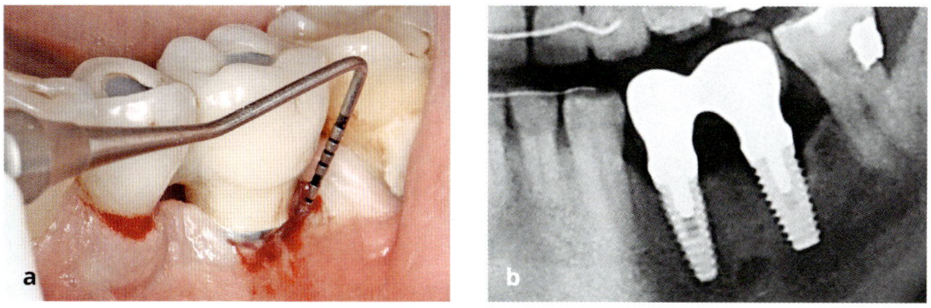

Figs 11-19a, b Clinical and radiographic images of peri-implantitis in an implant placed 7 years prior.

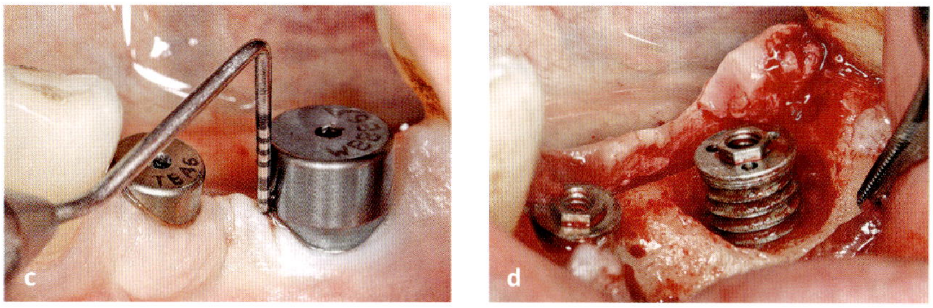

Figs 11-19c, d **(c)** After the inflammation control phase, which was performed according to the modification of the CIST protocol. **(d)** After elevation of a full-thickness flap and the removal of granulation tissue.

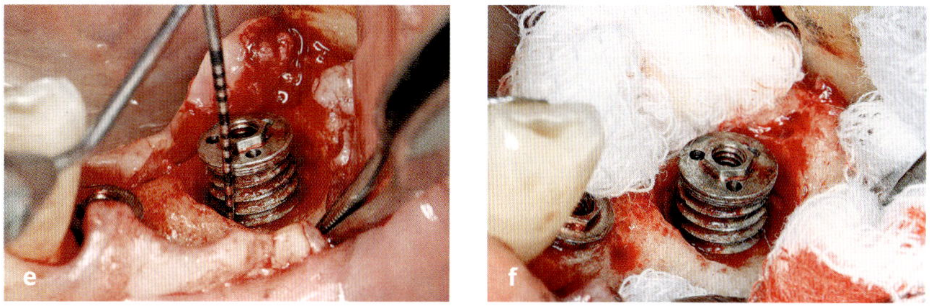

Figs 11-19e, f **(e)** A two-wall intraosseous defect was detected. **(f)** Gauzes were used to prevent dispersion of titanium particles in the surgical field.

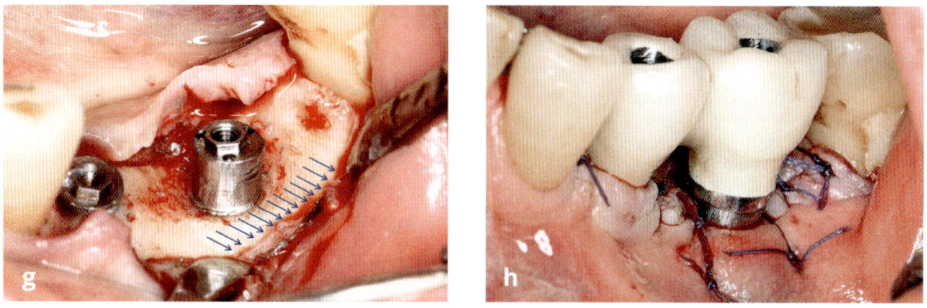

Figs 11-19 g, h **(g)** Thread smoothing and extensive bone surgery followed for better soft tissue adaptation and elimination of peri-implant pockets. The level of transition from a full-thickness to a partial-thickness flap (arrows) can be seen, showing the periosteum adhering to the bone. **(h)** Apical displacement and periosteal suturing.

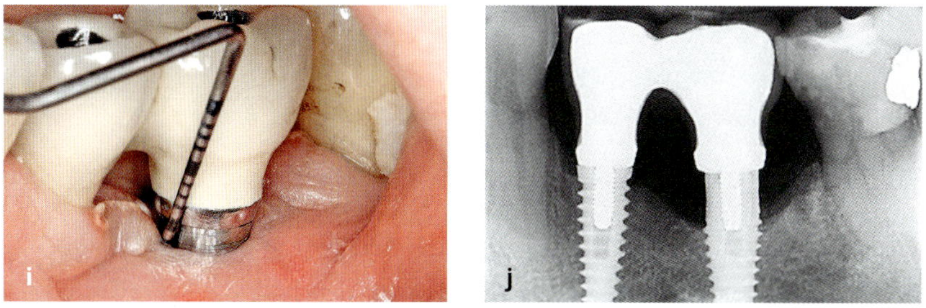

Figs 11-19i, j **(i)** Clinical picture 3 months after surgery. The pockets have disappeared. **(j)** The radiograph shows the smooth implant surface coronal to the bone, which has maintained its osseointegration.

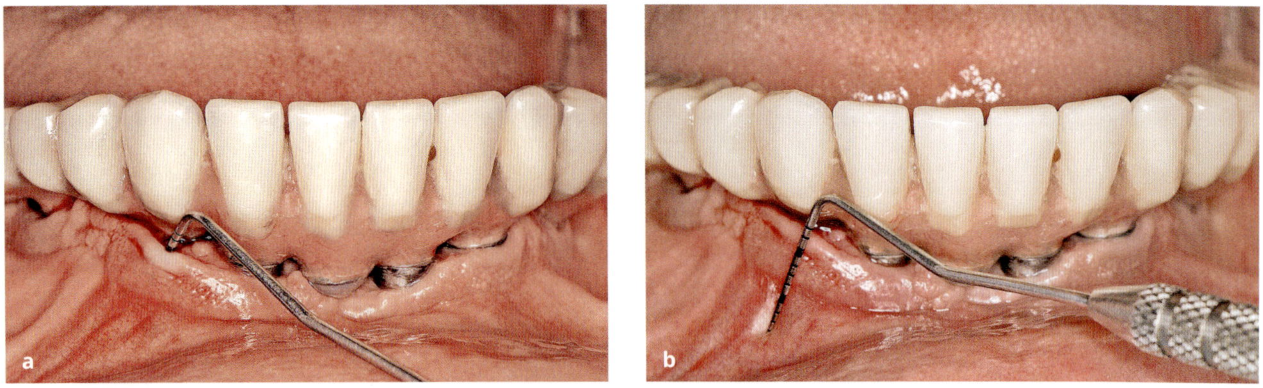

Figs 11-20a, b Clinical pictures of a patient with peri-implantitis with deep pockets. The pocket in implant site no. 43 reached a depth of 10 mm.

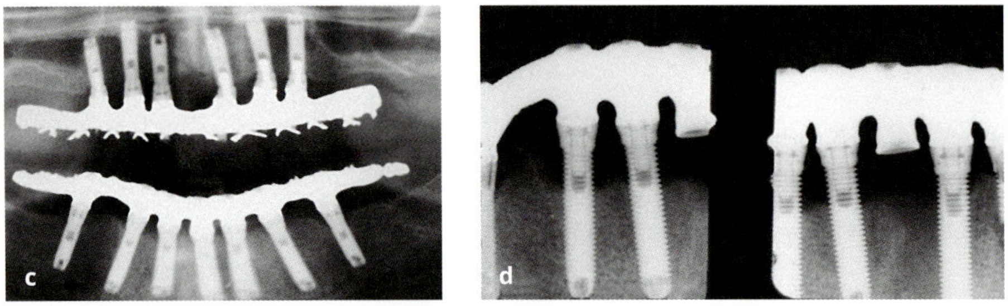

Figs 11-20c, d **(c)** Radiographic image of the patient after placement of the prosthetic restoration. **(d)** Radiographic image 10 years later. It was preceded by loss of the implant in position no. 31. Bone loss and implant threads no longer covered by bone were detected.

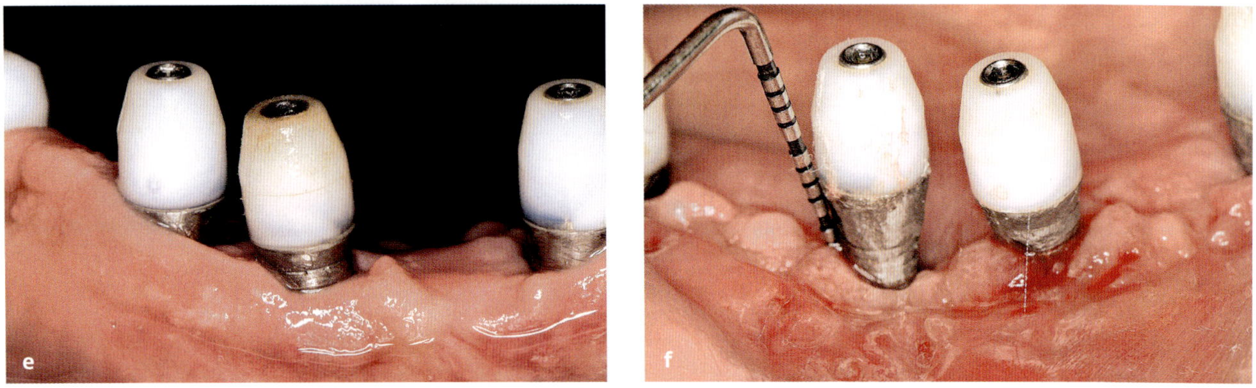

Figs 11-20e, f **(e)** The area from no. 45 to no. 31 before surgery. A flap was elevated, initially with full and then partial thickness, followed by implant thread smoothing and osteoplasty. **(f)** Immediately after suture remova, which took place after 10 days. Apical displacement of the peri-implant mucosa and elimination of the pockets can be observed.

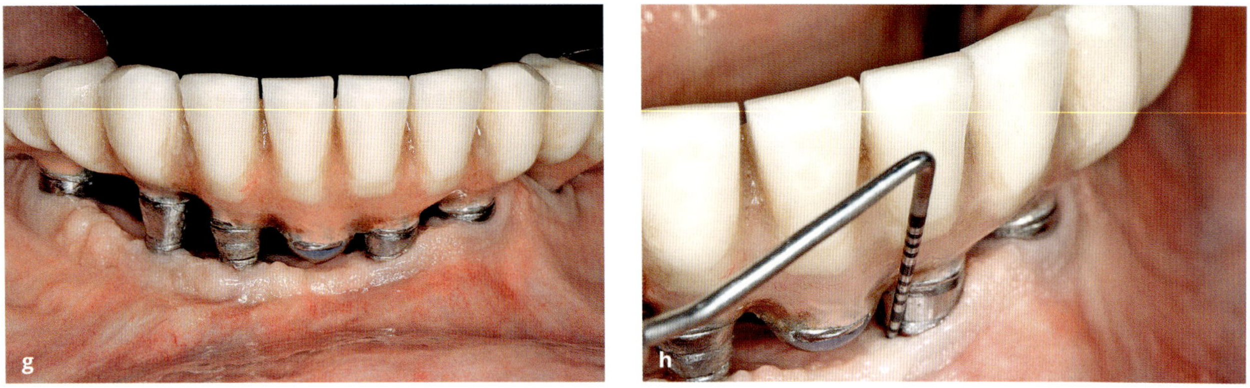

Figs 11-20g, h Clinical images 9 years later, where the absence of peri-implant pockets deeper than 4 mm was ascertained.

11.1.6 Implant thread smoothing and polishing (implantoplasty)

This technique is applied in combination with an access flap, an apically repositioned flap, or regenerative techniques. Application of this method began in 2007[18] when a clinical study found that in the group of patients who, in addition to undergoing resective surgery, had the surface of their implants smoothed, the results of treatment were significantly better compared to the group of patients who did not have their implant threads smoothed.

This is a demanding procedure in which the titanium surface is smoothed with the help of special burs, such as diamond, Arkansas, and tungsten carbide. The aim is to change the topography and eliminate the macroscopically visible protrusions that are typical of implant threads. By applying burs with gradually reduced roughness and completing the process with Arkansas burs, an attempt is made to make the surface of the affected implant as smooth as possible. The result is not always ideal, depending on the anatomy and peculiarities of the area. Another important concern is the difficulty of preventing the spread of titanium particles in the surrounding soft tissue and bone. To avoid this phenomenon, surgery should be performed under very strong surgical suction and, if possible, with the help of two surgical nurses. Isolation of areas other than the surgical field with gauzes impregnated with saline is clinically relevant. In any case, after the procedure is completed, visible particles may be removed with ultrasonic instruments, AIRFLOW, and strong suction.

However, thread smoothing and polishing of implant surfaces is important. Until another more predictable procedure has been devised, the present author believes that thread polishing should be selected and applied when access is needed or in the case of apically repositioned flaps. Use in bone regenerating surgery should be avoided, provided it is possible to disinfect the implant surface with air debriding decontamination.

The main disadvantage of this technique is the level of difficulty and the surgical skills required for its correct application (Figs 11-21a–f).

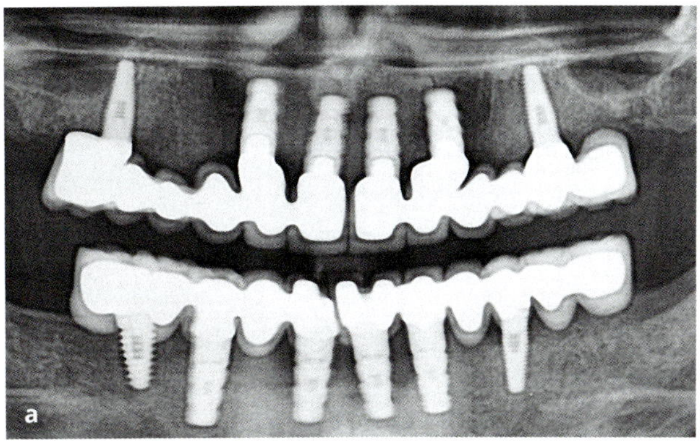

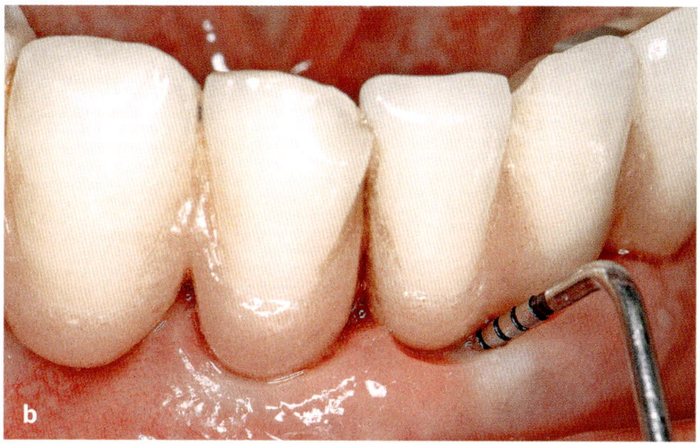

Figs 11-21a, b (a) Radiographic image of a patient with peri-implantitis. **(b)** The clinical picture shows the existence of deep peri-implant pockets reaching 10 mm.

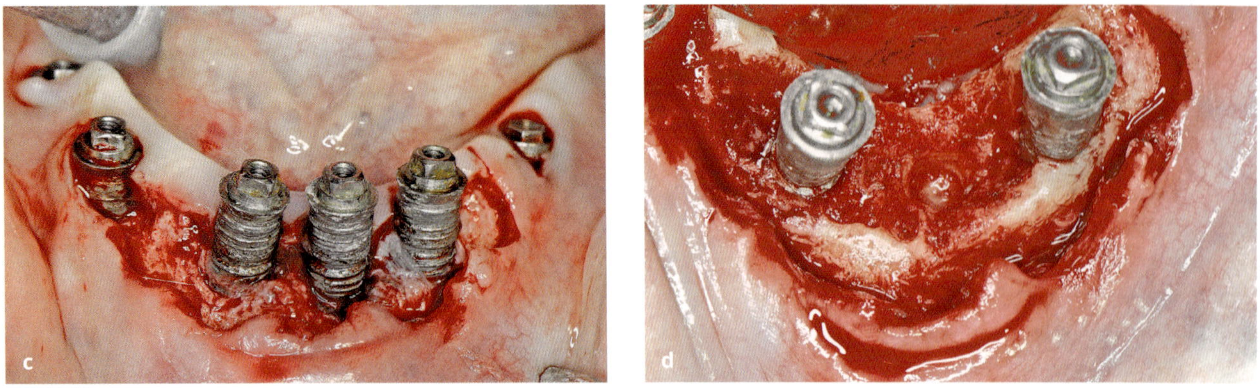

Figs 11-21c, d (c) After elevation of a full- and then partial-thickness mucoperiosteal flap, the implant threads were smoothed and polished. (d) Clinical picture after polishing and explantation of the misplaced implants nos. 31 to 41.

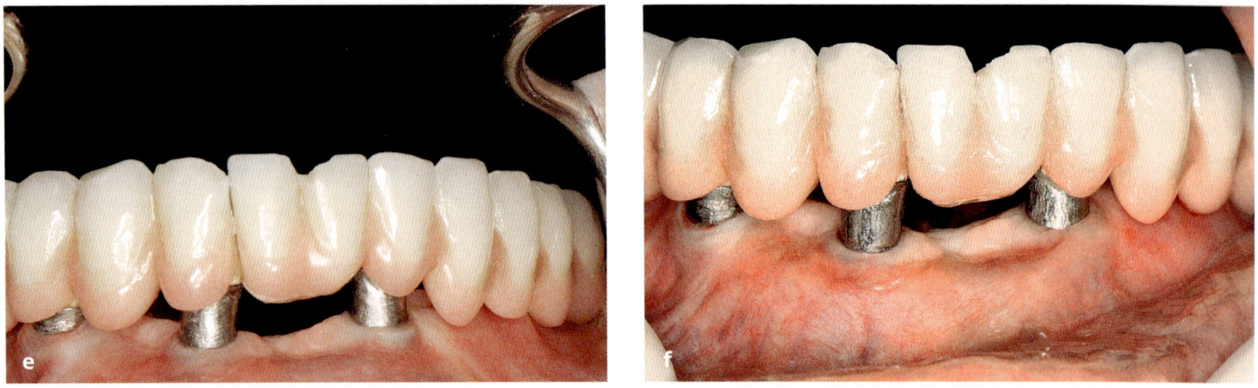

Figs 11-21e, f (e) Clinical picture of the patient when they arrived for their quarterly visit, 1 year after the elevation of an apically repositioned flap. (f) Clinical picture 9 years after surgery. The health and stability of the peri-implant tissues are evident.

References

1. Gupta S, Kaushik M. Peri-implantitis Management from Periodontal Perspective. Saarbrücken: LAP LAMBERT Academic Publishing, 2016.
2. Persson LG, Berglundh T, Lindhe J, Sennerby L. Re-osseointegration after treatment of peri-implantitis at different implant surfaces. An experimental study in the dog. Clin Oral Implants Res 2001;12:595–603.
3. Steinemann SG, Eulenberge J, Maeusli PA, Schroeder A. Adhesion of bone to titanium: biological and biomechanical performance of biomaterials. In: Christel P, Meunier Lee AJC (eds). Advances in Biomaterials. Amsterdam: Elsevier Science Publishers, 1986:409–414.
4. Renvert S, Samuelsson E, Lindahl C, Persson G. Mechanical non-surgical treatment of peri-implantitis: a double-blind randomized longitudinal clinical study. I: clinical results. J Clin Periodontol 2009;36:604–609.
5. Salvi GE, Ramseier CA. Efficacy of patient-administered mechanical and/or chemical plaque control protocols in the management of peri-implant mucositis. A systematic review. J Clin Periodontol 2015;42:187–201.
6. Birang E, Talebi Ardekani MR, Rajabzadeh M, Sarmadi G, Birang R, Gutknecht N. Evaluation of effectiveness of photodynamic therapy with low-level diode laser in nonsurgical treatment of peri-implantitis. J Lasers Med Sci 2017;8:136–142.
7. Yan M, Liu M, Wang M, Yin F, Xia H. The effects of Er:YAG on the treatment of peri-implantitis: a meta-analysis of randomized controlled trials. Lasers Med Sci 2015;30:1843–1853.
8. Sahm N, Becker J, Santel T, Schwarz F. Non-surgical treatment of peri-implantitis using an air-abrasive device or mechanical debridement and local application of chlorhexidine: a prospective, randomized, controlled clinical study. J Clin Periodontol 2011;38:872–878.
9. Schwarz F, Becker K, Bastendorf K-D, et al. Recommendations on the clinical application of air polishing for the management of peri-implant mucositis and peri-implantitis. Quintessence Int 2016;47:293–296.
10. Carcuac O, Derks J, Charalampakis G, Abrahamsson I, Wennström J, Berglundh T. Adjunctive systemic and local antimicrobial therapy in the surgical treatment of peri-im-

plantitis: a randomized controlled clinical trial. J Dent Res 2016;95:50–57.

11. Cha JK, Lee JS, Kim CS. Surgical therapy of peri-implantitis with local minocycline: a 6-month randomized controlled clinical trial. J Dent Res 2019;98:288–295.
12. Heitz-Mayfield LJA, Salvi GE, Mombelli A, Faddy M, Lang NP. Anti-infective surgical therapy of peri-implantitis. A 12-month prospective clinical study. Clin Oral Implants Res 2012;23:205–210.
13. Øen M, Leknes, KN, Lund B, Bunæs DF. The efficacy of systemic antibiotics as an adjunct to surgical treatment of peri-implantitis: a systematic review. BMC Oral Health 2021;21:666.
14. Shibli JA, Ferrari DS, Siroma RS, Figueiredo LC, Faveri M, Feres M. Microbiological and clinical effects of adjunctive systemic metronidazole and amoxicillin in the non-surgical treatment of peri-implantitis: 1 year follow-up. Braz Oral Res 2019;33(suppl 1):e080.
15. Berglundh T, Wennström JL, Lindhe J. Long-term outcome of surgical treatment of peri-implantitis. A 2-11-year retrospective study. Clin Oral Implants Res 2018;29:404–410.
16. Carcuac O, Derks J, Abrahamsson I, Wennström JL, Petzold M, Berglundh T. Surgical treatment of peri-implantitis: 3-year results from a randomized controlled clinical trial. J Clin Periodontol 2017;44:1294–1303.
17. Chan H-L, Lin G-H, Suarez F, MacEachern M, Wang H-L. Surgical management of peri-implantitis: a systematic review and meta-analysis of treatment outcomes. J Periodontol 2014;85:1027–1041.
18. Romeo E, Lops D, Chiapasco M, Ghisolfi M, Vogel G. Therapy of peri-implantitis with resective surgery. A 3-year clinical trial on rough screw-shaped oral implants. Part II: radiographic outcome. Clin Oral Implants Res 2007;18:179–187.
19. Khoury F, Buchmann R. Surgical therapy of peri-implant disease: a 3-year follow-up study of cases treated with 3 different techniques of bone regeneration. J Periodontol 2001;72:1498–1508.
20. Buser D, Dahlin C, Shenk RK. Guided bone regeneration in implant dentistry. Chicago: Quintessence Publishing, 1994.
21. Buser D, Dahlin C, Schenk R. 20 years of guided bone regeneration in implant dentistry in implant dentistry. Chicago: Quintessence Publishing, 2009.
22. Tomasi C, Regidor E, Ortiz-Vigón A, Derks J. Efficacy of reconstructive surgical therapy at peri-implantitis-related bone defects. A systematic review and meta-analysis. J Clin Periodontol 2019;46(suppl 21):340–356.
23. Isler SC, Soysal F, Ceyhanlı T, Bakırarar B, Unsal B. Regenerative surgical treatment of peri-implantitis using either a collagen membrane or concentrated growth factor: a 12-month randomized clinical trial. Clin Implant Dent Relat Res 2018;20:703–712.
24. Renvert S, Roos-Jansåker AM, Persson GR. Surgical treatment of peri-implantitis lesions with or without the use of a bone substitute—a randomized clinical trial. J Clin Periodontol 2018;45:1266–1274.
25. Roccuzzo M, Bonino F, Bonino L, Dalmasso P. Surgical therapy of peri-implantitis lesions by means of a bovine-derived xenograft: comparative results of a prospective study on two different implant surfaces. J Clin Periodontol 2011;38:738–745.
26. Roccuzzo M, Pittoni D, Roccuzzo A, Charrier L, Dalmasso P. Surgical treatment of peri-implantitis intrabony lesions by means of deproteinized bovine bone mineral with 10% collagen: 7-year-results. Clin Oral Implants Res 2017;28:1577–1583.
27. Roos-Jansåker A-M, Persson GR, Lindahl C, Renvert S. Surgical treatment of peri-implantitis using a bone substitute with or without a resorbable membrane: a 5-year follow-up. J Clin Periodontol 2014;41:1108–1114.
28. Schwarz F, Sahm N, Schwarz K, Becker J. Impact of defect configuration on the clinical outcome following surgical regenerative therapy of peri-implantitis. J Clin Periodontol 2010;37:449–455.
29. Schwarz F, Sahm N, Iglhaut G, Becker J. Impact of the method of surface debridement and decontamination on the clinical outcome following combined surgical therapy of peri-implantitis: a randomized controlled clinical study. J Clin Periodontol 2011;38:276–284.
30. Wetzel AC, Vlassis J, Caffesse RG, Hämmerle CH, Lang NP. Attempts to obtain re-osseointegration following experimental peri-implantitis in dogs. Clin Oral Implants Res 1999;19:111–119.
31. Hämmerle CH, Chiantella GC, Karring T, Lang NP. The effect of deproteinized bovine bone mineral on bone regeneration around titanium dental implants. Clin Oral Implants Res 1998;9:151–162.
32. Roccuzzo A, Stähli A, Monje A, Sculean A, Salvi GE. Peri-implantitis: a clinical update on prevalence and surgical treatment outcomes. J Clin Med 2021;10:1107.
33. Bertl K, Stavropoulos A. A mini review on non-augmentative surgical therapy of peri-implantitis—What is known and what are the future challenges? Front Dent Med 2021;2:659361.
34. Sykaras N, Triplett RG, Nunn ME, Iacopino AM, Opperman LA. Effect of recombinant human bone morphogenetic protein-2 on bone regeneration and osseointegration of dental implants. Clin Oral Implants Res 2001;12:339–349.
35. Roffi A, Filardo G, Kon E, Marcacci M. Does PRP enhance bone integration with grafts, graft substitutes, or implants? A systematic review. BMC Musculoskelet Disord 2013;14:330.
36. Weibrich G, Hansen T, Kleis W, Buch R, Hitlerd WE. Effect of platelet concentration in platelet-rich plasma on peri-implant bone regeneration. Bone 2004;34:665–671.
37. Petkovic-Curcin A, Zeljic K, Cikota-Aleksic B, Dakovic D, Tatic Z, Magic Z. Association of cytokine gene polymorphism with peri-implantitis risk. Int J Oral Maxillofac Implants 2017;32:e241–e248.
38. Barfeie A, Wilson J, Rees J. Implant surface characteristics and their effect on osseointegration. Br Dent J 2015;218:E9.
39. Novaes AB Jr, de Souza SL, de Barros RRM, Pereira KKY, Iezzi G, Plattelli A. Influence of implant surfaces on osseointegration. Braz Dent J 2010;21:471–481.

40. Dank A, Aartman IHA, Wismeijer D, Tahmaseb A. Effect of dental implant surface roughness in patients with a history of periodontal disease: a systematic review and meta-analysis. Int J Implant Dent 2019;5:12.
41. Papadopoulos CA, Vouros I, Menexes G, Konstantinidis A. The utilization of a diode laser in the surgical treatment of peri-implantitis. A randomized clinical trial. Clin Oral Investig 2015;19:1851–1860.
42. Ashnagar S, Nowzari H, Nokhbatolfoghahaei H, Yaghoub Zadeh B, Chiniforush N, Choukhachi Zadeh N. Laser treatment of peri-implantitis: a literature review. J Lasers Med Sci 2014;5:153–162.
43. Bach G, Neckel C, Mall C, Krekeler G. Conventional versus laser-assisted therapy of peri-implantitis: a five-year comparative study. Implant Dent 2000;9:247–251.
44. Grzech-Leśniak K, Sculean A, Gašpirc B. Laser reduction of specific microorganisms in the periodontal pocket using Er:YAG and Nd:YAG lasers: a randomized controlled clinical study. Lasers Med Sci 2018;33:1461–1470.
45. Świder K, Dominiak M, Grzech-Leśniak K, Matys J. Effect of different laser wavelengths on periodontopathogens in peri-implantitis: a review of in vivo studies. Microorganisms 2019;7:189.
46. Takei HH, Han TJ, Carranza FA Jr, Kenney EB, Levkowic V. Flap technique for periodontal bone implants. Papilla preservation technique. J Periodontol 1985;56:204–210.
47. Cortellini P, Prato GP, Tonetti MS. The modified papilla preservation technique. A new surgical approach for interproximal regenerative procedures. J Periodontol 1995;66:261–266.
48. Vrotsos IA, Karoussis IK. Peridodontology-Implantology. Athens: BETA Publications, 2016.
49. Mann M, Parmar D, Walmsley AD, Lea SC. Effect of plastic-covered ultrasonic scalers on titanium implant surfaces. Clin Oral Implants Res 2012;23:76–82.
50. De Tapia B, Valles C, Ribeiro-Amaral T, et al. The adjunctive effect of a titanium brush in implant surface decontamination at peri-implantitis surgical regenerative interventions: a randomized controlled clinical trial. J Clin Periodontol 2019;46:586–596.
51. Valderrama P, Wilson TG Jr. Detoxification of implant surfaces affected by peri-implant disease: an overview of surgical methods. Int J Dent 2013;2013:740680.
52. Romanos G, Ko H-H, Froum S, Tarnow D. The use of CO_2 laser in the treatment of peri-implantitis. Photomed Laser Surg 2009;27:381–386.
53. Romanos GE, Nentwig GH. Regenerative therapy of deep peri-implant infrabony defects after CO_2 laser implant surface decontamination. Int J Periodontics Restorative Dent 2008;28:245–255.
54. Kreisler M, Götz H, Duschner H. Effect of Nd:YAG Ho:YAG, Er:YAG, CO_2, and GaAIAs laser irradiation on surface properties of endosseous dental implants. Int J Oral Maxillofac Implants 2002;17:202–211.
55. Fekrazad R, Karamifar K, Bahador A. Comparison of antibacterial effect of photodynamic therapy using indocyanine green (Emundo) with 2% metronidazole and 2% chlorhexidine gel on Porphyromonas gingivalis (an in-vitro study). Photodiagnosis Photodyn Ther 2016;15:28–33.
56. Chiang C-P, Hsieh O, Tai W-C, Chen Y-J, Chang P-C. Clinical outcomes of adjunctive indocyanine green-diode lasers therapy for treating refractory periodontitis: a randomized controlled trial with in vitro assessment. J Formos Med Assoc 2019;119:652–659.
57. Chala M, Anagnostaki E, Mylona V, Chalas A, Parker S, Lynch E. Adjunctive use of lasers in peri-implant mucositis and peri-implantitis treatment: a systematic review. Dent J 2020;8:68.
58. Sarmiento HL, Norton M, Korostoff J, Ko KI, Fiorellini JP. Surgical Alternatives for Treating Peri-implantitis. Int J Periodontics Restorative Dent 2018;38:665–671.
59. Reddy VK, Parthasarathy H, Lochana P. Evaluating the clinical and esthetic outcome of apically positioned flap technique in augmentation of keratinized gingiva around dental implants. Contemp Clin Dent 2013;4:319–324.

12 Corrective Phase of Therapy: Regenerative Techniques

S. Sylvestros, I.K. Karoussis

Regeneration of peri-implant hard and soft tissues lost as a result of peri-implantitis improves the prognosis of both implants and implant restorations. It is usually esthetically advantageous compared to the surgical techniques mentioned in Chapter 11 and is the ultimate goal of therapeutic approaches.[1]

Regeneration is defined as "the healing mechanism by which the damaged tissue is replaced by new tissue, identical in morphology and function with the lost one".[2]

Most interventions and techniques applied in peri-implantitis treatment, whether surgical or nonsurgical, lead to healing patterns of repair. The latter is healing whereby damaged tissue is replaced by tissue with a different morphology, which does not perform the desired function of its damaged predecessor. It is usually healing by scar tissue.[2]

After the trauma caused during surgery, erosion of blood vessels leads to bleeding and blood clot formation. Activation of different cells within the wound and adjacent tissues begins immediately. The order and control of the following procedures, such as chemotaxis, proliferation, differentiation, and synthesis of intercellular fluids, are determined by growth factors. The effect of those in the healing process are the same for all tissues.[2]

The goals of regenerative procedures in the treatment of peri-implantitis are:[3]

- accessibility for the most efficient removal of biofilms from the surface of the implant and subsequent elimination of inflammation;
- improvement of clinical attachment levels;
- reduction of peri-implant pocket depth;
- partial or complete bone filling of peri-implant defects;
- ideally, reestablishment of osseointegration.

Today, the formation of a new attachment with the application of guided bone regeneration (GBR) in periodontal three- or four-wall intrabony defects is a predictable procedure.[4] On the other hand, reestablishment of osseointegration is not predictable and needs further research.[5]

In surgical procedures aimed at the regeneration of peri-implant tissues, the following are included:[6,7]

- bone grafts;
- GBR;
- autologous platelet concentrates;
- combinations of the above (Fig 12-1).

The effectiveness of regenerative procedures is evaluated both clinically, with assessment of the clinical attachment level, and radiographically, by comparing the level of presumptive bone–implant contact with radiographs taken before surgery and at least 6 months thereafter. The ideal method of evaluating effectiveness is through histology. However, this can only be used in research studies. It is clear that the improvement of clinical parameters does not necessarily imply regeneration at the histologic level. Indications are shown in Fig 12-2 and are as follows:[8]

- circumferential four-wall intrabony defects;
- three-wall intrabony defects;
- existence of bone dehiscence (Fig 12-3a–i).

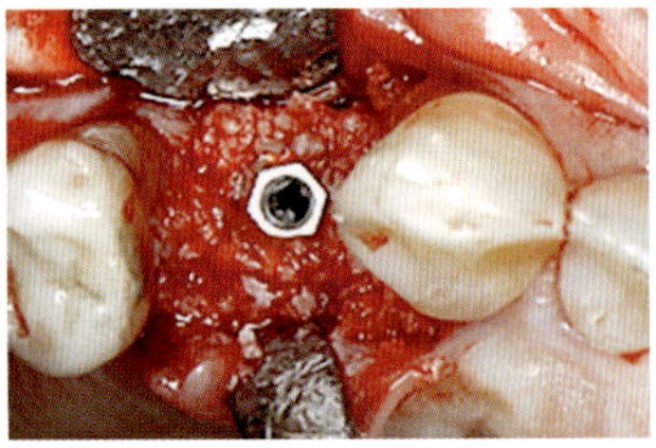

Fig 12-1 Mixed xenograft with autologous platelet concentrate ("sticky bone").

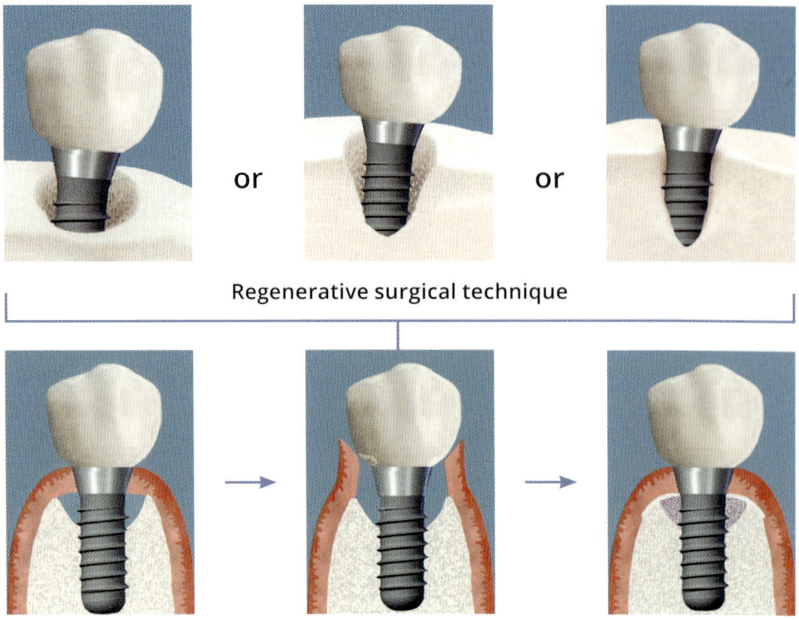

Fig 12-2 In intrabony defects with three or four walls, the regenerative technique includes full-thickness flap elevation, removal of dental biofilm, placement of bone graft and membrane, which may require stabilization with titanium pins or sutures, and finally suturing.

Contraindications include the following[8]:

- one- or two-wall intrabony defects;
- intrabony defects with shallow depth (< 4 mm) or wide angles (> 25 degrees);
- implant mobility; in this case, the implant must be removed;
- inability to completely remove biofilms and eliminate inflammation;
- patients with limited ability to cooperate and low oral hygiene levels;
- heavy smokers;
- uncontrolled diabetes mellitus.

Preoperative and presurgical care includes the following:

- performance of stages A and B of the cumulative interceptive supportive therapy protocol (oral hygiene instructions, AIRFLOW and PERIOFLOW (EMS Dental, Nyon, Switzerland), mechanical biofilm removal) or use of laser for bactericidal control prior to GBR. The latter should be performed at least 2 weeks before the day of surgery so that the tissues have been given time to heal from cause-related therapy;
- checking of the effectiveness of oral hygiene;
- removal of implant-supported prosthetic restoration when feasible;
- radiographic examination and evaluation of the morphology of the defect.

12.1 Operative and surgical phase

After administration of local anesthesia, which is done as for the apically repositioned flap, intrasulcular incisions are made with a no. 15 or 15c scalpel or ophthalmic blades, retaining all the soft tissues buccally, and lingually and palatally. Maintenance of the interdental papillae is essential. When repositioning the flap, complete covering of the regenerated area and achievement of healing by primary intention are anticipated. An Orban knife (Hu-Friedy, Chicago, IL, USA) is used to separate soft tissues with junctional epithelium on the one hand and connective tissue on the other. The incision starts from the most distal point of the defect and is directed toward the mesial aspect. In flaps without vertical incisions, an envelope flap is prepared. The flap should be extended approximately to a distance of two teeth mesial and distal to the area to be regenerated. This flap design ensures an adequate field of vision and easy handling, and avoids tearing of the flap during surgical manipulations, which may create flap dehiscence, with consequent bleeding, postoperative pain, and swelling, thus jeopardizing the outcome of the regenerative procedure.

To achieve better access to the area, a vertical incision may be prepared. In the anterior maxilla, a vertical incision is made distally and always only on the buccal aspect to avoid injury to the greater

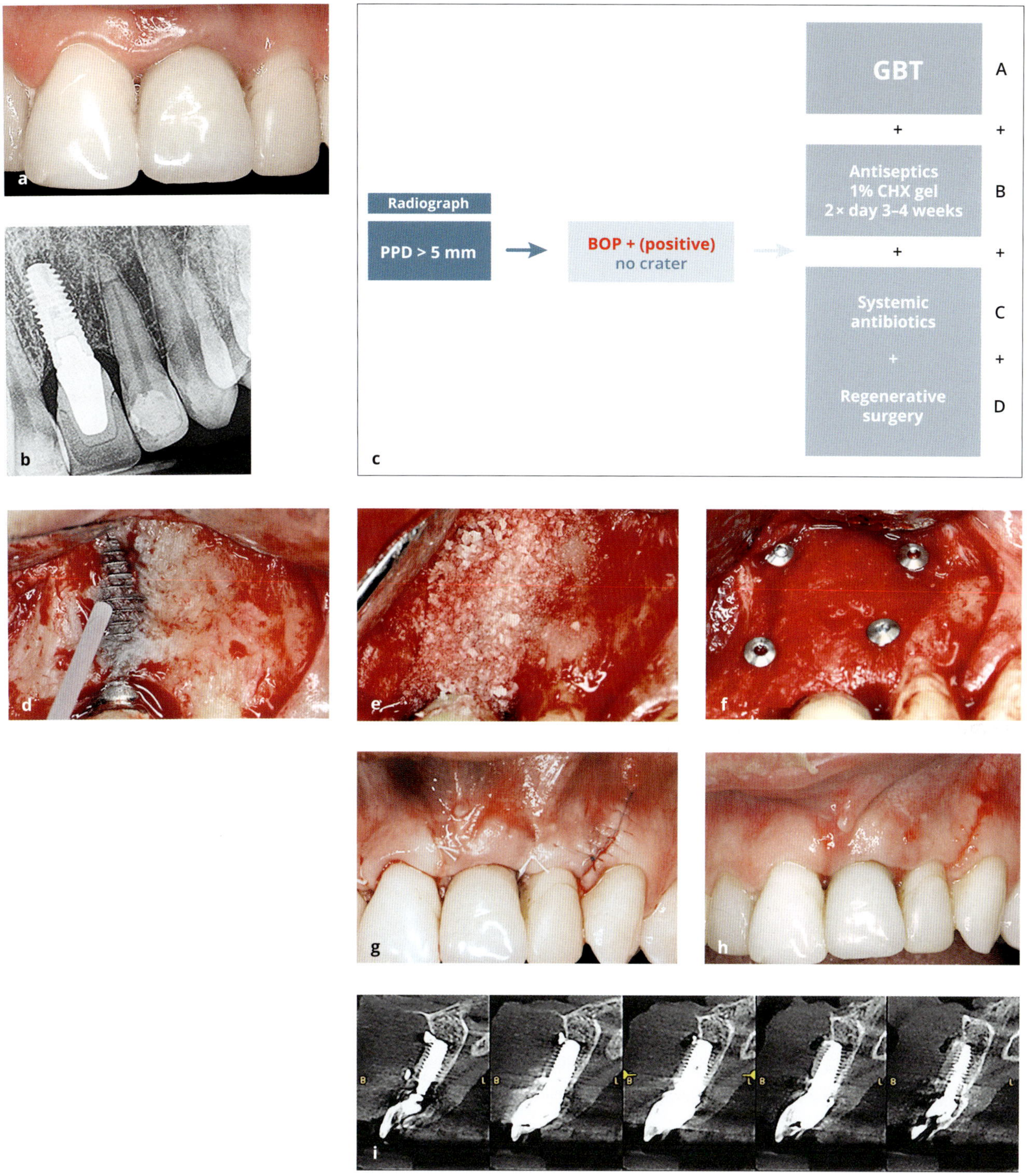

Figs 12-3a–i (a and b) Initial clinical and radiographic images of implant no. 21 where a peri-implant pocket was found on the buccal surface. **(c)** Proposed approach to cases suitable for bone regeneration according to clinical data. **(d)** After flap elevation, bone dehiscence was observed. Disinfection of the implant surface was performed using an Er:YAG laser (2,940 nm) in 40 mJ (pulse) and 20 Hz (control) settings. Bioactivation was carried out with the same laser to increase cell proliferation and productivity of osteoblasts, with settings of 300 mJ and 20 Hz. **(e)** Placement of the xenograft was followed by covering of the bony defect. **(f)** The implant was covered with a resorbable collagen membrane, which was stabilized with titanium pins. **(g)** Suturing of the flap was performed with external horizontal 4-0 polytetrafluoroethylene mattress sutures and 6-0 polyamide single sutures. **(h)** Buccal view of the area after suture removal, 2 weeks after surgery. **(i)** Radiographic image of the defect 6 months after surgery. Note the buccal surface of the implant covered with bone. BOP, bleeding on probing; CHX, chlorhexidine; GBT, guided biofilm therapy; PPD, pocket probing depth.

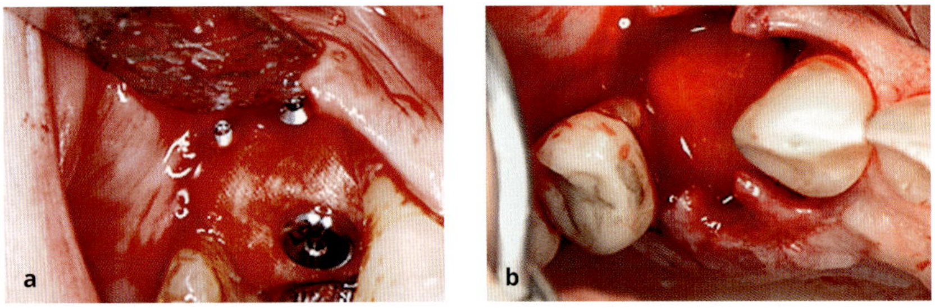

Figs 12-4a, b (a) The xenograft was covered with a resorbable collagen membrane. The membrane was fixed with a cover screw and titanium pins. **(b)** The regenerative materials were covered with membranes from autologous platelet concentrate. The photographs are the continuation of Fig 12-1.

palatine nerve. The vertical incision is made respective to a tooth or implant distal to the last element designed for regeneration. The vertical incision is made as previously described in the apically repositioned full-thickness flap. This is followed by flap elevation, complete removal of granulation tissue, and disinfection of the implant surface. Ideally, this is accomplished using AIRFLOW, or other mechanical means.[9,10] Regardless of the type of technique the clinician employs, the area should be rinsed with sterile saline. If the implant prosthesis is to be removed at this stage, after disinfecting the implant surfaces, a cover screw will be placed.

The bone graft is then prepared by mixing it with saline or with autologous platelet concentrate. The result is a thick mixture known as sticky bone. For bone graft placement, a Lucas surgical curette or a P24G elevator (Hu-Friedy) are used. Any quantity left after the bone graft has been placed is pressed lightly with a bone condenser of appropriate size, depending on the defect, to achieve condensation. The defect is filled up to the alveolar crest. Then, the membrane is prepared to cover the entire bony defect and extend at least 3 mm around its borders. The membrane should be at least 1 mm from the adjacent teeth. Membranes that may be used are:[3,11]

- resorbable collagen membranes;
- nonresorbable polytetrafluoroethylene (PTFE) membranes (expanded PTFE or high-density PTFE) with titanium reinforcement;
- nonresorbable expanded PTFE or high-density PTFE without titanium reinforcement;
- titanium membranes;
- membranes derived from the autologous platelet concentrate alone or in combination with saline (Figs 12-4a, b).

The membrane is placed so that it covers the bone graft and defect; thus, cells from the soft tissues (connective tissue and epithelium) cannot colonize the area of the defect. Membrane stabilization is achieved with titanium or absorbable pins by suturing the palatal flap, or whenever feasible, with the cover screw or healing abutment. A periosteal incision is made to cut the muscle fibers to mobilize the flaps and achieve as much coronal displacement as possible. Finally, the flap is sutured so that it completely covers the membrane. Whenever possible, the implant with its cover screw is fully covered to achieve submucosal healing.[12] In these cases, before the procedure, a provisional restoration has been manufactured (Figs 12-5a–j).

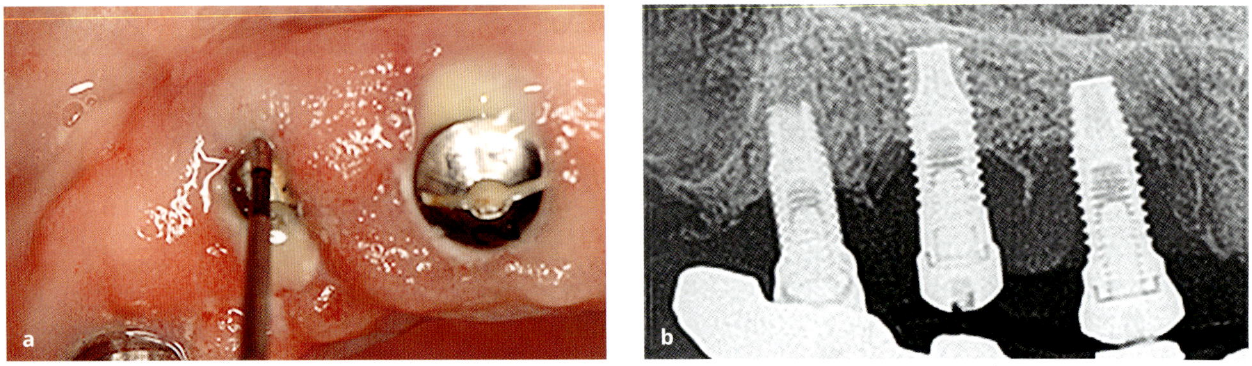

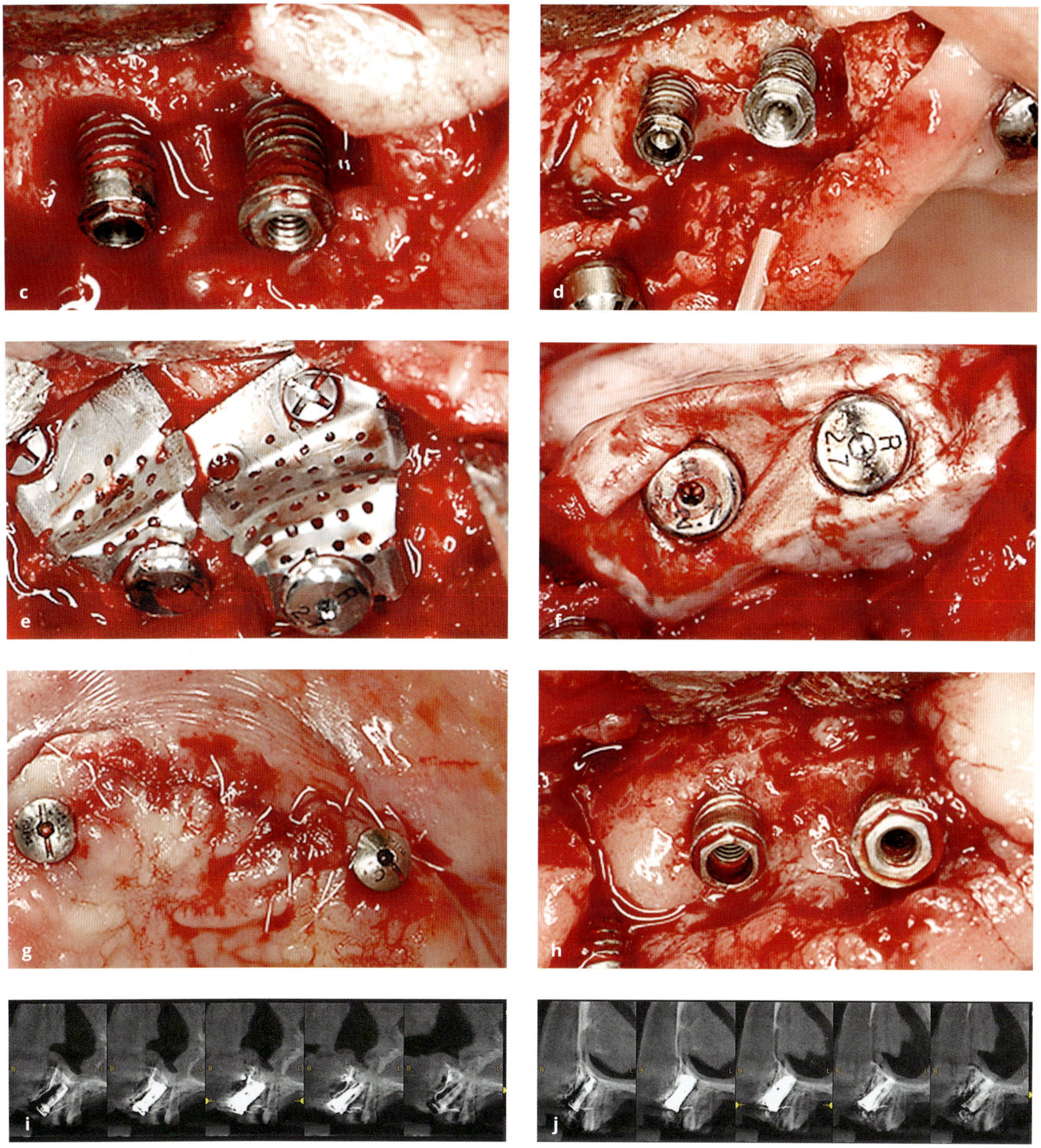

Figs 12-5a–j **(a)** Clinical picture of implants nos. 12 and 13, with exudate and increased pocket depth. Removal of the implant-supported partial denture had already taken place. **(b)** Initial radiograph of implants nos. 12 and 13, where significant bone loss is evident. **(c)** After flap elevation and removal of the healing abutments. Significant bone loss had occurred and many threads had been exposed to the pocket environment. **(d)** After removal of the granulation tissue, the surface of implants was disinfected. A bone defect is not ideal for guided bone regeneration because there is insufficient support for a membrane unless it is a titanium or titanium-reinforced membrane. **(e)** Xenograft placement followed, and a nonresorbable titanium membrane was placed in each implant. Membranes were fixed with the help of titanium pins and cover screws. **(f)** After placement of a second resorbable collagen membrane to cover the nonresorbable membranes. The membrane was fixed again using cover screws. **(g)** This was followed by suturing of the flap with external horizontal mattress and single sutures with 4-0 polytetrafluoroethylene sutures. **(h)** Buccal view of the area after flap elevation to remove the nonresorbable titanium membranes and pins. Note the newly formed tissue. **(i)** Computed tomography scan immediately after surgery. The membrane and titanium pins can be distinguished. **(j)** Computed tomography scan 8 months after surgery. Newly formed bone can be seen on the buccal surface.

In the middle of the flaps, a horizontal mattress suture is used to bring the bases of the flaps together and, at the same time, to achieve coronal displacement with a 4-0 suture. Then, modified vertical mattress sutures are placed mesially and distally; modified horizontal mattress sutures are used in edentulous ridges, with 5-0 sutures. The vertical incisions are sutured with 5-0 or 6-0 sutures (Figs 12-6a–j).

Monofilament sutures are advantageous; the options of choice are nonresorbable PTFE (Cytoplast, Osteogenics, Lubbock, TX, USA), polyamide (Seralon, Serag-Wiessner, Naila, Germany), or resorbable polydioxanone monofilament sutures (Monosorb, Yavo, Belchatow, Poland). With regard to braided sutures, those most commonly used are resorbable ones made from polylactic acid (Stoma, Emmingen-Liptingen, Germany) (Figs 12-7a, b). Finally, the provisional restoration is placed if submucosal healing has been achieved.

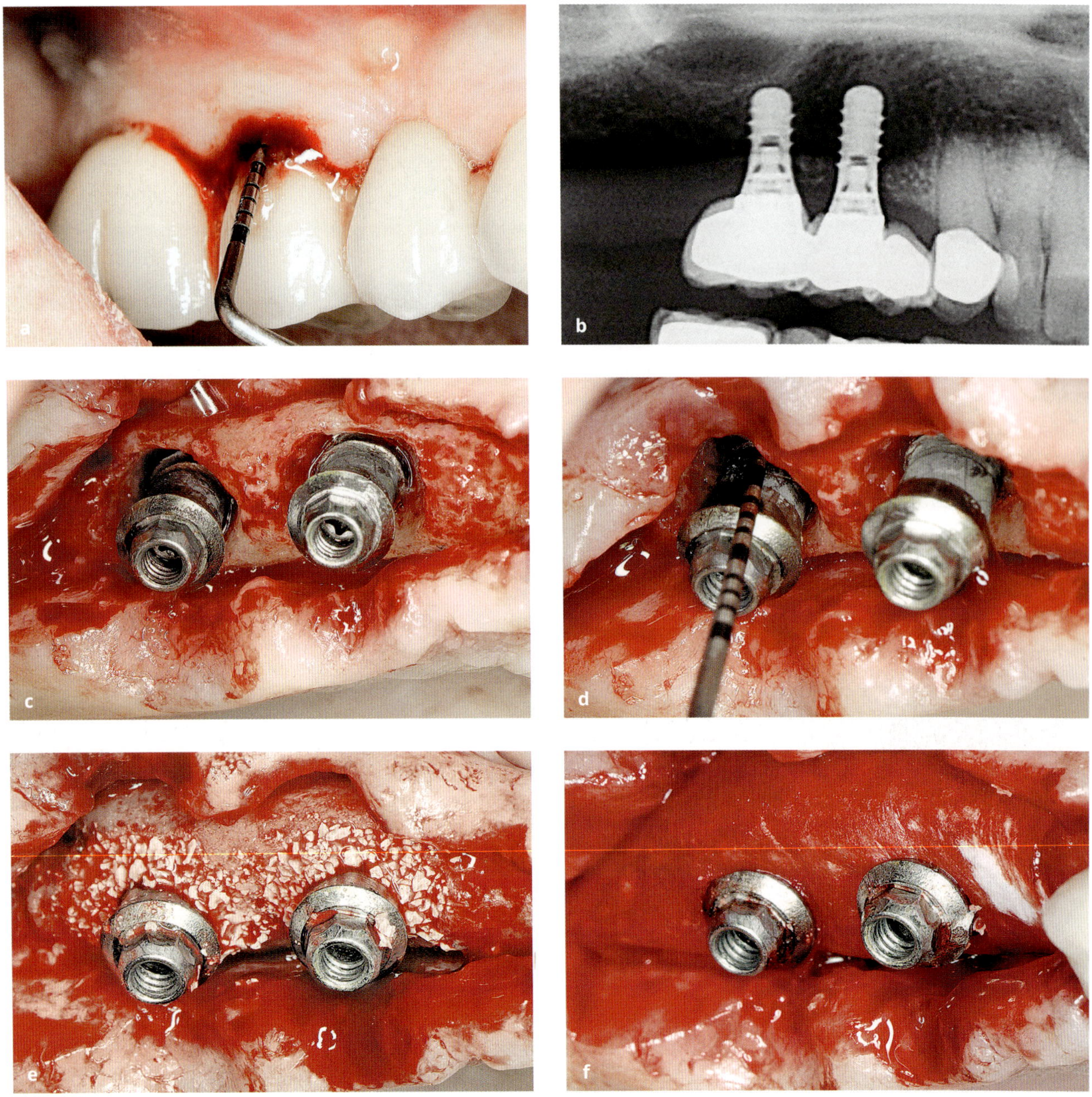

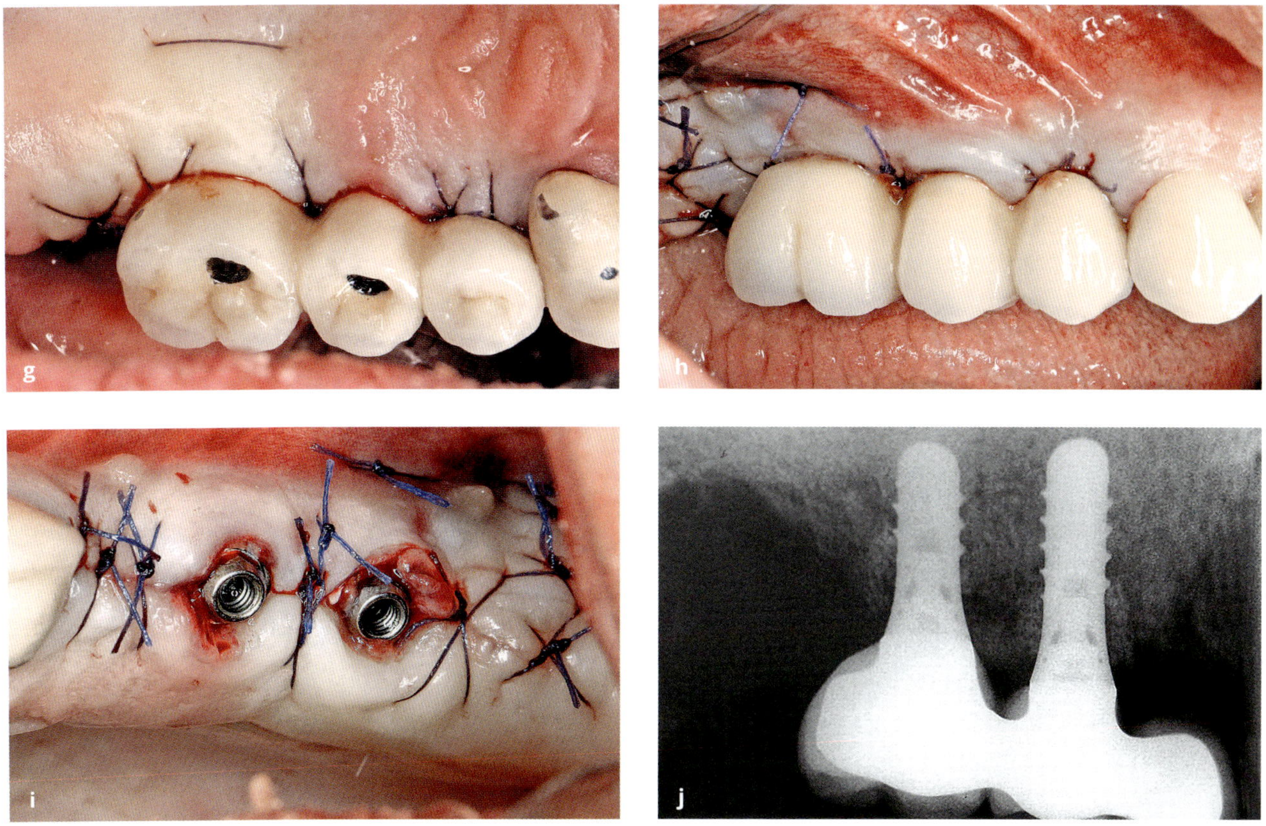

Figs 12-6a–j **(a)** Clinical picture of peri-implantitis. Peri-implant pockets and bleeding on probing were diagnosed. **(b)** Radiographic examination showed bone loss and saucer-shaped defects. **(c)** One month after the application of steps A and B, after flap elevation and under perioperative antibiotic coverage of amoxicillin and 625 mg clavulanate three times daily for 7 days; the exposed threads are visible. **(d)** Intrabony defects (four walls with sufficient depth) direct the selected surgical technique. **(e and f)** A bovine xenograft and a collagen membrane were placed. **(g to i)** After suturing. The horizontal mattress suture can be seen at the base of the flaps; it moves and holds the soft tissues coronally. **(j)** Radiographic image of the defect 6 months after surgery.

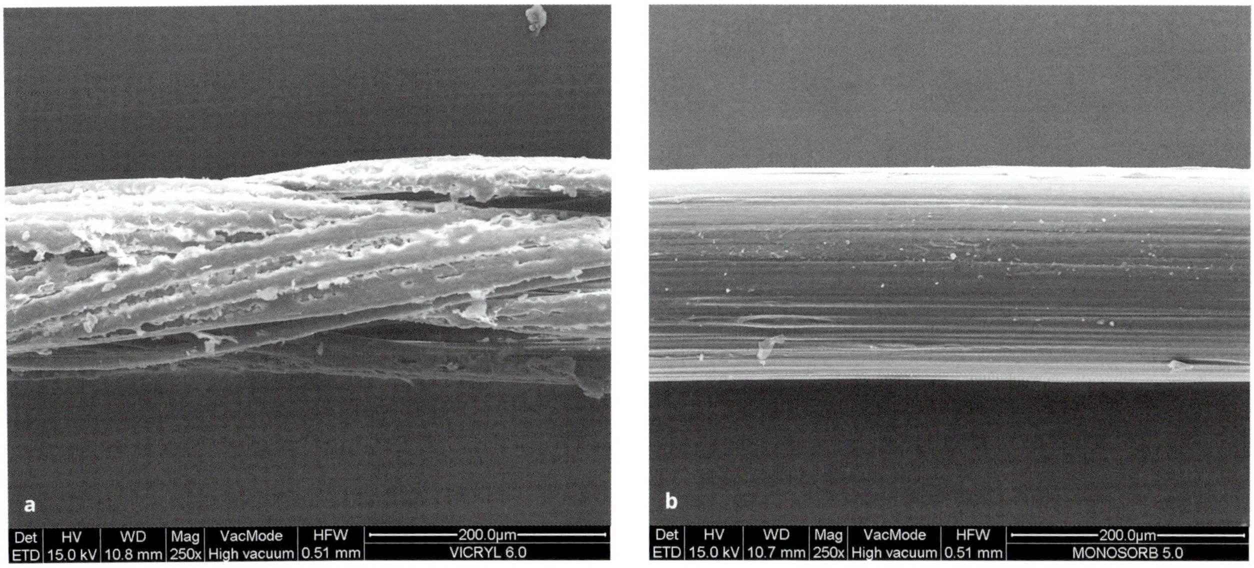

Figs 12-7a, b Because of their microstructure, braided sutures lead to higher bacterial concentration compared to monofilament sutures.

12.2 Postoperative and postsurgical care

The administration of perioperative antibiotics may be necessary in regenerative procedures.[13] The present authors recommend administering amoxicillin and clavulanic acid (625 mg). The patient receives a loading dose of 1,250 mg 1 hour before surgery followed by 62 mg every 8 hours for 7 days. In patients with a penicillin allergy, a broad-spectrum alternative is administered, preferably clindamycin. In this case, the loading dose is 600 mg 1 hour before surgery and then 300 mg every 6 hours for 7 days.

Painkillers are recommended on the first day and then as needed by the patient. The administration of anti-inflammatory analgesics provides significant assistance, preventing the appearance of swelling or pain. The present authors recommend using 0.1% to 0.2% chlorhexidine solution twice per day for 4 weeks. The patient should then apply 1% chlorhexidine gel to the area operated on for another 4 weeks.

Patients are reexamined every week for the first 2 months, and then once per month for the next 6 months. At each visit, dental biofilms are removed with AIRFLOW if transmucosal healing was planned. Alternatively, biofilm can be removed with special ultrasonic polyetheretherketone tips. Sutures are removed after 2 weeks.

If a nonreworkable membrane was used, it is removed 4 to 6 weeks after its placement. The procedure for its removal is performed with a small incision and careful handling, so as not to injure the newly formed tissue under the membrane.

A periodontal probe may be used 6 months after the procedure. Bleeding on probing, pocket depth, and clinical attachment levels are assessed. Radiographically, the result of the regenerative process is also evaluated, comparing the bone–implant contact before and after regeneration. If submucosal healing was planned, a small incision is made in the ridge to expose the implant and replace the cover screw with a healing abutment. After 10 days, the restoration is placed or initiation of a new prosthetic reconstruction begins, depending on the overall treatment plan.

12.3 Effectiveness and limitations of regenerative procedures

Studies comparing nonsurgical and surgical treatment of peri-implantitis show that the latter is advantageous in eliminating inflammation, reducing pocket depth, and gaining clinical attachment level. Regenerative procedures, in turn, have an advantage over other surgical techniques in bone filling when applied to deeper intraosseous defects with three or four bony walls.[3,13–18]

Limitations of regenerative techniques include:

- inability to use the technique for every peri-implant defect;
- inability to completely regenerate peri-implant tissues;
- lack of predictability of reestablishment of osseointegration.

12.4 Factors that determine the success of regenerative procedures

The success of regenerative procedures in the treatment of peri-implantitis is determined by the interaction of various factors.

12.4.1 Factors related to the bone graft

These include the following:

- ability of the graft to be osteoconductive;
- ability of an autogenous bone graft to maintain the vitality of its cells;
- possibility for biologic absorption and replacement to be performed with bone tissue (bone remodeling);
- ability to easily obtain a sufficient amount of bone graft;
- being biologically compatible, immunologically acceptable, and safe to rule out transmission of infectious diseases;
- minimal or no absorption in the early stages of postoperative healing;
- particle size that favors placement and healing;
- porous texture and sufficient size of pores and canals that connect the particles between them. More specifically, small particle size and the many pores and canals of the graft increase the area

around and inside them. This increased area provides a wide surface for absorption, leading to the freeing of morphogenetic proteins that will interact with the organic matrix. The pores and canals that connect the particles must be large enough to allow the bone to expand into them. A pore size of about 200 µm, with intermediate 100-µm-wide channels, may favor bone expansion.

Several different bone grafts have been used for regenerative procedures in peri-implantitis.[3,19–21]

The autogenous cancellous bone graft obtained from the maxillary tuberosity or from the mandible, is preferred among graft materials in terms of the rate at which it matures at the recipient site. An obvious disadvantage of autogenous cancellous bone graft is the second surgical wound; thus, it is not the first choice of bone graft for peri-implantitis treatment. Another disadvantage of a graft from the maxillary tuberosity is the volumetric absorption that occurs during its maturation phase due to the high cancellous bone content compared to bone grafts from the mandible. The problem of absorption can be compensated by using bovine xenografts. The use of autogenous cancellous bone grafts provides:

- osteogenesis directly from transplanted osteoblasts, which immediately begin to produce and deposit the bone matrix at the recipient site;
- osteoinduction from the local release of bone morphogenetic proteins (BMPs) that induce progenitor cells carried to the area of the defect through a network of newly formed capillaries to differentiate into osteoblasts;
- osteoconduction, which is created by the microscopic texture of the graft, which acts as a scaffold and supports fibroplasty and angiogenesis. The newly formed capillaries carry growth factors and progenitor cells to the regenerative area.

Allogenic bone grafts are the most common choice for peri-implantitis treatment. These are human bone grafts obtained from cadavers. They are treated to ensure the absence of antigenicity and to eliminate transmission of infectious diseases (such as hepatitis V, hepatitis C, and human immunodeficiency virus). In some countries they are commercially available in granular form (cancellous, cortical, and corticocancellous). The most commonly used is demineralized freeze-dried bone allograft. This is because demineralization causes the release of BMPs from the bone graft, thus amplifying its osteoinductive ability.

Another choice for bone regeneration in three- or four-wall bony defects is xenograft. It undergoes appropriate processing to keep only the inorganic phase of the bone, to be fully inactivated in terms of antigenicity and prions. Therefore, elimination of possible infectious diseases is ascertained (such as spongiform encephalopathy). The xenograft is only osteoconductive, acting as a scaffold. It is composed of deproteinized bovine bone mineral (DBBM), with a particle size of 0.25 to 1.00 mm. DBBM particles are only slowly replaced by bone.

From a technical point of view, the use of allografts or bovine xenografts in peri-implantitis treatment is a simple and safe procedure. The advantage of allografts or xenografts is the reduction in intraoperative and postoperative morbidity, as there is no need for a second surgical wound. In every case of GBR, allografts or xenografts should be covered by a membrane, usually resorbable, to avoid a second surgery to remove it.

12.4.2 Factors related to the membranes

These include the following:

- ability to create a barrier around and in the bone defect;
- selective permeability, which allows cellular colonization of the defect from the alveolar bone;
- ability to create space around the implant for coronal displacement of the desired cells and maintenance of this space for a long time;
- flexibility but also stability as the membrane does not recede into the bony defect.

12.4.3 Factors related to the bony defect

The success of regenerative procedures is greater in circumferential shallow and narrow intrabony defects than in shallow and wide defects. The greater the number of bony walls in the defect, the greater the predictability (success) of the technique. A greater number of bony walls indicates the existence of a sufficient amount of bony tissue and hence undifferentiated mesenchymal cells. Another positive prognostic factor for the success of the technique is the narrow radiographic angle of the bony defect.[8]

12.4.4 Factors related to the soft tissues covering the bony defect

These include:

- soft tissues with sufficient thickness. According to studies, when the thickness of soft tissue is greater than 1 mm, postoperative recession is significantly smaller. Many authors have suggested additional soft tissue surgery after the regenerative procedure to increase the thickness of keratinized tissues[22];
- ability to achieve full coverage of regenerative materials with the flap.

12.4.5 Factors related to the surgical technique

These are:

- The flap must be designed in such a way as to achieve maximum soft tissue preservation.
- Thorough removal of biofilms from the implant surface and granulation tissue from the bone defect is needed, especially from the bottom, before placing the regenerative materials.
- The shape of the membrane should be adjusted so that no sharp edges are left, which predispose the flap to dehiscence and tissue necrosis postoperatively.
- Bone defects should be completely covered with the membrane, which should be extended by at least 3 mm beyond the bone defect, while being at a distance of 1 mm from the adjacent teeth.
- Regenerative materials should be completely covered with the surgical flap so that no tension is applied to the flap.

12.4.6 Factors related to the surface of the implant

Implants with a rough surface retain more microbial plaque when they are exposed to a peri-implant pocket environment. However, they support postoperative clot formation better after a regenerative procedure, thus promoting bone healing.[5,23]

12.4.7 Factors related to the postoperative compliance of the patient

These are:

- The patient should abstain from mechanical removal of biofilms (toothbrush, interdental brushes) until the nonresorbable membrane is removed. The same applies for 4 weeks when resorbable membranes are used. During this time, chemical biofilm control is applied using antimicrobial agents (mainly chlorhexidine in solution for the first 4 weeks and gel for the next 4 weeks). In addition, effective daily mechanical biofilm removal after this healing period is of utmost importance.
- The patient should be consistent in attending regular recall visits to assess the progress of healing and, later on, the outcome of the therapeutic result.
- The patient should abstain from heavy smoking.

References

1. Kormas I, Pedercini C, Pedercini A, Raptopoulos M, Alassy H, Wolff LF. Peri-implant diseases: diagnosis, clinical, histological, microbiological characteristics and treatment strategies. A narrative review. Antibiotics 2020;9:835.
2. Dentino A, Lee S, Mailhot J, Hefti AF. Principles of periodontology. Periodontol 2000 2013;61:16–53.
3. Khoury F, Keeve PL, Ramanauskaite A, et al. Surgical treatment of peri-implantitis—Consensus report of working group 4. Int Dent J 2019;69(suppl 2):18–22.
4. Nibali L, Koidou VP, Nieri M, Barbato L, Pagliaro U, Cairo F. Regenerative surgery versus access flap for the treatment of intra-bony periodontal defects: a systematic review and meta-analysis. J Clin Periodontol 2020;47(suppl 22): 320–351.
5. Madi M, Htet M, Zakaria O, Alagl A, Kasugai S. Re-osseointegration of dental implants after periimplantitis treatments: a systematic review. Implant Dent 2018;27:101–110.
6. Daugela P, Cicciù M, Saulacic N. Surgical regenerative treatments for peri-implantitis: meta-analysis of recent findings in a systematic literature review. J Oral Maxillofac Res 2016;7:e15.
7. Strauss FJ, Stähli A, Gruber R. The use of platelet-rich fibrin to enhance the outcomes of implant therapy: a systematic review. Clin Oral Implants Res 2018;29(suppl 18):6–19.
8. Mordini L, Sun N, Chang N, De Guzman J-P, Generali L, Consolo U. Peri-implantitis regenerative therapy: a review. Biology 2021;10:773.
9. Yamamoto A, Kubota T, Komatsu Y, et al. Efficacy of erbium:YAG laser for regenerative surgical treatment of peri-implantitis: clinical, microbiological, and biomarker analyses. Int J Periodontics Restorative Dent 2021;41: 187–192.
10. Dhaliwal JS, Abd Rahman NA, Ming LC, Dhaliwal SKS, Knights J, Albuquerque RF Jr. Microbial biofilm decontamination on dental implant surfaces: a mini review. Front Cell Infect Microbiol 2021;11:736186.

11. Isler SC, Soysal F, Ceyhanlı T, Bakırarar B, Unsal B. Regenerative surgical treatment of peri-implantitis using either a collagen membrane or concentrated growth factor: a 12-month randomized clinical trial. Clin Implant Dent Relat Res 2018;20:703–712.
12. Wen SC, Barootchi S, Huang W-X, Wang H-L. Surgical reconstructive treatment for infraosseous peri-implantitis defects with a submerged healing approach: a prospective controlled study. J Periodontol 2022;93:195–207.
13. Carcuac O, Derks J, Abrahamsson I, Wennström JL, Petzold M, Berglundh T. Surgical treatment of peri-implantitis: 3-year results from a randomized controlled clinical trial. J Clin Periodontol 2017;44:1294–1303.
14. Heitz-Mayfield LJA, Mombelli A. The therapy of peri-implantitis: a systematic review. Int J Oral Maxillofac Implants 2014;29(suppl):325–345.
15. Chan H-L, Lin G-H, Suarez F, MacEachern M, Wang H-L. Surgical management of peri-implantitis: a systematic review and meta-analysis of treatment outcomes. J Periodontol 2014;85:1027–1041.
16. Claffey N, Clarke E, Polyzois I, Renvert S. Surgical treatment of peri-implantitis. J Clin Periodontol 2008;35(8, suppl): 316–332.
17. Renvert S, Polyzois I. Treatment of pathologic peri-implant pockets. Periodontol 2000 2018;76:180–190.
18. Berglundh T, Wennström JL, Lindhe J. Long-term outcome of surgical treatment of peri-implantitis. A 2-11-year retrospective study. Clin Oral Implants Res 2018;29:404–410.
19. Roccuzzo M, Pittoni D, Roccuzzo A, Charrier L, Dalmasso P. Surgical treatment of peri-implantitis intrabony lesions by means of deproteinized bovine bone mineral with 10% collagen: 7-year-results. Clin Oral Implants Res 2017;28:1577–1583.
20. Artas G, Gul M, Acikan I, et al. A comparison of different bone graft materials in peri-implant guided bone regeneration. Braz Oral Res 2018;32:e59.
21. Yamada M, Egusa H. Current bone substitutes for implant dentistry. J Prosthodont Res 2018;62:152–161.
22. Sanz-Martín I, Cha J-K, Sanz-Sánchez I, Figuero E, Herrera D, Sanz M. Changes in peri-implant soft tissue levels following surgical treatment of peri-implantitis: a systematic review and meta-analysis. Clin Oral Implants Res 2021;32(suppl 21): 230–244.
23. Botticelli D, Berglundh T, Persson LG, Lindhe J. Bone regeneration at implants with turned or rough surfaces in self-contained defects. An experimental study in the dog. J Clin Periodontol 2005;32:448–455.

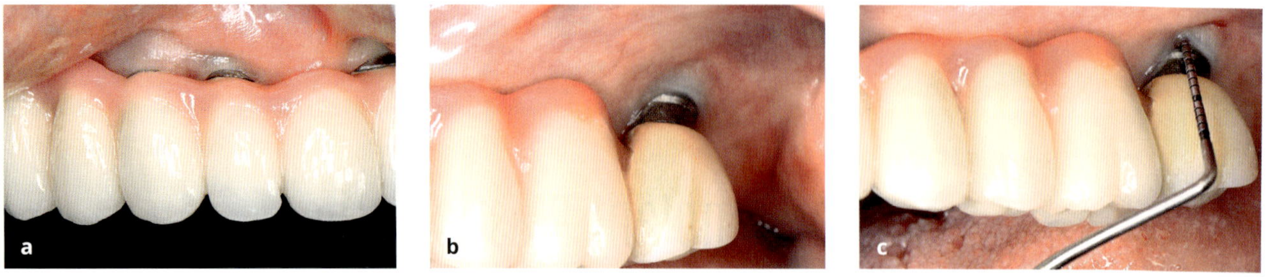

Figs 13-2a–c Clinical images of a compliant patient who attended the maintenance care appointments for 7 years after implant placement. Despite the absence of keratinized mucosa, the health of the peri-implant tissues was maintained.

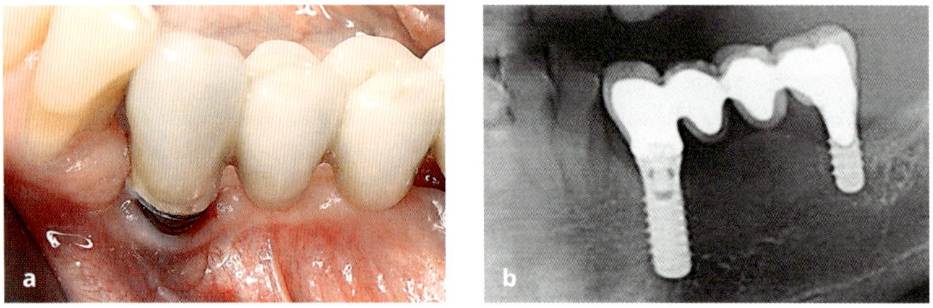

Figs 13-3a, b Clinical and radiographic images of an implant with a minimal zone of free keratinized mucosa. Minimal bleeding could be observed after the application of AIRFLOW (EMS Dental, Nyon, Switzerland). The patient was compliant with the maintenance care program for 15 years and applied daily effective oral hygiene practices.

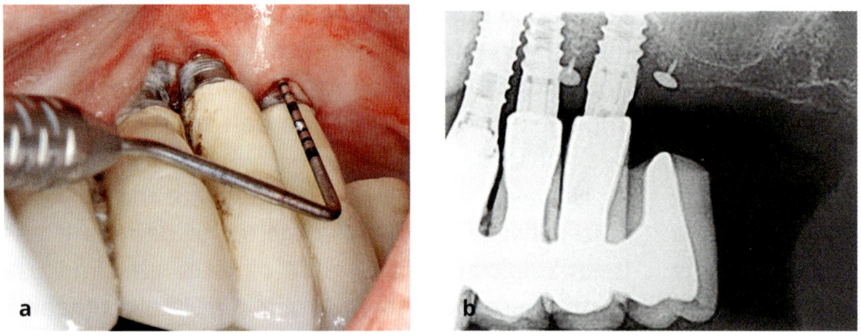

Figs 13-4a, b **(a)** Clinical picture of a patient 6 years after implant placement. An absence of keratinized peri-implant mucosa, pocket probing on implant no. 25, and exposed threads on implants nos. 23 and 24 may be seen. The patient was in pain when applying oral hygiene. The accumulation of biofilm is obvious. **(b)** The radiograph revealed significant bone loss. Note the pins remaining from previous guided bone regeneration.

provided that effective daily oral hygiene is practiced and patients are enrolled in personalized maintenance care programs (Figs 13-2a–c and 13-3a, b).[12,13]

Indeed, the width and thickness of keratinized tissue around implants does not affect biofilm retention. Therefore, an inadequate width of keratinized mucosa may not be a risk factor for the development of peri-implantitis.[12] However, in the absence of keratinized mucosa, a possible change of the anatomy may be encountered due to resorption of the alveolar ridge before implant placement. Patients can sometimes cause trauma to the peri-implant mucosa by using ineffective hygiene practices.[14,15] Thus, biofilms increase the likelihood of peri-implant mucositis, which, if poorly handled, may later evolve into peri-implantitis (Figs 13-4a, b).[16]

The use of peri-implant plastic surgery to increase the width and thickness of keratinized tissues is beneficial in inhibiting the progression of peri-implantitis.[17,18]

To increase the keratinized peri-implant mucosa and treat peri-implant soft tissue defects, several plastic surgery techniques have been advocated.[19] Those most commonly applied are placement of a free gingival (mucosal) graft[20] or of a subepithelial connective tissue graft (Figs 13-5a–n).[21]

As there are no conclusive data on the most effective surgical technique for the treatment of soft tissue defects at implants, the choice is based on the following parameters:

- the thickness of the mucosa at the implant site;
- the thickness of the mucosa at the donor site;
- the depth of the vestibule;
- the height of the smile line if the operation involves the esthetic zone.[22–24]

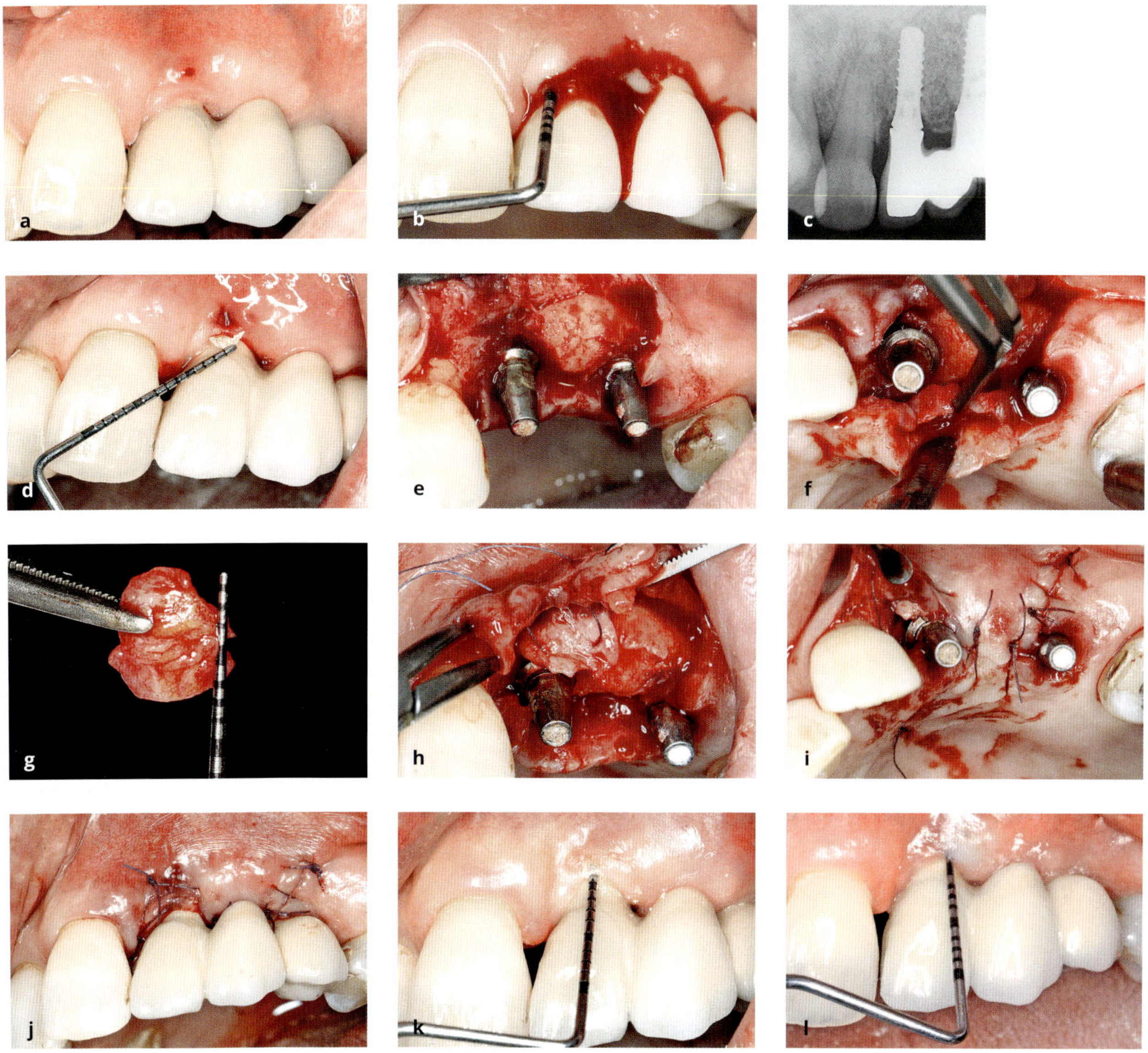

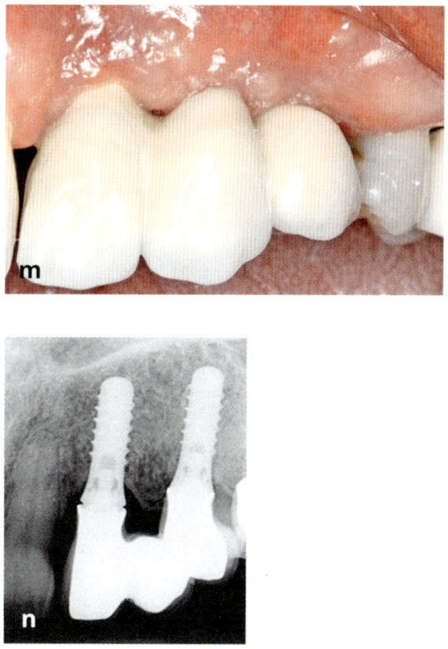

Figs 13-5a–n **(a)** Peri-implant abscess and fistula 8 years after implant placement and 1 month after decementation and recementation of the implant-supported partial denture. **(b)** Bleeding on probing (BOP) and pus formation may be seen, as well as a pocket at the buccal site of implant no. 22. **(c)** Radiography did not reveal bone loss. However, a poorly fitting prosthetic restoration can be observed. **(d)** After drainage of the abscess, cement residue was found and removed. The mucosal defect can be seen. **(e)** Full-thickness flap elevation and removal of granulation tissue. No threads were exposed to the pocket environment; the pus was collected subperiosteally and the periodontal probe was directed there. **(f)** Preparation of a connective tissue graft from the palate to close the fistula and increase the thickness of the peri-implant mucosa at implant no. 22. **(g)** The connective tissue graft. **(h)** Graft sutured at the area of the fistula. **(i)** Sutures stabilizing the graft at the buccal area. **(j)** After flap suturing. **(k)** 6 months later, the peri-implant tissues appear healthy and no peri-implant pockets and BOP were detected. **(l and m)** Two years after surgery, the therapeutic result had been maintained. Note the absence of pockets and BOP. **(n)** Radiographic image 2 years after surgery.

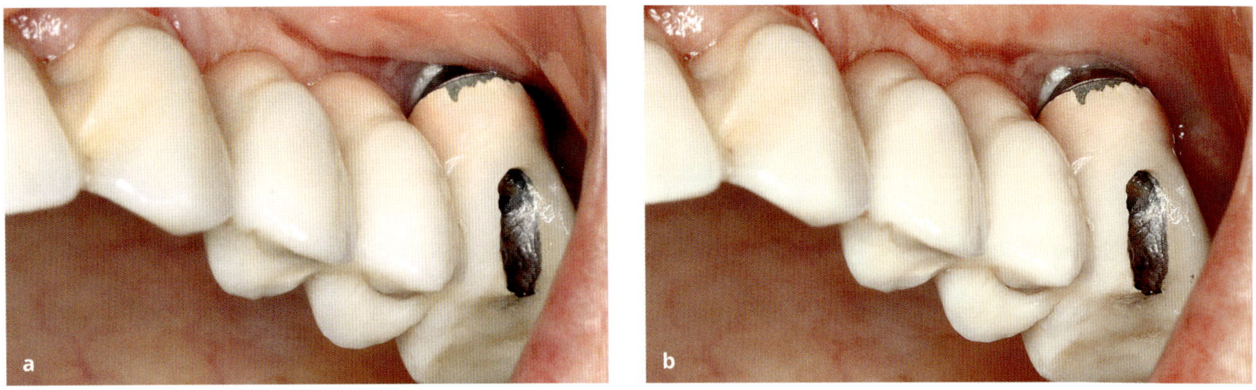

Figs 13-6a, b (a) Clinical picture of a patient with peri-implantitis. Steps A and B of the cumulative interceptive supportive therapy (CIST) protocol have been completed. Mucosal folding may be observed. **(b)** The buccal mucosa needed to be pulled strongly to reveal the neck of the implant. This, in combination with the complete lack of keratinized peri-implant mucosa, made the application of oral hygiene ineffective and biofilm accumulation can be observed.

13.1 Free mucosal grafts

Free mucosal grafts consist of epithelium and connective tissue. The graft is taken from one area (the donor site) and placed into another area (the recipient site). The free gingival graft technique was first described by Younger[25] in 1904. In 1963, Björn[26] documented its use to increase the width of keratinized tissues, while in 1966, Nabers[27] applied it for the first time to achieve root coverage and treat gingival recession.

The technique initially involved removal of the epithelium from the surface of the peri-implant mucosa at the recipient site.[24] In essence, a partial-thickness flap is prepared to reveal the underlying connective tissue onto which the free graft will be sutured. The palate serves as the donor site of the graft. Alternatively, the graft may be harvested from the posterior region of the maxillary third molar or from an edentulous part of the maxillary alveolar ridge. The graft is placed in contact with the exposed connective tissue bed of the recipient site, where it is sutured to the periosteum.

If the mucosa at the recipient site is too thin to make the preparation of a partial-thickness flap possible, the free mucosal graft may be placed onto the bone and immobilized to the adjacent tissues using suturing. This technique may increase the width and thickness of the keratinized peri-implant mucosa with substantial predictability.[20]

In 1973, Bernimoulin[28] described a two-step approach. First, a free gingival graft is placed, then later, a coronally repositioned flap is raised to achieve root coverage. At implant sites, when a lack of keratinized mucosa is combined with exposure of the implant neck,[29,30] the graft is initially placed to increase the thickness and width of the keratinized mucosa; after at least 2 months, a coronally repositioned flap is raised.[31] However, the technique does not lead to complete coverage of the exposed surface of the implant. Treatment of peri-implant mucosal recession is, in general, much less predictable[30,32,33] than periodontal recession coverage.[34–36] The main disadvantage of the combined technique is that additional surgery is required. Indications include:

- insufficient thickness or width of the keratinized mucosa in areas where dental implants will be placed before implantation;
- when application of effective oral hygiene is jeopardized because of insufficient thickness or width of the keratinized peri-implant mucosa;
- in combination with other surgical techniques to treat peri-implantitis when the keratinized peri-implant mucosa is insufficient. In these cases, graft placement usually precedes resective surgery (Figs 13-6a–r) or follows regenerative surgery (Figs 13-7a–n).

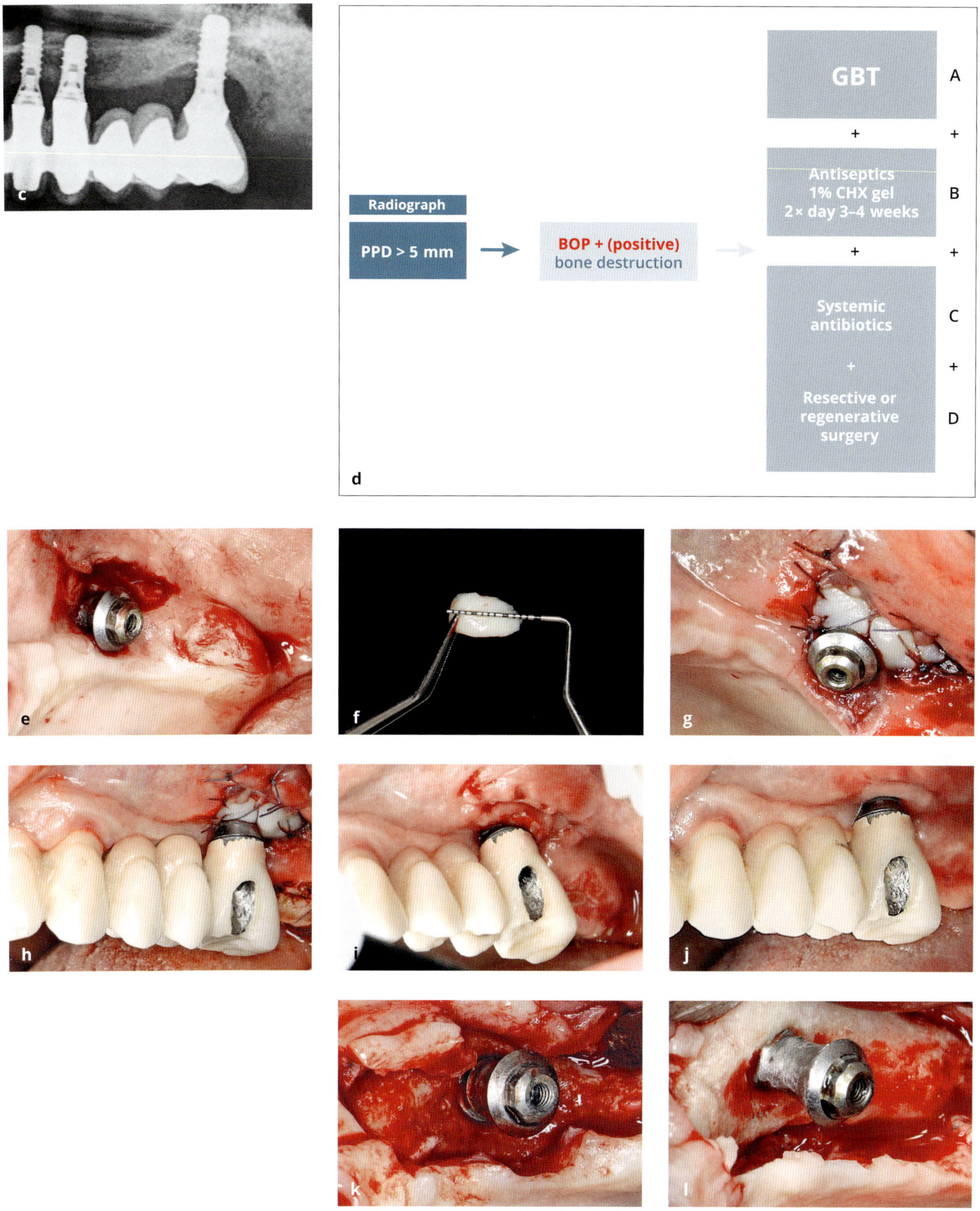

Figs 13-6c–l **(c)** A radiograph revealed bone loss. The morphology of the bony defect is not an indication for reconstructive surgery. **(d)** Proposed approach according to the current data. **(e)** Preparation of a partial-thickness flap buccally to the implant. **(f)** Harvesting of a free gingival graft from the posterior molar region. **(g and h)** Graft placement and suturing. **(i)** Suture removal after 10 days. **(j)** The area after 8 weeks. **(k and l)** After flap elevation, exposed implant thread polishing and bone surgery were performed. BOP, bleeding on probing; CHX, chlorhexidine; GBT, guided biofilm therapy; PPD, periodontal probing depth.

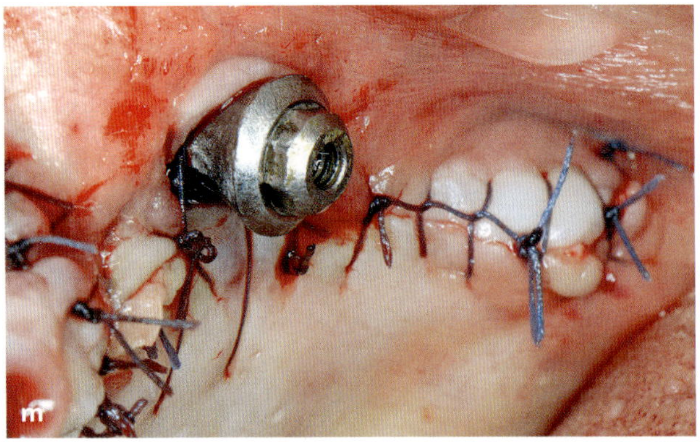

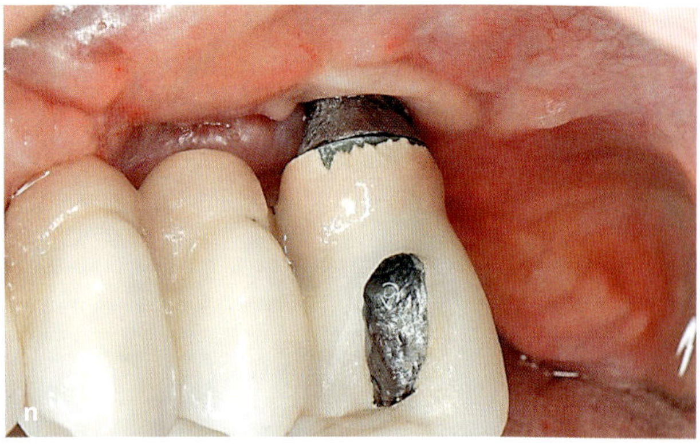

Figs 13-6m, n **(m)** Suturing. **(n)** Three weeks after surgery.

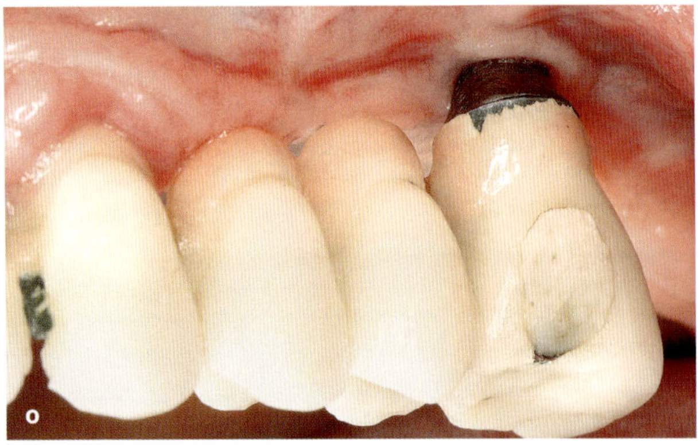

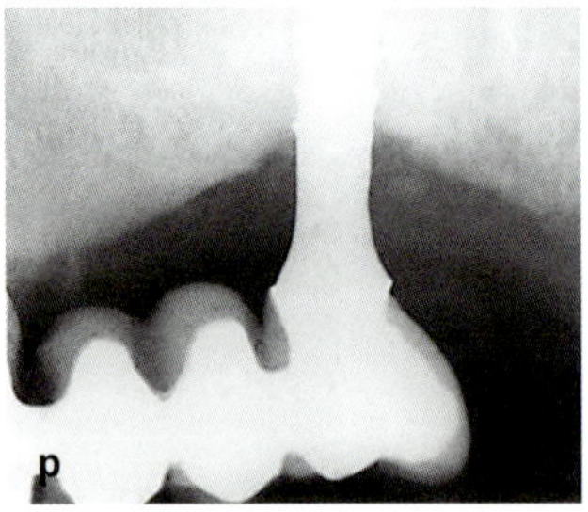

Figs 13-6o, p Clinical and radiographic images 2 years after the treatment of peri-implantitis. Stability and maintenance of peri-implant tissue health was established.

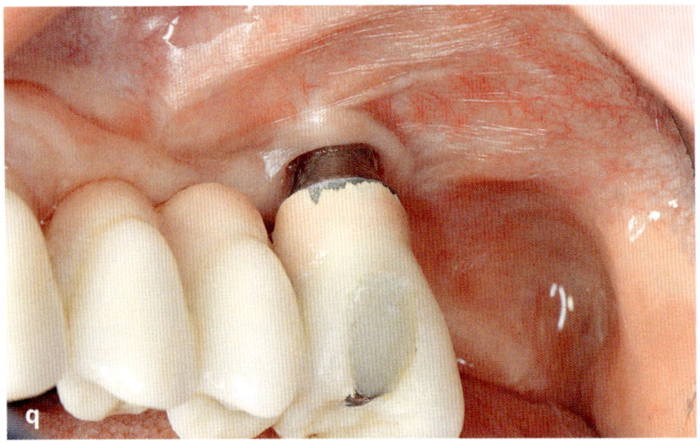

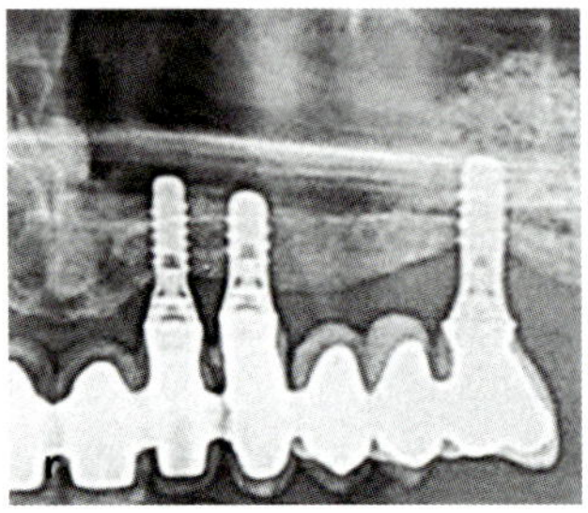

Figs 13-6q, r Clinical and radiographic images 6 years after peri-implantitis treatment.

Contraindications for this surgery are:

- inability to obtain a graft because of extremely thin palatal soft tissue volume or a flat, shallow palate;
- a high smile line due to esthetic color disharmony.

Generally, however, this is an easier technique than connective tissue grafting, but disadvantages include the following:

- it requires special skills and training;
- it leaves a second surgical site;
- at the donor site, there is healing by secondary intention;
- the graft may shrink up to 50%;
- there is a lack of satisfactory esthetic results due to the white shade of the grafted area.

Preoperative care involves meticulous implementation of steps A and B of the cumulative interceptive supportive therapy (CIST) protocol.

The surgical phase consists of the following:

- Recipient site: surgery is initiated from the recipient site to achieve hemostasis until suturing of the graft. Accordingly, the time from obtaining the graft to its placement at the recipient site is

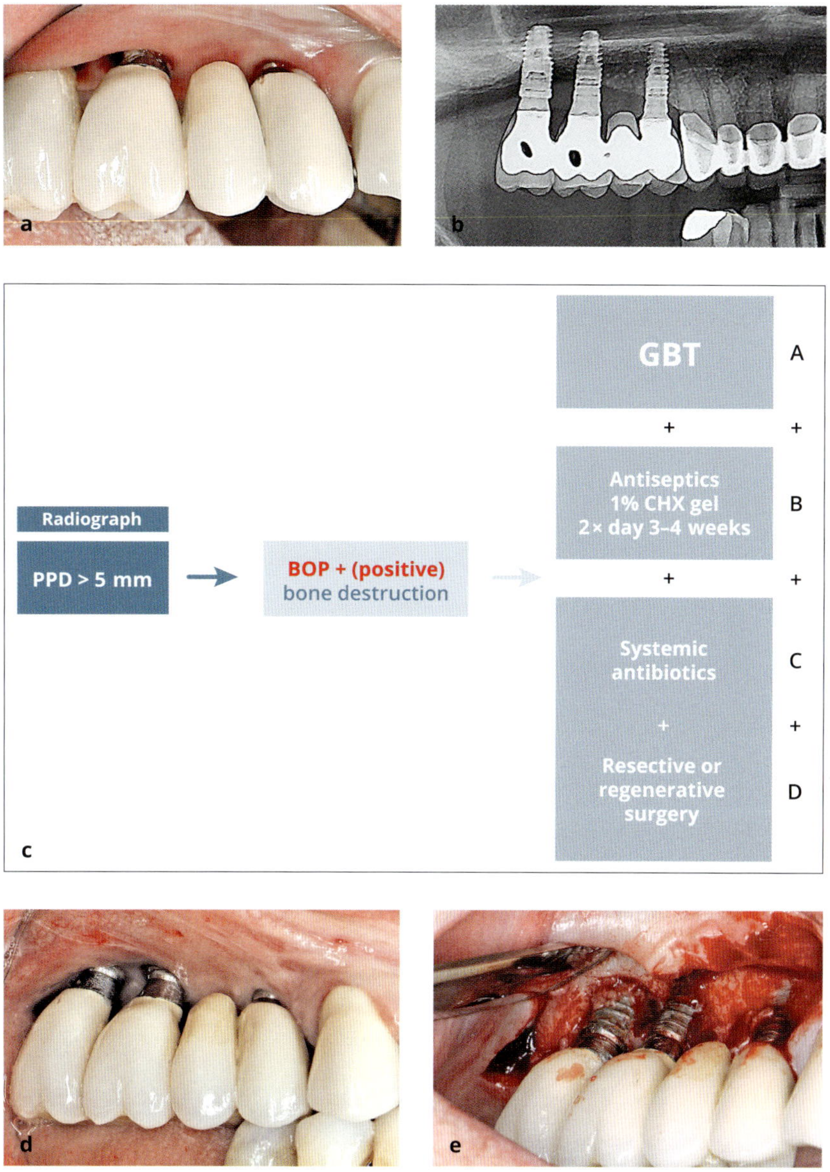

Figs 13-7a–e (a) A mucosal fold over implant no. 17 can be seen due to the absence of keratinized mucosa. **(b)** Radiography revealed the severity of bone loss. The combination of clinical and radiographic data led to the possibility of intrabony defects. **(c)** Proposed approach for corresponding cases according to the current data. **(d)** Significant force was exercised to reveal the neck area. The difficulty of applying effective oral hygiene is clear. **(e)** After flap elevation. BOP, bleeding on probing; CHX, chlorhexidine; GBT, guided biofilm therapy; PPD, periodontal probing depth.

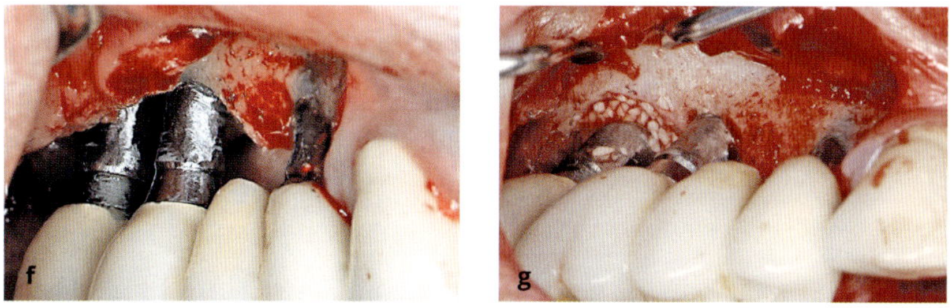

Figs 13-7f, g (f) Polishing of the supracrestal part of the exposed implant threads. **(g)** Filling of the intraosseous portion of the defect.

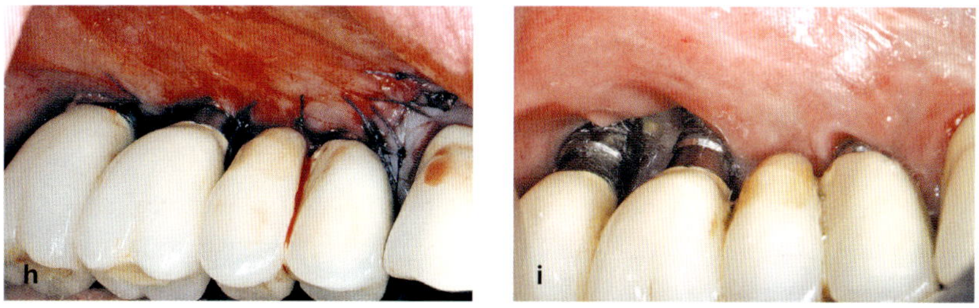

Figs 13-7h, i (h) Flap suturing. **(i)** Clinical image after suture removal.

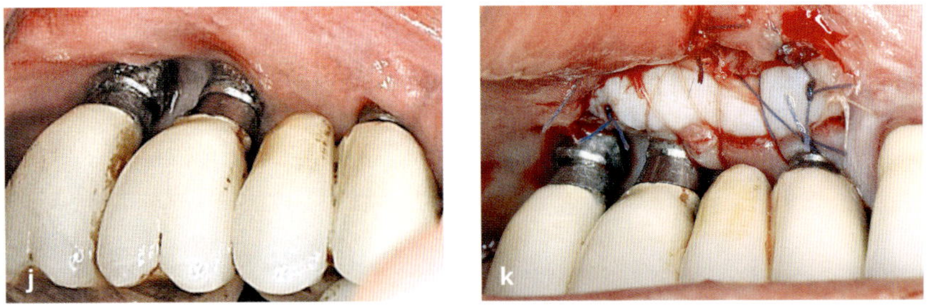

Figs 13-7j, k (j) Clinical image 2 months after the first surgery and before the placement of a free mucosal graft. **(k)** Graft suturing. The graft is not sufficient to cover the buccal area of implant no. 17.

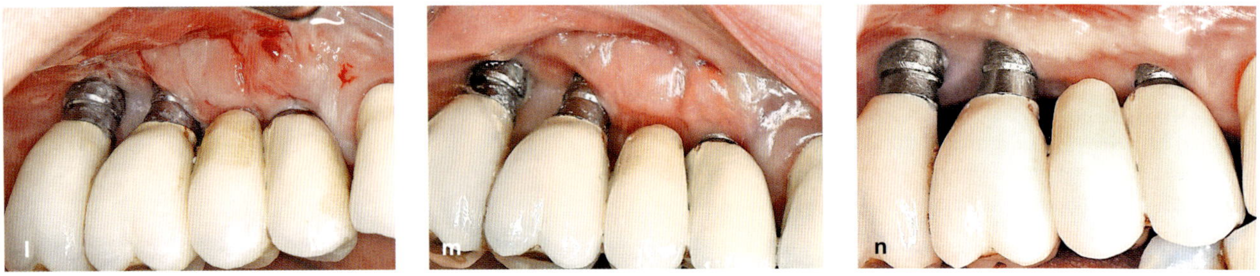

Figs 13-7l–n (l) Suture removal 11 days after graft placement. **(m)** Two weeks later. **(n)** Three months after graft placement. Shrinkage is evident.

reduced. Initially, local anesthesia is administered with a vasoconstrictor. A partial-thickness flap is prepared at the recipient site with a no. 15 or 15c scalpel or an ophthalmic blade. The prepared recipient site should always be slightly larger than the dimensions of the graft. The purpose is to achieve contact of the entire graft surface with the underlying periosteum. Therefore, anastomosis formation of the vessels throughout the length of the graft allows better perfusion. The preparation is made so that a smooth cut surface remains at the recipient site. Sufficient thickness of connective tissue should remain above the periosteum to achieve better vascularization of the graft.

- Donor site: the area from where the graft will be obtained is selected. This is followed by local anesthesia with a vasoconstrictor peripheral to the area from where the graft will be taken. Then, the dimensions of the recipient site are measured and the size of the graft to be harvested is decided. The incision is made with a no. 15 or 15c scalpel or an ophthalmic blade. The graft includes the epithelium and connective tissue. Graft thickness should be between 1.5 and 2.0 mm and of an even nature throughout. If the graft is thicker than desired, it is thinned by removing parts of the connective tissue before its placement. To control bleeding at the donor site, a Hawley retainer may be used as a pressure splint to hold the surgical dressing in place. Alternatively, hemostasis may be induced using a diode (810 or 940 or 980 nm) or Nd:YAG laser (1,064 nm). The high absorption of radiation by hemoglobin leads to complete thrombosis of the capillaries in the area. More simply, bleeding can be stopped by applying pressure, placing a few stitches, or using a periodontal dressing (Figs 13-8k, l).

The graft is then placed in the recipient site. Its dimensions are checked and shaped so that it does not overlap the prepared surgical bed. After this, it is sutured with interrupted polydioxanone or polyglactin 910 or polyglycolic acid 5-0 resorbable sutures and an atraumatic 16-mm needle. Multiple incisions should be avoided to prevent decreasing perfusion. Two or three sutures placed coronally to the graft and two placed apically are sufficient to hold it in place. A modified Malament suture may be placed for better graft fixation. Gentle pressure is then applied with a saline-soaked gauze to reduce the volume of the clot formed between the graft and the underlying connective tissue at the recipient site. A large clot may prevent perfusion. It is feasible, but not necessary, to place a surgical dressing. If the latter is used, it will be removed after 7 to 8 days. The patient is prescribed 0.1% to 0.2% chlorhexidine rinses to use twice daily, for 1 minute, and is instructed to avoid brushing the operated areas during this period (Figs 13-8a–q).[37,38]

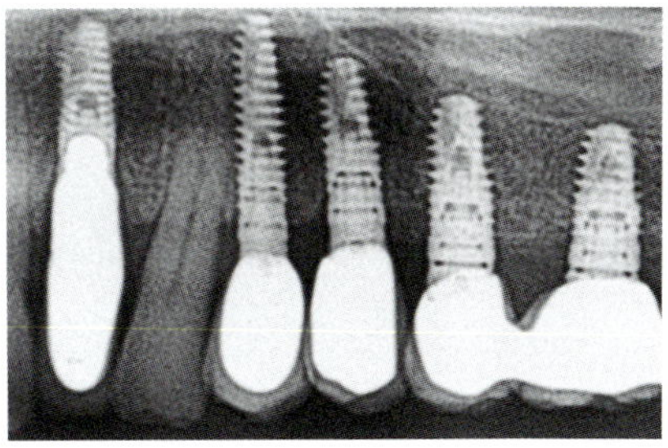

Fig 13-8a Radiographic image of a patient (smoker) who had implants for 15 years. There was some bone loss at implant no. 25, which may have resulted from the placement of a wide implant in a narrow alveolar ridge or from the incorrect placement of the neck of the implant in a position above the edge of the alveolar ridge.

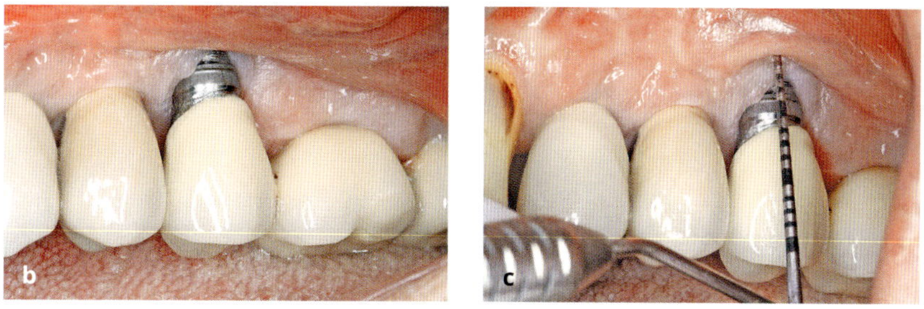

Figs 13-8b, c (b) Clinical examination revealed peri-implant soft tissue recession. However, no signs of inflammation are visible. The mucogingival junction and a mucosal fold, due to muscle tension, are prominent, thus restricting the administration of oral hygiene. This case is suitable for the application of vestibuloplasty, that is, surgery with an apically repositioned partial thickness flap in combination with a free mucosal graft. **(c)** The narrow zone of the free keratinized peri-implant mucosa is distinguished when the cheek is pulled upward .

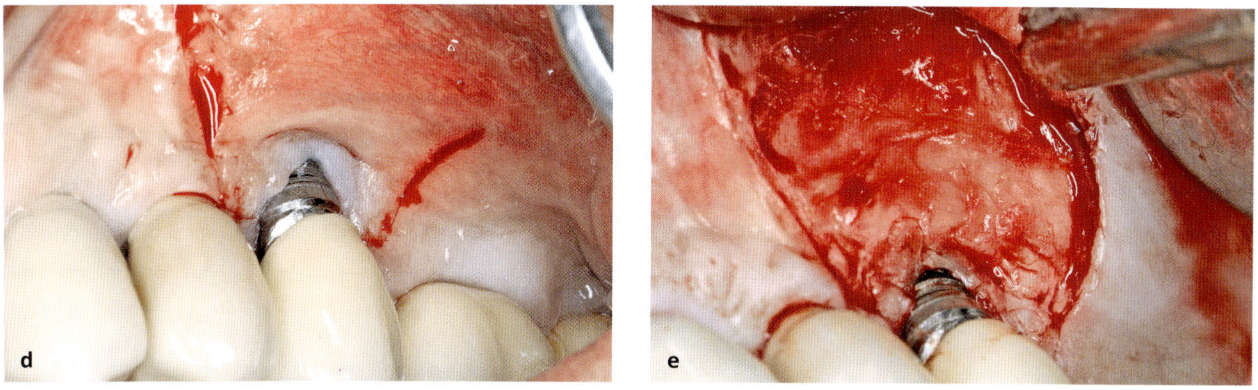

Figs 13-8d, e (d) Preparation of a trapezoidal partial-thickness flap. The flap will be repositioned and sutured apically to the free mucosal graft to limit the area to be left for secondary healing. At the same time, this design provides a vestibular deepening to correct the folding of the mucosa, to facilitate oral hygiene. **(e)** After flap elevation, the remaining part of the connective tissue and underlying periosteum may be seen. Above them, the free mucosal graft was sutured.

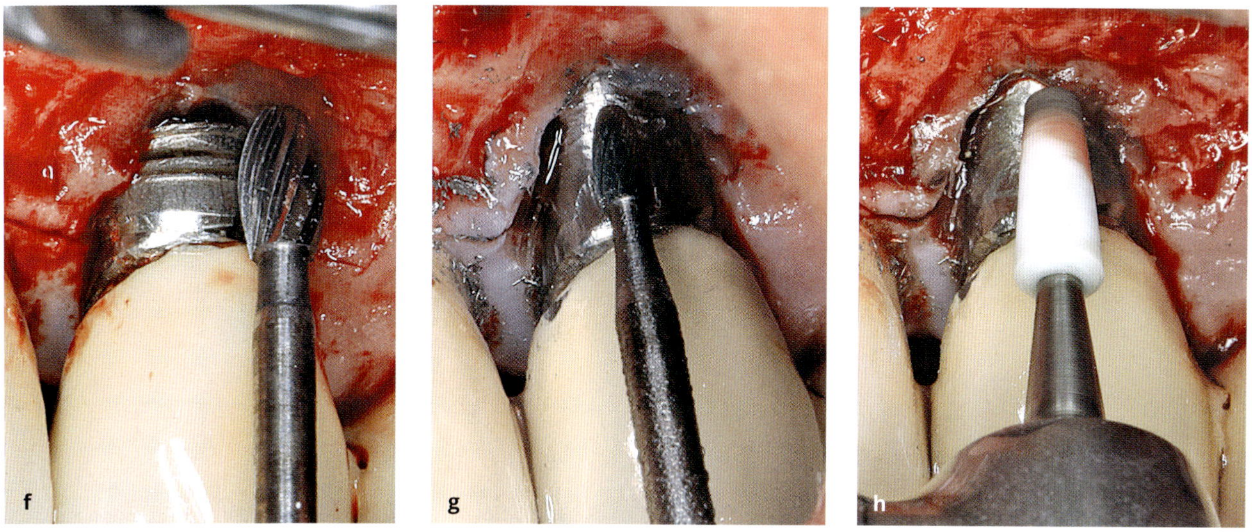

Figs 13-8f–h The use of sequentially grooved burs for the smoothening of exposed threads and completion of polishing with Arkansas stone burs.

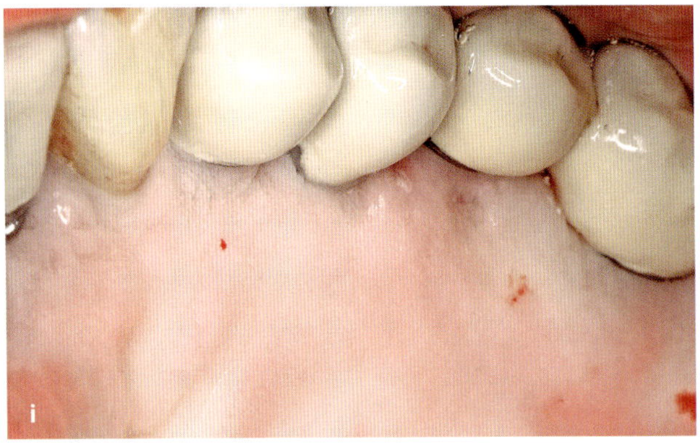
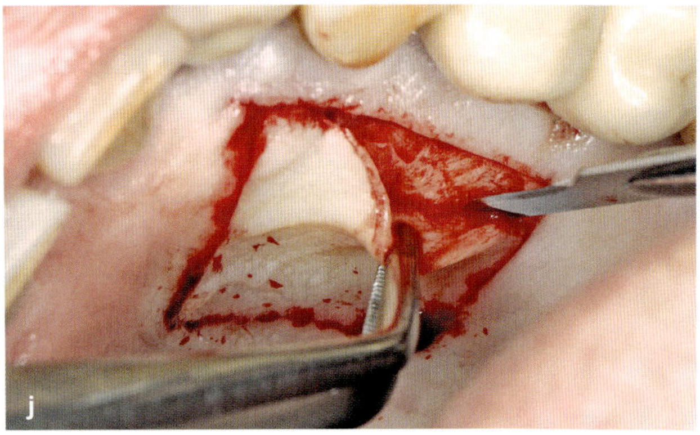

Figs 13-8i, j **(i)** The area of the palate from which the graft will be harvested. **(j)** Preparation of the free mucosal graft with a no. 15 scalpel.

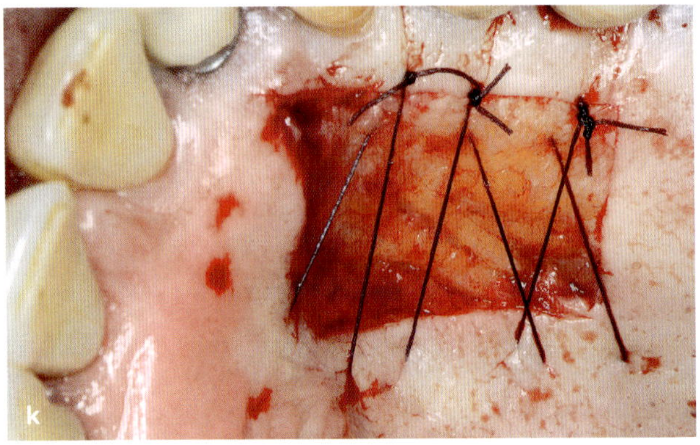
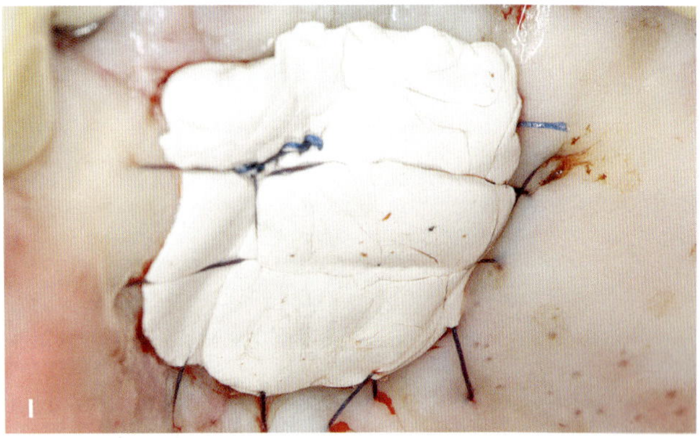

Figs 13-8k, l **(k)** Suturing for retention of the periodontal dressing. **(l)** Placement of a periodontal dressing that did not fully cover the sutures, so that they could be safely removed, and a horizontal mattress suture to stabilize the dressing.

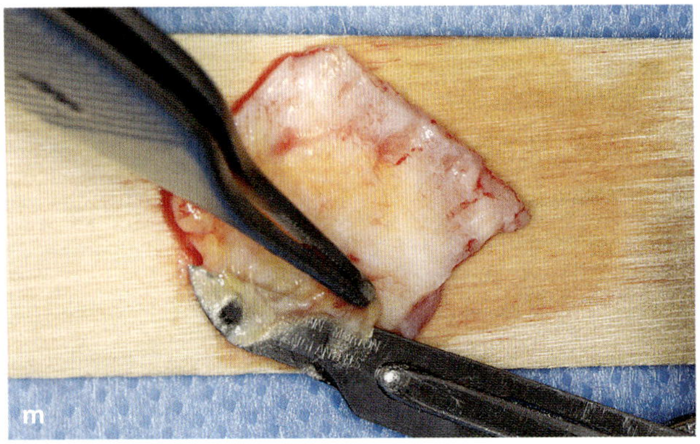
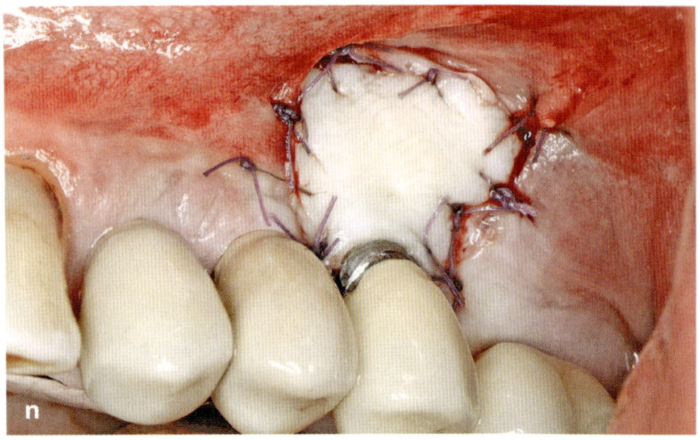

Figs 13-8m, n **(m)** Thinning of the graft so that it acquired a uniform thickness. **(n)** Placement and suturing of the graft and apical suturing of the prepared partial-thickness flap to limit the surface exposed to secondary healing. A deepening of the vestibulum and absence of mucosal folding can also be seen.

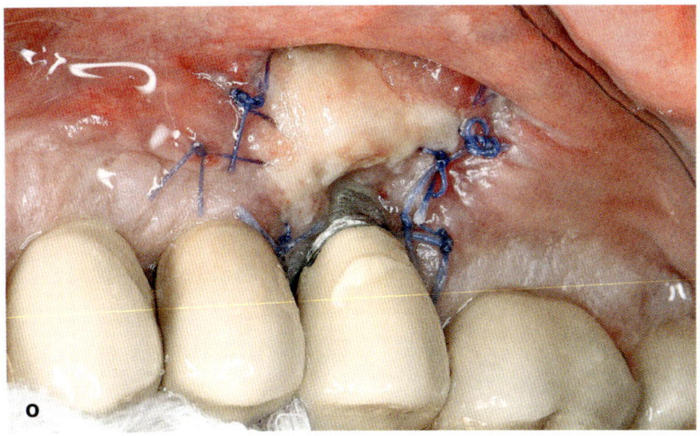

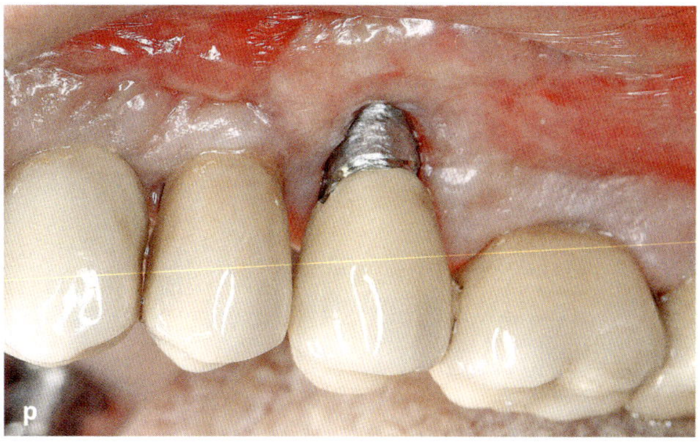

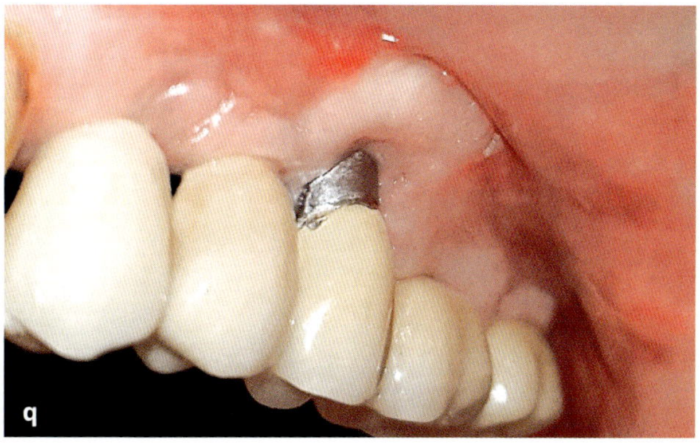

Figs 13-8o–q **(o)** Eight days after vestibuloplasty surgery. Effective growth of the keratinized mucosa may be seen. **(p)** Two weeks after placement of the free gingival graft. Deepening of the vestibulum, adequate keratinized mucosa, and absence of inflammation were noted. **(q)** Four weeks after placement of the free mucosal graft. With a simple pull of the cheek, the mucosal fold is no longer visible.

During the postoperative phase:

- The patient may report discomfort at the donor or the recipient site (or both).
- 0.1% to 0.2% chlorhexidine should be used for 1 minute twice daily and mechanical oral hygiene in the operated areas should be avoided for 2 weeks.
- Sutures are removed after 7–10 days. If periodontal dressings have been used, care must be taken when they are removed so that they do not rip a suture embedded in them. This is important at the recipient site, where the dressing has been deliberately pressed with the retaining sutures. In this case, the sutures are removed first before the dressing.
- After the sutures have been removed, periodontal dressings may be placed in the recipient area for a second week after the operation.
- If no periodontal dressing has been applied, or after it is removed, laser application may be recommended for biostimulation. This helps speed up healing. Biostimulation is the process by which radiation leads to an increase in cell proliferation and differentiation that can be achieved in the postoperative period. For best results, radiation from a distance of 0.5 to 1.0 cm is recommended, for 60 to 120 s/cm^2 of the operated surface, every 2 to 3 days, starting immediately after graft placement.

13.2 Subepithelial connective tissue graft

The connective tissue graft was first described in 1974 by Edel[39] to increase the width of attached gingiva. In 1980, Langer and Calagna[40] suggested this technique to increase the volume of the alveolar ridge and applied a connective tissue graft to cover the exposed root surfaces.[41] The connective tissue graft, unlike the free gingival graft, does not include the epithelium from the donor site but only the connective

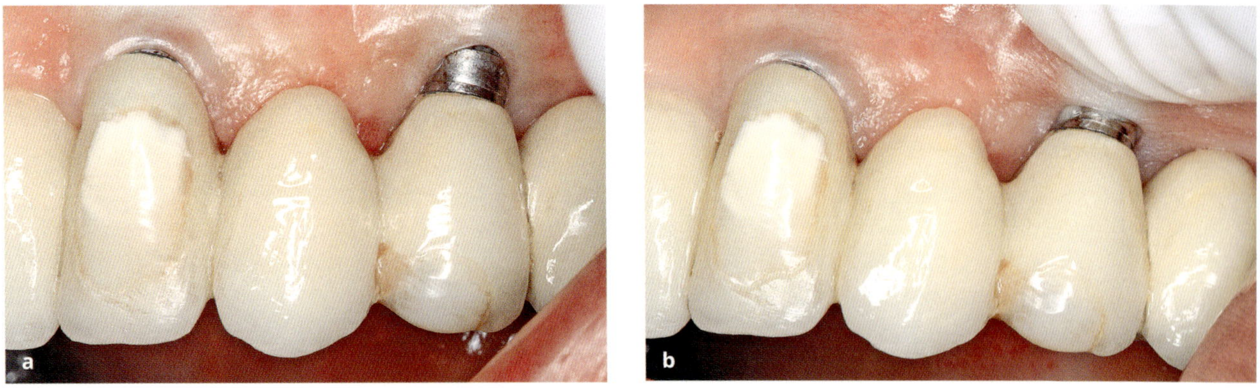

Figs 13-9a, b **(a)** Clinical image of a patient with recession and exposure of the neck of implant no. 24. **(b)** Simple finger pressure reveals that the mucosa is loose and does not adapt to the underlying bone.

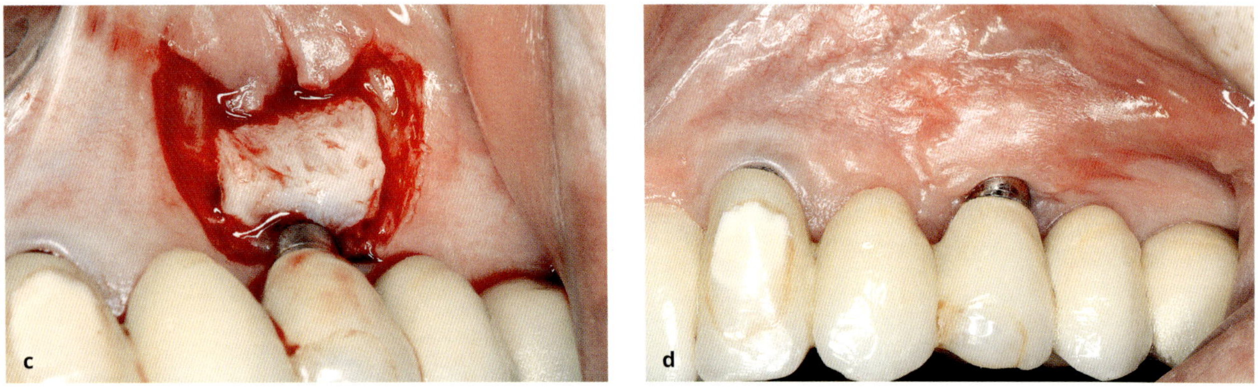

Figs 13-9c, d **(c)** Connective tissue graft placed at the implant site to increase the thickness of the keratinized tissues. **(d)** Note the increase in the thickness and width of the keratinized mucosa (continuation of the case shown in Figs 11-8a–e).

tissue. For this reason, it offers better color harmony and more favorable esthetic results. The part of the hard palate corresponding to the maxillary premolars up to the first molars is usually chosen as the donor site. Alternately, if conditions allow, it may be harvested from the maxillary tuberosity or from any edentulous area of the maxillary alveolar ridge. Several surgical techniques for obtaining a connective tissue graft have been described:[37,38]

- With a horizontal incision at a distance of about 4 to 5 mm from the margin of the free gingiva. The graft is harvested through this slit as an envelope graft.
- With two parallel horizontal incisions. The first is like the one mentioned above. A second horizontal incision is made, parallel to the first and at a distance of about 2 mm from it. From the apically placed incision, a partial-thickness flap is prepared parallel to the outer surface and the coronally placed incision at a depth of about 2 mm. Finally, incisions are made under the partial-thickness flap perpendicular to the bone to obtain an equilateral graft that resembles a rectangle.
- By preparing a square partial-thickness flap and then thinning it.

The last of these approaches is the simplest, The product resulting from the thinning of the palatal flap consists of periosteum and part of the connective tissue. The result at the recipient site is an increase in the thickness and width of the keratinized mucosa. Differentiation of the covering epithelium is determined by the thickness of the underlying connective tissue. There is evidence that the deeper layer of connective tissue of the palate does not have enough potential to induce keratinization of the epithelium.

Indications include insufficient width or thickness (or both) of the keratinized mucosa in areas where dental implants will be placed, and the exposed neck of dental implants in an esthetic area (Figs 13-9a–d).

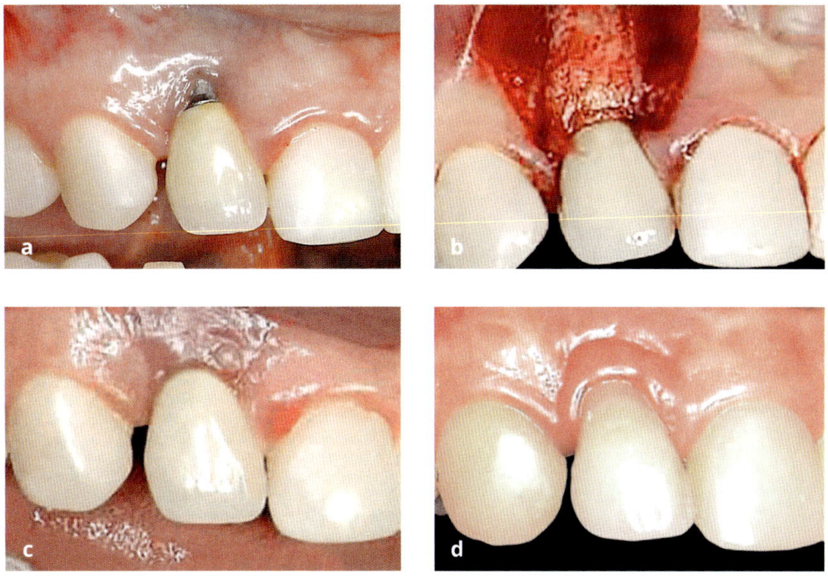

Figs 13-10a–d **(a)** Clinical image of recession at implant no. 12. **(b)** Preparation of a partial-thickness flap and placement of a connective tissue graft. **(c)** The area 5 years after surgery. **(d)** The area 8 years after plastic peri-implant soft tissue surgery. An improvement in the clinical situation was observed over time. Esthetic intervention was performed in crown no. 13 and replacement of the implant crown in no. 12.

A contraindication is insufficient soft tissue thickness in the hard palate. Attempting to obtain a connective tissue graft with any technique carries the risk of tearing the flap and an increased chance of mucosal necrosis at the donor site. The same result may be observed when a thin flap remains at the donor site. Eventually, wound healing by secondary intention will occur.

Advantages of the technique include:

- better color performance;
- avoidance of secondary wound healing in the palate, as is the case with a free mucosal graft;
- less inconvenience for the patient (Figs 13-10a–d and 13-11a–h).

The preoperative phase includes case evaluation and determination of the graft donor and recipient sites, and meticulous application of steps A and B of the CIST protocol.

For the surgical phase, local anesthesia is administered in the area where the graft will be placed and in the area from where it will be harvested. Block of the greater palatine nerve has an advantage over supraperiosteal injections throughout the palate because it avoids extensive vasoconstriction; hence, perfusion of the graft is not impaired. Initially, one intrasulcular and two vertical incisions are made at the recipient site on either side of the implant where the keratinized tissues will be augmented. The vertical incisions are made so that they do not reach the bone; they are made first in order to prepare the partial-thickness flap. The vertical parts form a flap, which will eventually have a trapezoidal shape. Next, the flap is prepared with a no. 15c scalpel or an ophthalmic blade, which must extend beyond the mucogingival junction. Disinfection of the exposed surface of the implant with AIRFLOW and erythritol is mandatory. It is often possible to smoothen the threads to better adapt the graft and enable better access of the PERIOFLOW nozzle during the maintenance care phase. To mobilize the flap, it can be repositioned coronally without exercising tension during suturing.

With a no. 15 or 15c scalpel or an ophthalmic blade, the graft is prepared using one of the techniques mentioned. The palatal flap is sutured either with polytetrafluoroethylene or polyamide nonresorbable single sutures, or with polydioxanone, polylactic acid, or polygalactin 910 resorbable sutures, and finally with 4-0 or 5-0 mm silk sutures and a 12-or 16-mm atraumatic needle.

The graft is placed and sutured in the underlying periosteum of the recipient site, with resorbable sutures, ideally 5-0 to 7-0 Monocryl (Ethicon, Raritan, NJ, USA), and a 12- or 16-mm atraumatic needle.

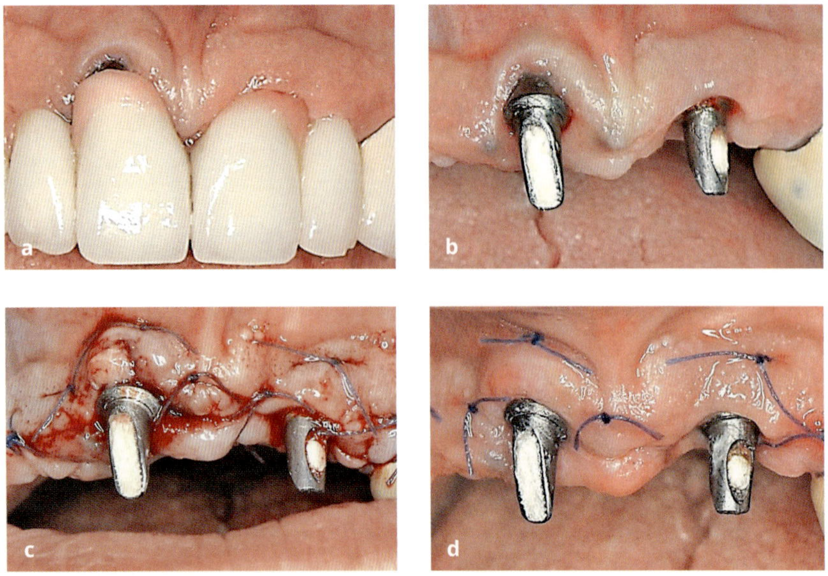

Figs 13-11a–d (a and b) Clinical image of a patient in need of peri-implantitis treatment in implant no. 21. **(c)** In the context of regenerative peri-implantitis treatment, the lack of keratinized soft tissues in implant no. 11 was also addressed with a connective tissue graft. **(d)** The area 10 days after surgery and before the removal of the sutures.

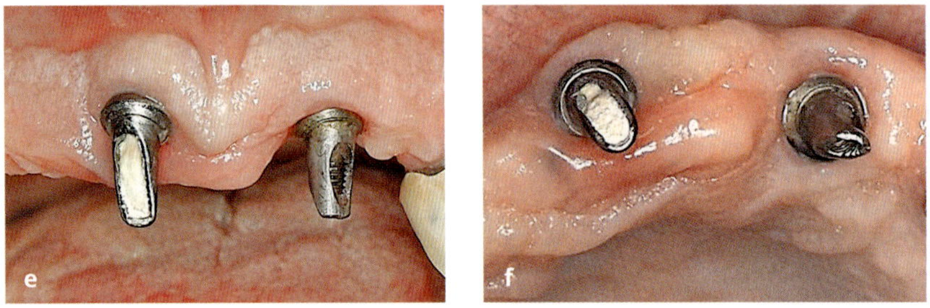

Figs 13-11e, f Sixteen months after surgery. Surgery was performed at the post-graduate Clinic of Periodontics, Dental School, National and Kapodestrian University of Athens, Athens, Greece.

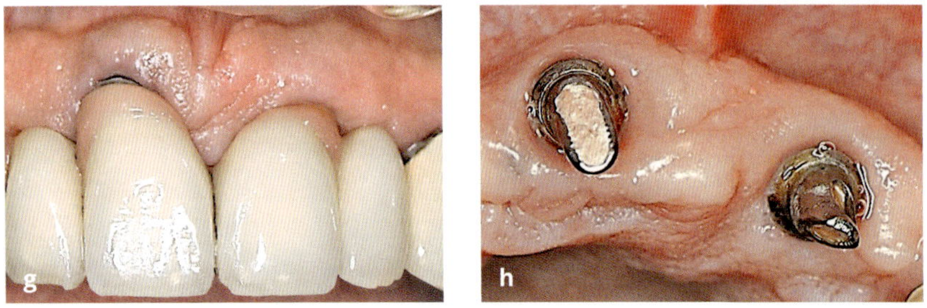

Figs 13-11g, h Ten years after surgery, the peri-implant soft tissues maintained their dimensions (images courtesy of Mr A. Gkogkos).

Finally, the flap is sutured with resorbable sutures to cover the graft. Although there is no research to confirm this, the result is proportional whether the flap completely covers the connective tissue graft, or whether part of it remains uncovered, because it will be epithelialized as healing progresses.

In peri-implant plastic surgery and in general periodontal surgery, the use of microsurgical instruments and optical aids, such as magnifying glasses, loupes, or surgical microscopes, offers greater precision and finer manipulation of tissues.[42]

Sutures are removed after 10 to 12 days. The patient should be warned in advance of any possible limitations that may arise from the placement of soft tissue grafts. Several factors may adversely affect the healing process of the peri-implant area, mainly because of the morphologic differences of the tissues surrounding the implants compared to natural teeth. Compared to the gingival anatomy, the mucosa around dental implants has reduced vascularity, and an increased ratio of collagen and decreased ratio of fibroblasts. The morphology of the soft peri-implant tissues has been compared with that of scar tissue after surgery, with structural support and vascularity coming solely from the underlying alveolar bone and not from a periodontal ligament (Figs 13-12a–h).

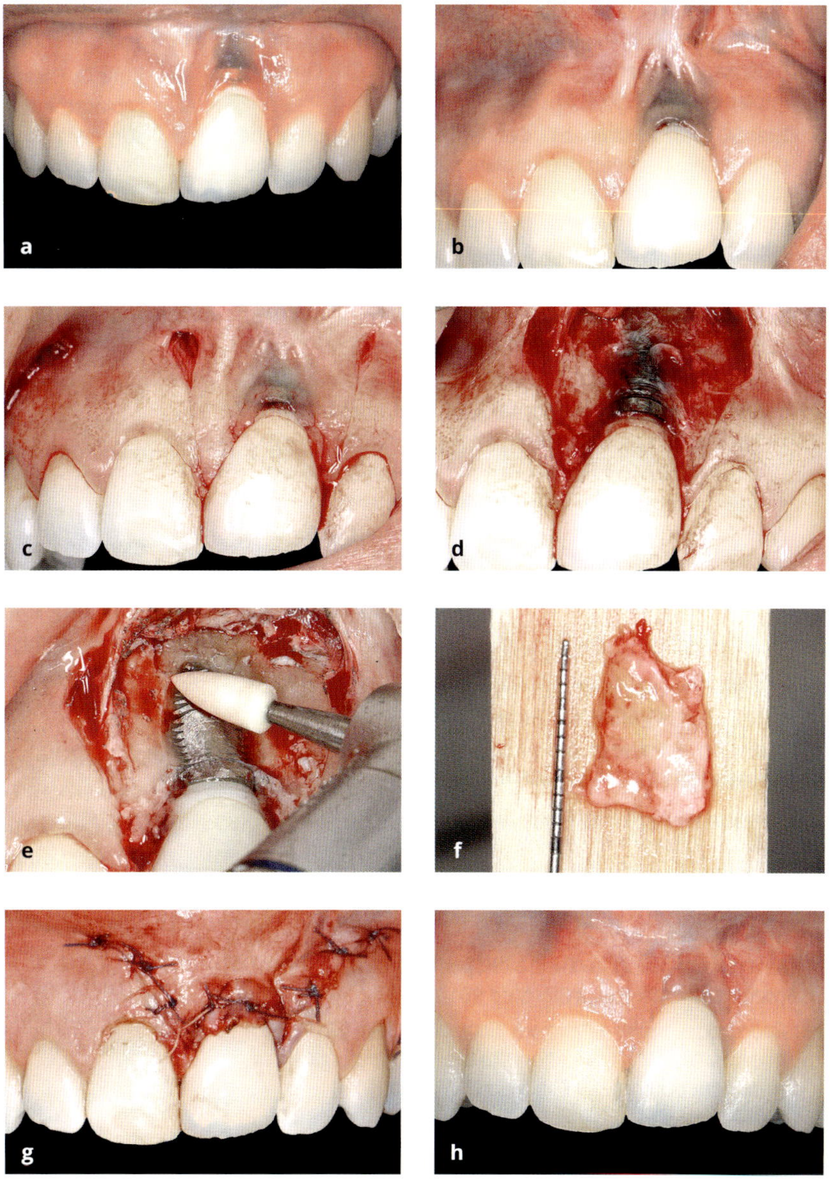

Figs 13-12a–h **(a)** The patient presented with the complaint of pain when administering oral hygiene. The implant in position no. 21 gives a gray shading to the mucosa, due to a lack of buccal bony plate. **(b)** Scar tissue had formed due to two previous surgeries for apicoectomy, which were painful. The patient did not consent to the removal of the implant, which was placed at great depth and in an exaggerated buccal position. **(c)** Plastic surgery aimed to increase the thickness of the soft tissues and correct the adhesions, to improve oral hygiene practices. An intrasulcular incision with vertical parts was prepared to design a trapezoidal flap. **(d)** After preparation of a partial-thickness flap. **(e)** After application of AIRFLOW (not shown), the part of the implant protruding from the buccal plate of the alveolar ridge was polished. **(f)** Connective tissue graft to increase the thickness of the keratinized mucosa. **(g)** The muscle fibers under the adhesions were released using a periosteal incision; after insertion of a connective tissue graft, the flap was repositioned and sutured coronally. **(h)** Clinical image 6 months after surgery. The increase in mucosal thickness and the elimination of tension from the adhesions are also clinically evident. In addition, the patient was able to perform oral hygiene.

References

1. Berglundh T, Lindhe J, Ericsson I, Marinello CP, Liljenberg B, Thomsen P. The soft tissue barrier at implants and teeth. Clin Oral Implants Res 1991;2:81–90.
2. Bouri A Jr, Bissada N, Al-Zahrani MS, Faddoul F, Nouneh I. Width of keratinized gingiva and the health status of the supporting tissues around dental implants. Int J Oral Maxillofac Implants 2008;23:323–326.
3. Buyukozdemir Askin S, Berker E, Akincibay H, et al. Necessity of keratinized tissues for dental implants: a clinical, immunological, and radiographic study. Clin Implant Dent Relat Res 2015;17:1–12.
4. Kungsadalpipob K, Supanimitkul K, Manopattanasoontorn S, Sophon N, Tangsathian T, Arunyanak SP. The lack of keratinized mucosa is associated with poor peri-implant tissue health: a cross-sectional study. Int J Implant Dent 2020;6:28.
5. Abrahamsson L, Berglundh T, Lindhe J. Soft tissue response to plaque formation at different implant systems. A comparative study in the dog. Clin Oral Implants Res 1998,9:73–79.
6. Berglundh T, Lindhe J, Ericsson I, Marinello CP, Liljenberg B. Soft tissue reactions to de novo plaque formation at implants and teeth. An experimental study in the dog. Clin Oral Implants Res 1992;3:1–8.

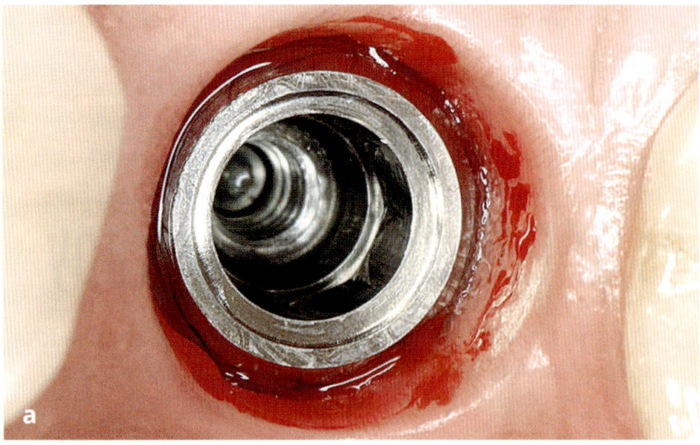

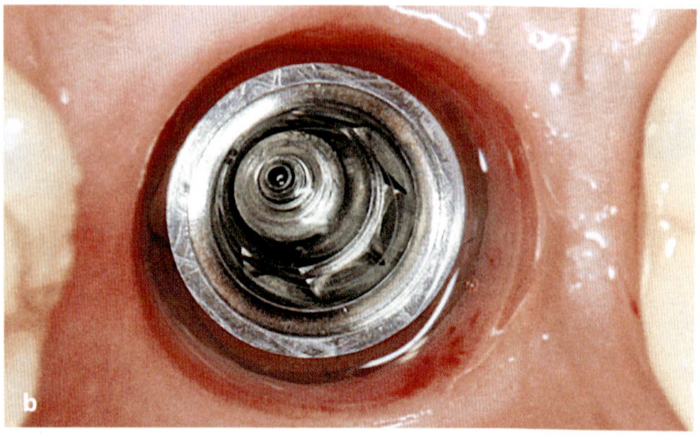

Figs 14-1a, b **(a)** Effectiveness of peri-implant mucositis treatment: after removal of the screw-retained crown from the implant before treatment of peri-implant mucositis. Inflammation and the bleeding surface of the peri-implant mucosa can be seen. **(b)** After inflammation was controlled, unscrewing of the crown revealed the health of the peri-implant tissues.

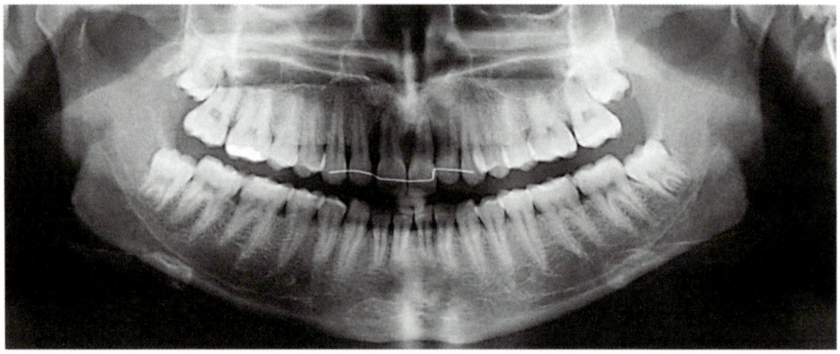

Fig 14-2a Radiographic image of a young patient, aged 16 years, with localized juvenile periodontitis (stage III, grade C).

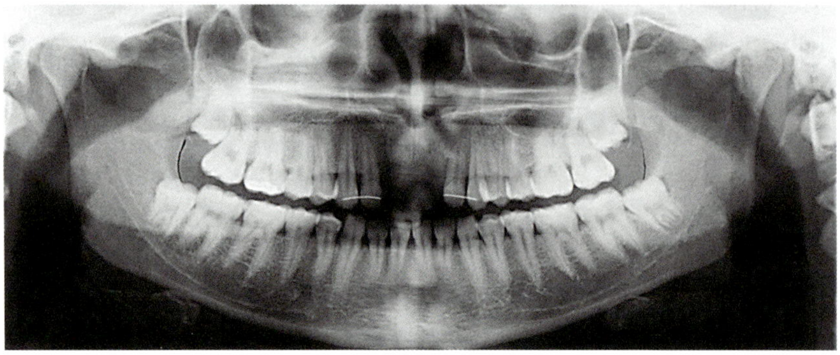

Fig 14-2b Tooth loss at the age of 18 years was treated with implant placement; the patient was told that she should be monitored by a periodontist to avoid the occurrence of peri-implant pathology.

difficult because of surface decontamination.[15–19] At the same time, ways of reshaping titanium layer oxides are being sought.[20] The question is how to deal with peri-implant pathology that will occur increasingly often in the future as the number of people with implants grows, and the number of implants that have already been placed worldwide is vast.

The Hippocratic approach is more relevant today than ever before. It advocates prevention as the best form of treatment. In the first instance, primary prevention is discussed through the identification of pathologic risk factors,[21] so that treatment plans can be individualized and include ways to deal with these. Secondary prevention focuses on the early diagnosis of diseases, eliminating etiological factors through effective and timely therapy. Thus, treatment of peri-implant mucositis is the best method of prevention for peri-implantitis (Figs 14-1a, b).

Finally, tertiary prevention must be introduced once the disease is established. To reduce damage and prevent further destruction, the most effective treatment is required (Figs 14-2a–q).

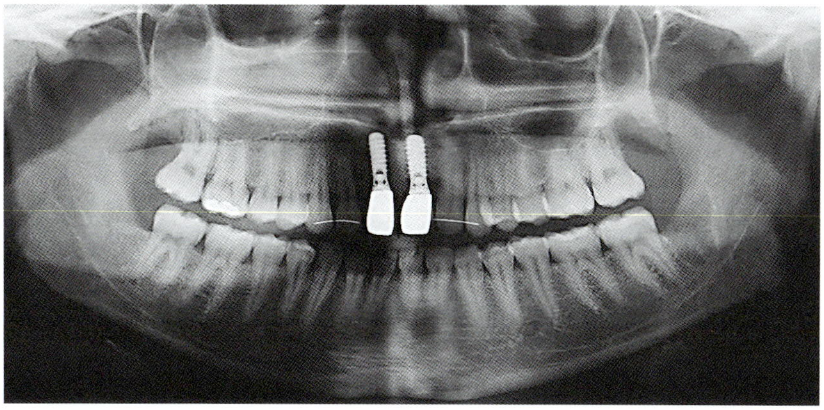

Fig 14-2c Radiographic image of the patient after completion of prosthetic rehabilitation.

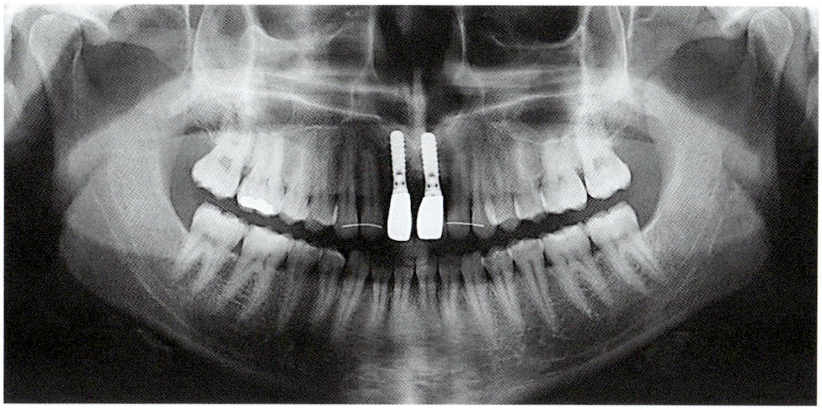

Fig 14-2d Radiographic image 11 years after implant placement. In the meantime, the patient had started smoking, but the therapeutic effect was maintained.

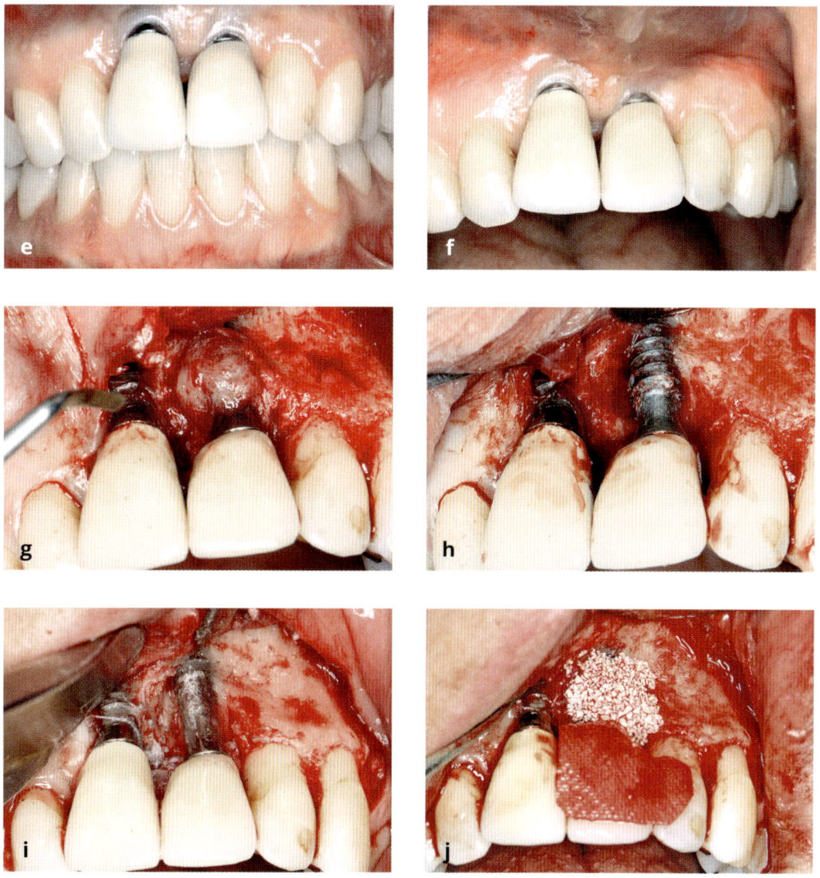

Figs 14-2e–j **(e)** Clinical situation 13 years after implant placement. **(f)** Fifteen years after placement and after a short period when the patient missed her supportive periodontal therapy sessions because of health problems, peri-implantitis was diagnosed. The patient had maintained her oral hygiene, but her tobacco consumption had increased significantly. There was a change in the clinical picture of the gingiva; 8-mm-deep peri-implant pockets were detected at implant no. 21 (not shown). **(g)** After elevation of a full-thickness flap, the granulation tissue surrounding the implant was displayed. **(h)** After removal of the granulation tissue and mechanical disinfection of the implant surface, the morphology and severity of the bony lesion were determined. A decision was made to smooth the threads above the bony crest and perform guided bone regeneration, as the patient was willing to quit smoking. **(i)** Area before the regeneration procedure. **(j)** Bone allograft placement.

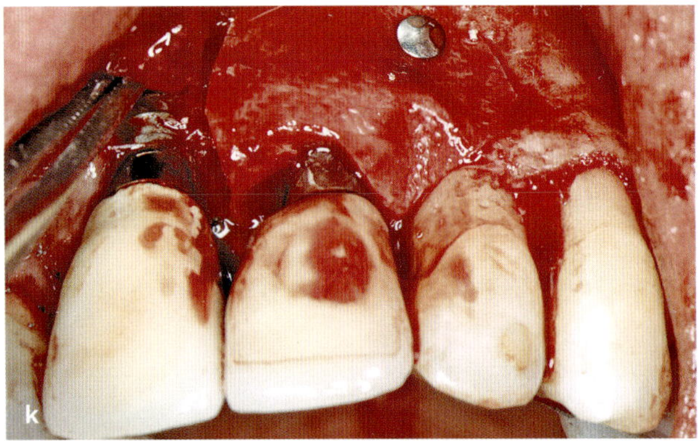

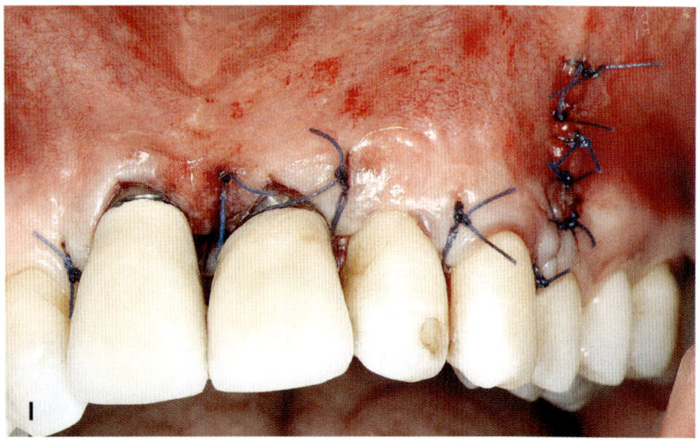

Figs 14-2k, l **(k)** Stabilization of the collagen membrane with titanium pins. **(l)** Flap suturing.

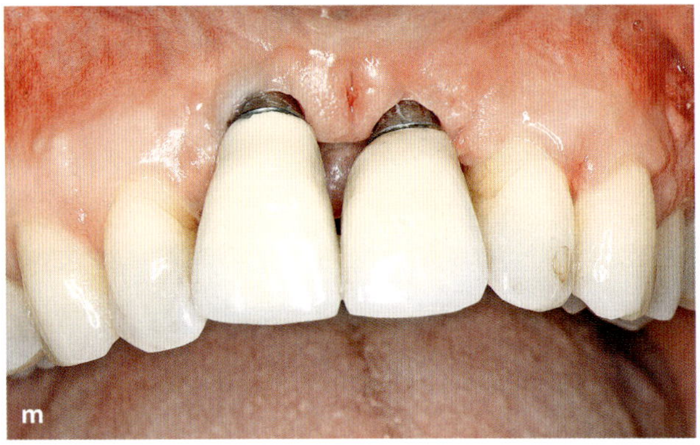

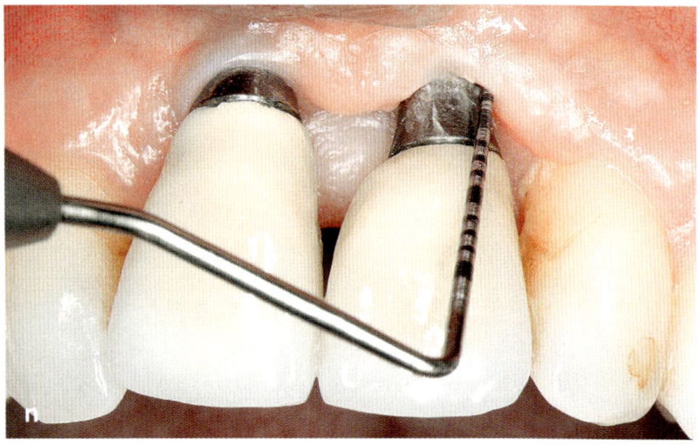

Figs 14-2m, n **(m)** Clinical situation of the site 14 days later and immediately after suture removal. There was a slight delay in healing between the two implants. **(n)** Two years after surgery. The impression on the interdental papilla was preserved, but the area remained relatively free of inflammation and pockets.

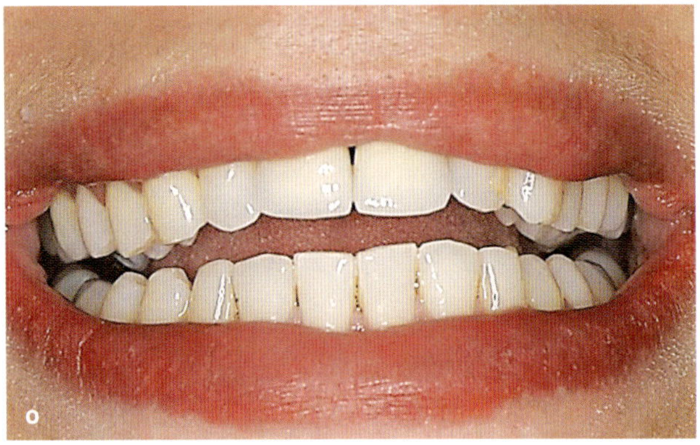

Fig 14-2o The patient's low smile line can be seen, which fortunately hides the metallic neck of the implants.

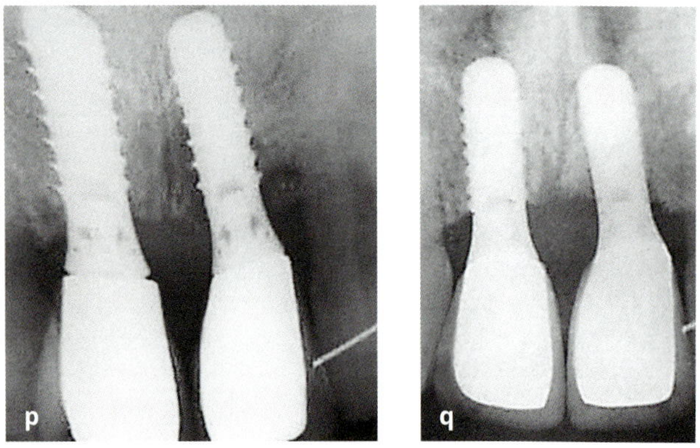

Figs 14-2p, q Radiographic images taken **(p)** before and **(q)** 2 years after peri-implantitis treatment. Smoothing of the threads can be seen, as well as filling of the endosseous defect. The titanium pin that held the membrane can also be seen.

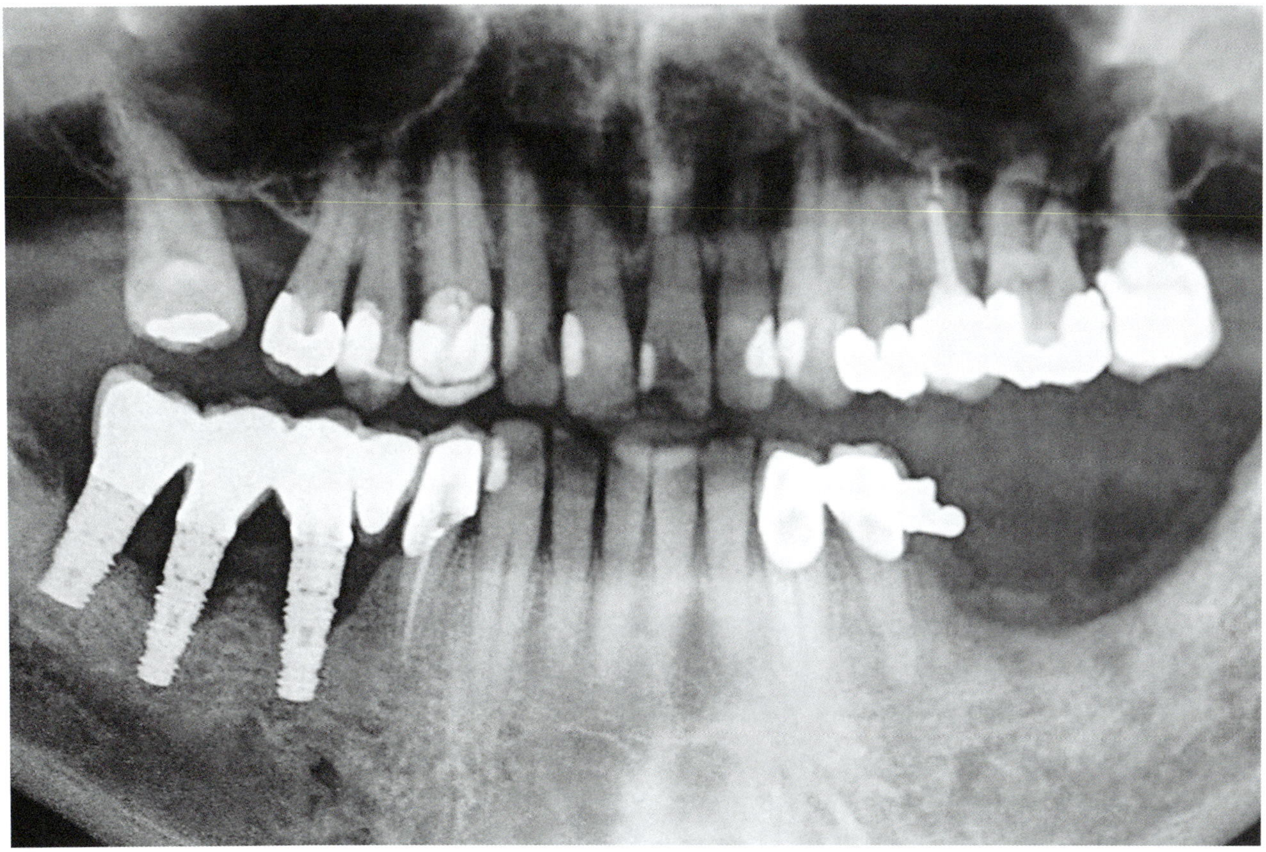

Fig 14-3a Radiographic image of a patient 8 years after implant placement. The patient developed periodontitis and peri-implantitis.

From research data to date, the following facts have emerged:

- Patient selection and control of known risk factors lead to significant improvements in outcomes, that is, the rate of achieving osseointegration, and significantly reduce the incidence of peri-implant lesions.
- Providing information in a timely manner and motivating and instructing patients with regard to performing oral hygiene, in combination with its effective implementation, significantly increase the percentage of cases that are disease-free.
- Patients should be enrolled in a strict maintenance care program that requires compliance with regular recall intervals and provided with supportive care.
- Patients with peri-implant mucositis should be diagnosed and treated immediately.
- Use of antimicrobial mouthrinses may help in combination with removal of the bacterial load.
- Administering systemic antibiotics in combination with mechanical removal of biofilms cannot replace optimal access to the contaminated surface or inhibit the progression of bone destruction.
- The effectiveness of nonsurgical approaches to peri-implantitis therapy is limited, regardless of the type of approach (Figs 14-3a–i).
- The lesser the bone loss at the diagnosis of peri-implantitis, the greater the chance that the therapeutic intervention will be effective in the long term.
- There is no specific surgical technique that is more advantageous over another in terms of clinical outcomes.
- All surgical techniques have limited success rates compared to when the same techniques are used to treat periodontitis.
- Peri-implantitis shows high rates of recurrence and retreatment is often necessary. For this reason, patients diagnosed with peri-implantitis should be informed accordingly and understand that the clinician's efforts are aimed primarily and realistically at extending the life expectancy of the implants affected by the disease (Figs 14-4a–h).

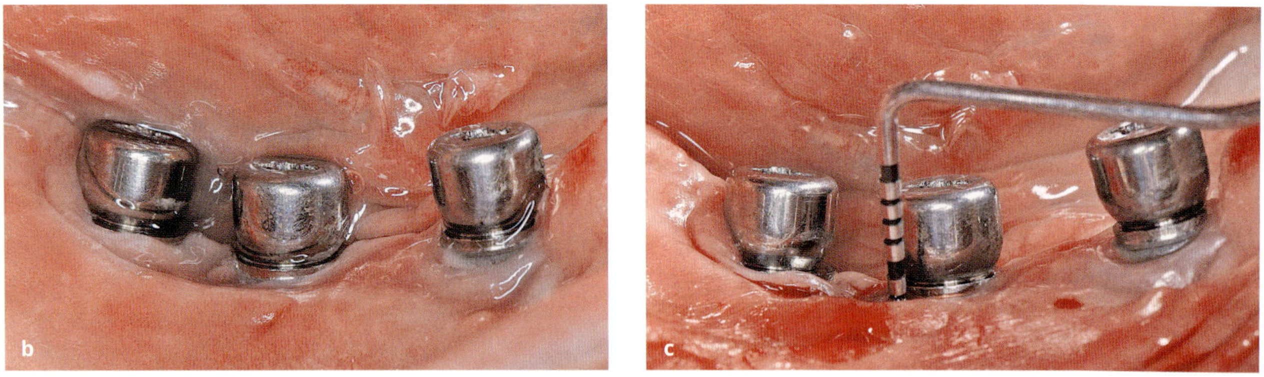

Figs 14-3b, c According to the patient, gingivectomy had been applied in the implant area; that is, the free peri-implant mucosa had been resected, apparently in an attempt to reduce the depth of the pockets. Mucosectomy was the wrong choice because it created additional mucosal problems, while the pockets remained during the initial examination.

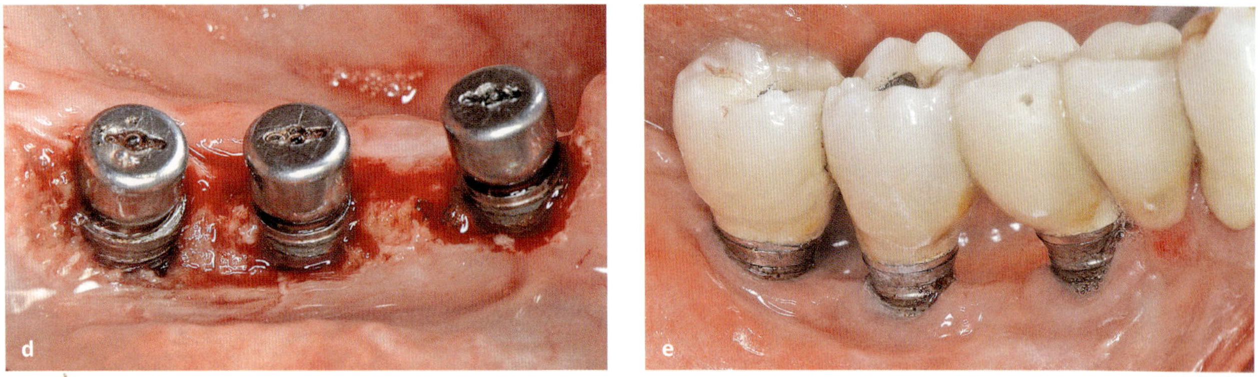

Figs 14-3d, e **(d)** The CIST protocol (steps A and B) was applied using a 980-nm diode laser. In addition, laser treatment was repeated every 2 months. **(e)** Two years after treatment, the condition had improved, with an increase in the width of the keratinized peri-implant mucosa and elimination of inflammation.

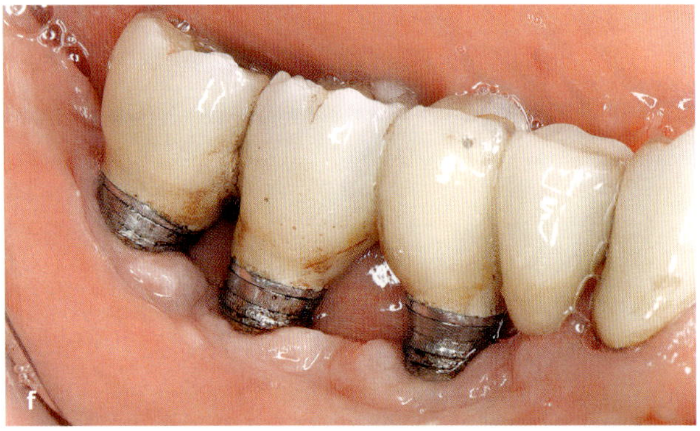

Fig 14-3f Seven years later, when the patient was receiving supportive periodontal therapy every 3 months. In each session, the CIST protocol was applied.

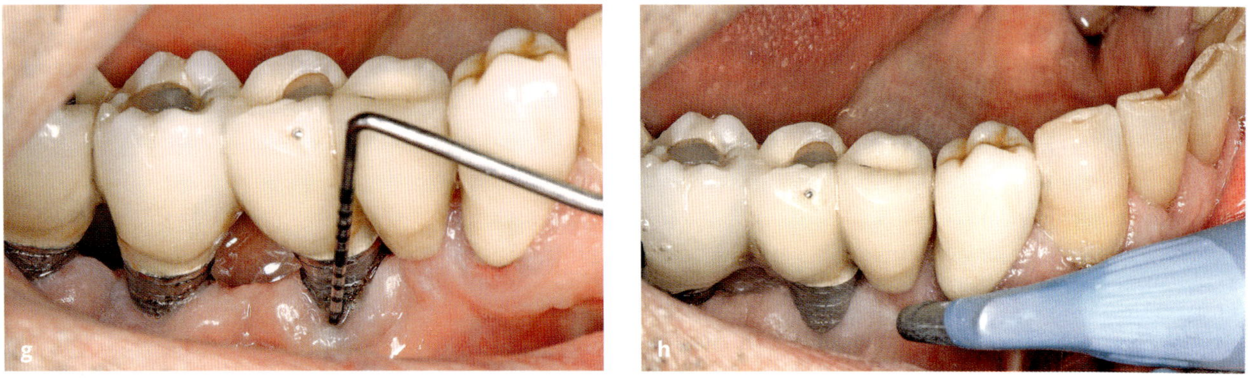

Figs 14-3g, h **(g)** Ten years after treatment of peri-implantitis and 18 years after implant placement. **(h)** In each supportive periodontal therapy session, guided biofilm therapy was applied.

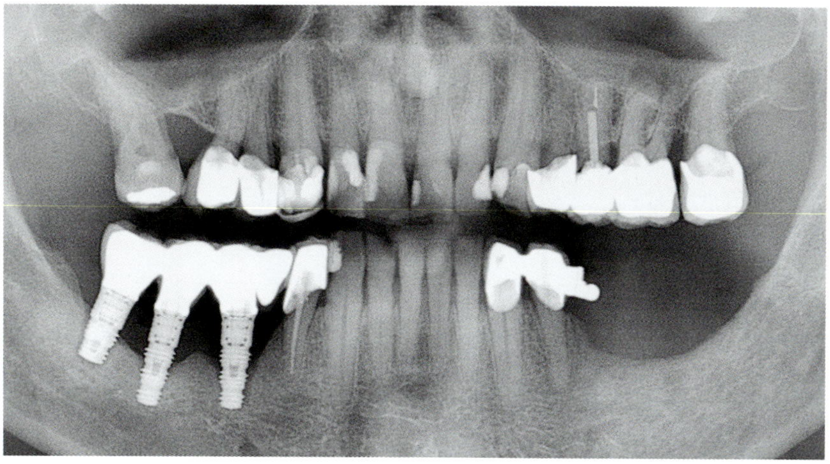

Fig 14-3i Radiographic image of the patient 18 years after implant placement and 10 years after the treatment of periodontitis and peri-implantitis. Effective oral hygiene, compliance with the supportive therapy protocol sessions, and the implementation of the CIST protocol, with amendments adopted over time, contributed to the preservation of teeth and implants in biologically, functionally, and esthetically acceptable conditions.

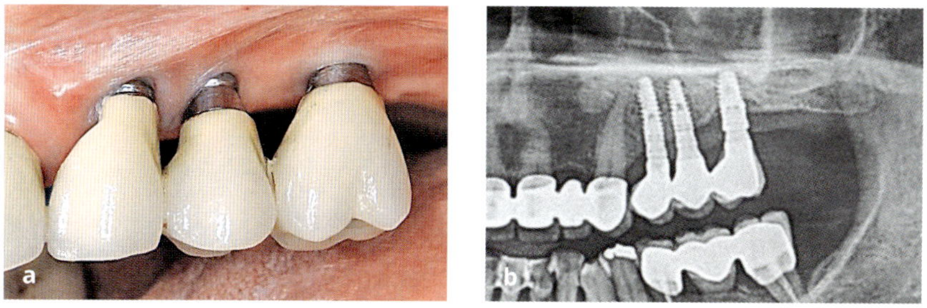

Figs 14-4a, b Clinical and radiographic images of a patient with peri-implantitis after completion of steps A and B of the CIST protocol.

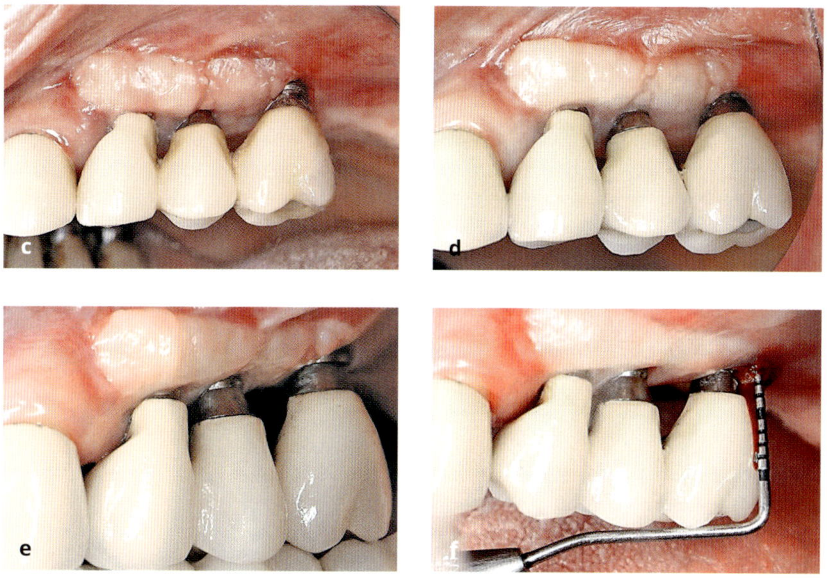

Figs 14-4c–f **(c)** Clinical picture 3 weeks after completion of treatment, which included an increase in the width of the keratinized mucosa. **(d)** Healing 1.5 months after placement of a free mucosal graft. **(e)** Six months after surgery. **(f)** One and a half years after completion of treatment, relapse was observed at implant no. 26, which was treated with control of inflammation (steps A and B).

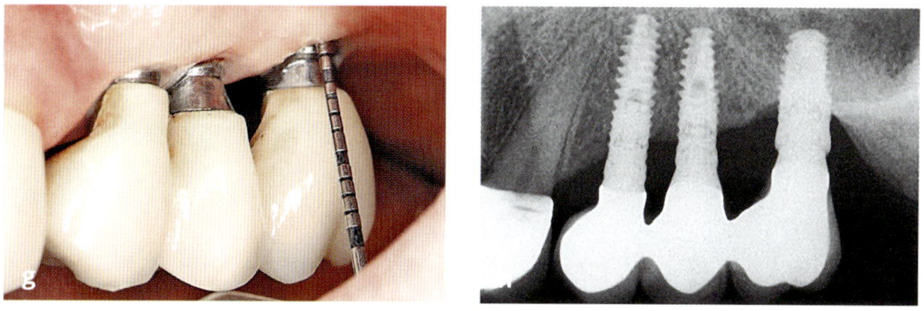

Figs 14-4 g, h Clinical and radiographic images 6 years after the onset of treatment and 4.5 years after treatment of the relapse. Note the preservation of implants in a healthy condition despite the need for a second treatment intervention.

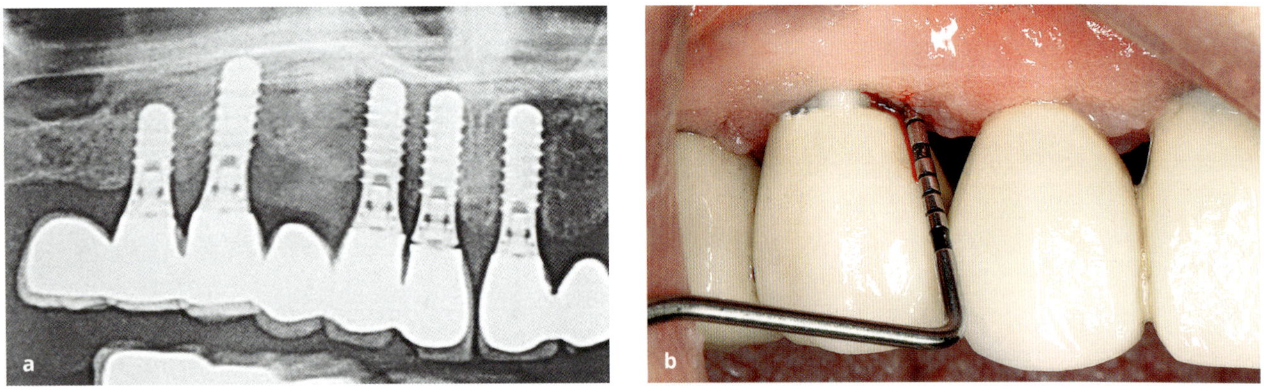

Figs 14-5a, b Clinical and radiographic images of a smoker with peri-implantitis at implant no. 14, 7 years after implant placement.

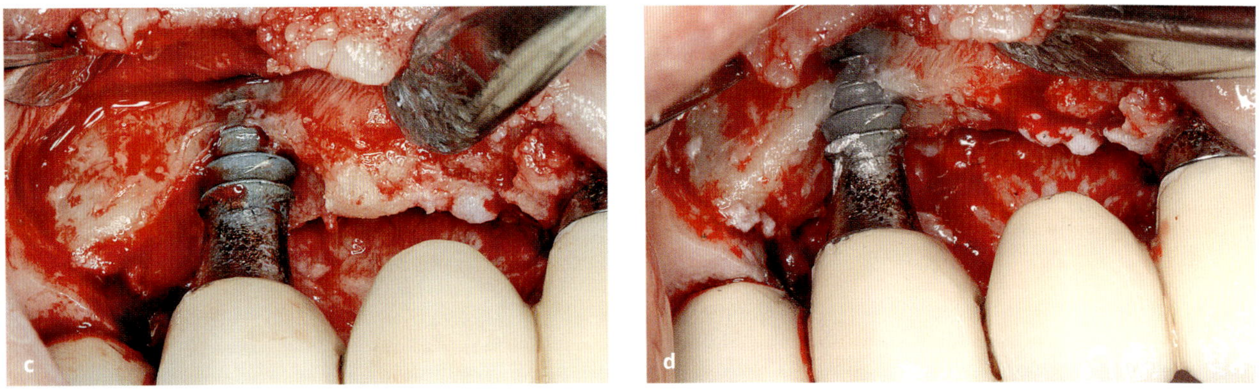

Figs 14-5c, d (c) Inflammation control was preceded by performing steps A and B (not shown), followed by surgery. After full-thickness flap elevation, the morphology of the intrabony lesion, which had two bony walls (one proximal and one distal) and a shallow depth, was disclosed. This is an indication for resective surgery. For implant no. 12, no bone destruction was noted. **(d)** Elimination of the lesion with osteoplasty after disinfection of the implant surface can be observed.

- The effectiveness of each individual treatment is determined by successful disinfection of the implant surface and reshaping of the morphology of the peri-implant defect, which may facilitate unobstructed oral hygiene practices.
- To date, no studies suggest that the prognosis of implants is better than that of periodontally treated teeth, even more so for healthy teeth.

The main difference in the treatment of peri-implant mucositis is the fact that removal of the cause leads to restoration of normal healthy tissues if inflammation is restricted to the mucosa. In peri-implantitis, however, the pocket and the implant surface will easily be recolonized even if bacteria were successfully removed from the pocket and implant surface.

To help the clinician choose the most appropriate treatment intervention depending on the requirements of each individual case, a special effort has been made to take into account as much scientific data as possible, to evaluate and incorporate it into a protocol suggested in this book.

In medicine in general, and specifically in dentistry, every therapeutic intervention aims to improve the quality of life and function of individuals with periodontal disease and maintain health (Figs 14-5a–t). Nevertheless, because treatment is combined with the most meaningful interventions, there is a significant number of problematic cases in which the disease may not be completely eliminated with the knowledge we have today (Figs 14-6a–d).

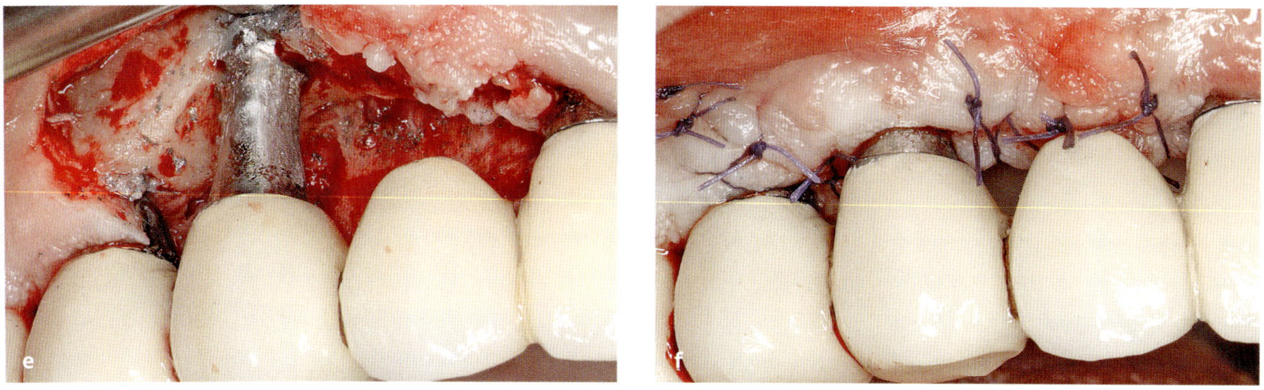

Figs 14-5e, f (e) The exposed threads were smoothed. **(f)** This was followed by apical displacement of the flap and suturing.

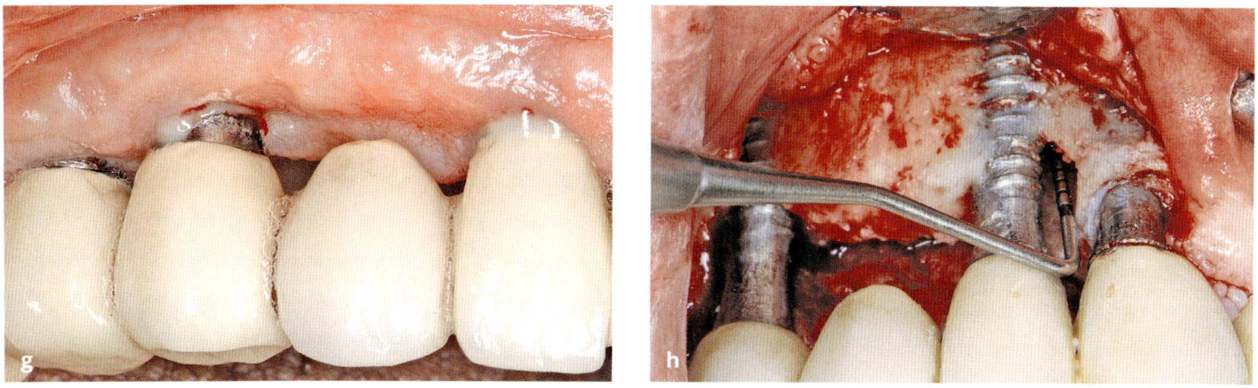

Figs 14-5 g, h (g) Two years after the operation, there was a recurrence of pockets (not shown), bleeding on probing, and pus exudation at implants nos.14 and 12. **(h)** After elevation of a full-thickness flap and removal of granulation tissue. Bone loss was found on the buccal surface of the implants, probably because during placement, the width of the alveolar ridge was thin and bone resorption had not been considered. However, peri-implantitis could be observed, as evidenced by extensive bone destruction in the adjacent areas. The intrabony lesion at no. 12 had a depth of 15 mm. The outcome of the smoothing of implant no. 14, which was done during the first operation, can now be seen.

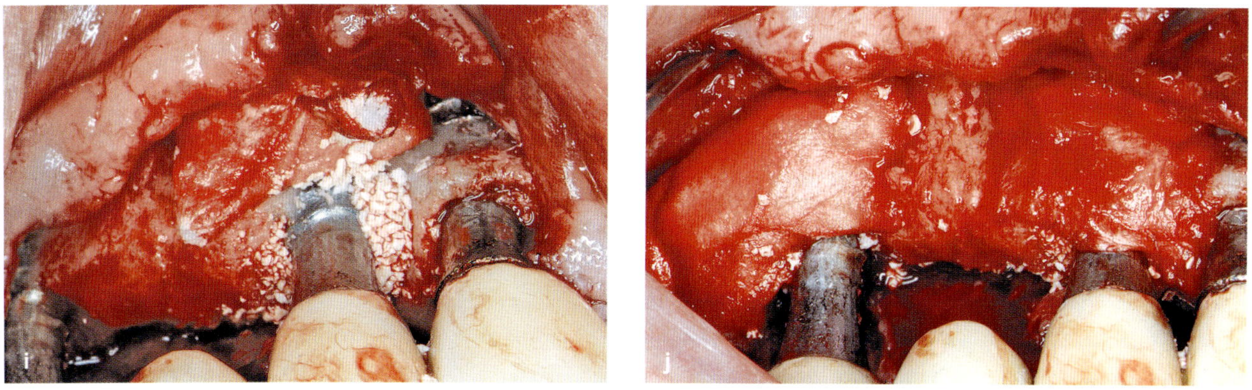

Figs 14-5i, j Bone graft placement and guided bone regeneration, first at implant no. 12 and then at implant no. 14. The patient agreed to quit smoking.

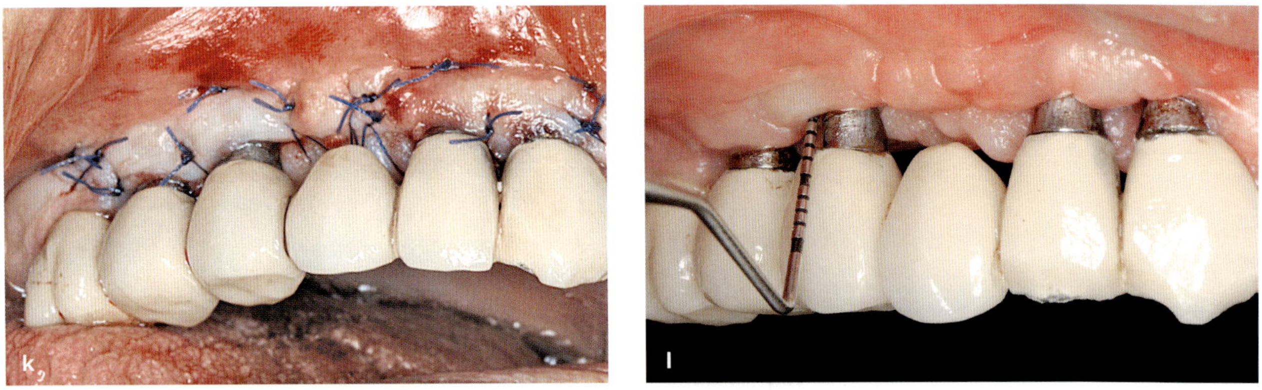

Figs 14-5k, l (k) Suturing of the flap. **(l)** Clinical situation 6 months after surgery. The goal was to eliminate inflammation and reduce pocket depth through regeneration of the peri-implant bone. Even though the patient denied quitting smoking, healing was observed.

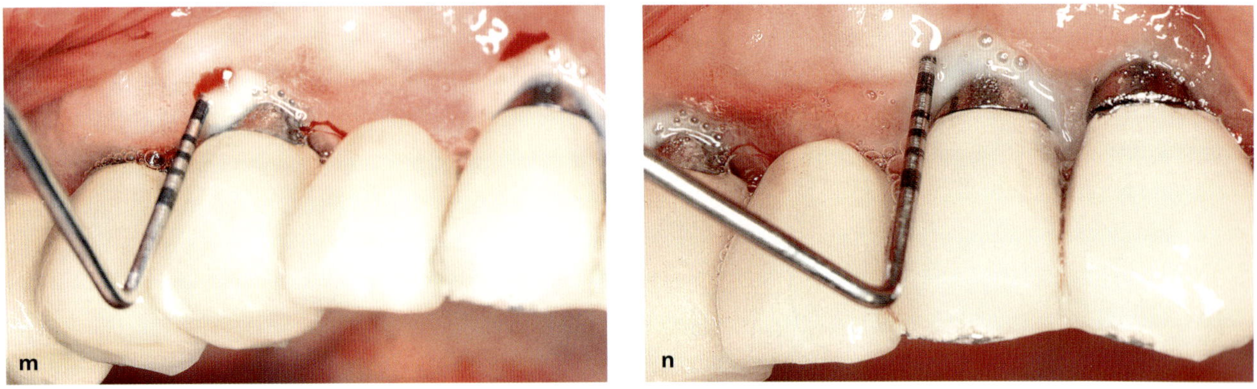

Figs 14-5m, n Three years later, recurrence of peri-implantitis was observed. Deepening of pockets, pus exudation, and bleeding on probing could be seen.

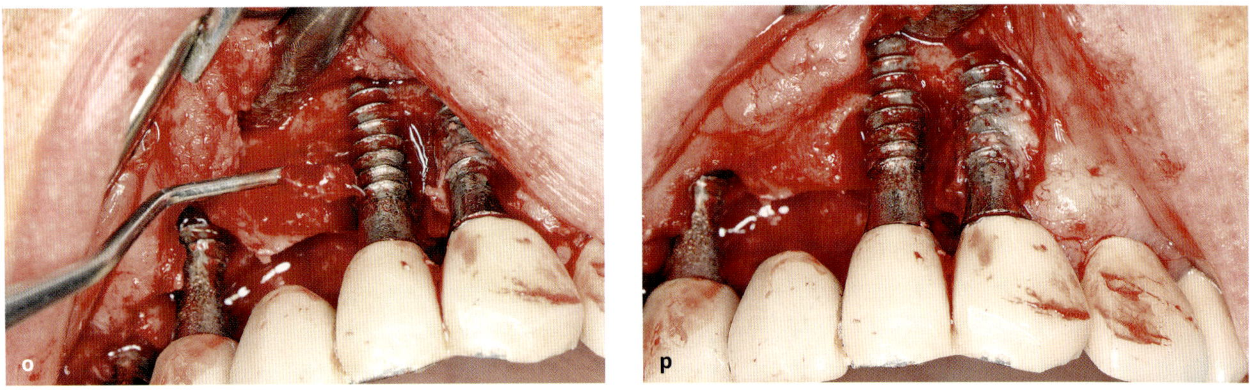

Figs 14-5o, p (o) During removal of granulation tissue, grains were found from the xenograft placed 3 years prior. **(p)** The morphology of the lesions was not suitable for use of regenerative techniques; on the other hand, the patient was not willing to try to quit smoking again. A decision was made to perform resective surgery. The clinical image of the implants revealed advanced and severe peri-implantitis. In the first quadrant, only implant no. 15 was not affected.

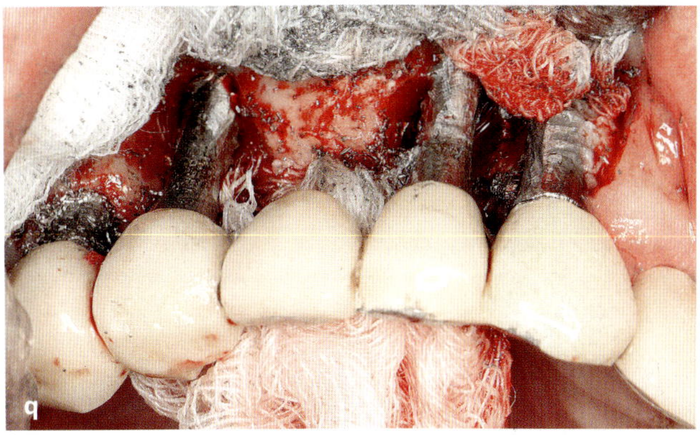

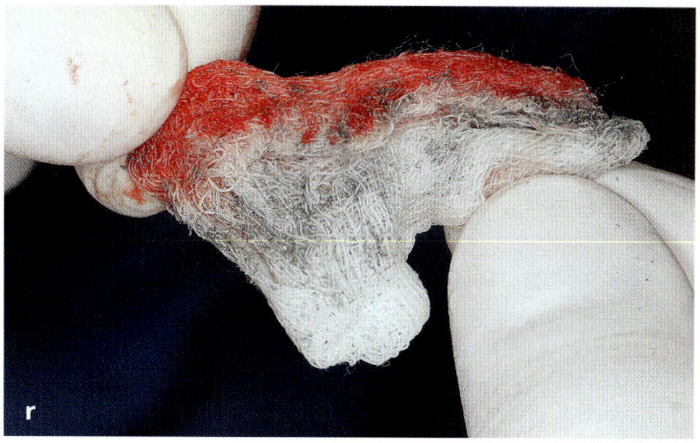

Figs 14-5q, r (q) Smoothing of the implant threads. A gauze was placed under the flaps to collect the shavings from grinding the titanium threads. **(r)** The mass of the shavings was significant, as shown by the gray color of the gauze.

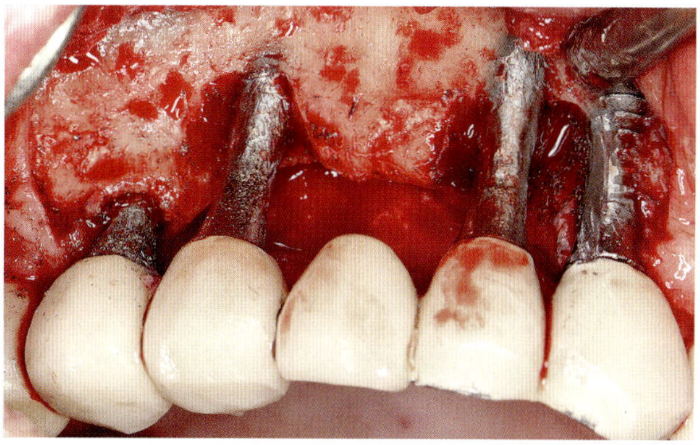

Fig 14-5s During smoothing of the threads and before completion of bone surgery. Ultrasonic cleaning was used to remove as much of the titanium shavings as possible.

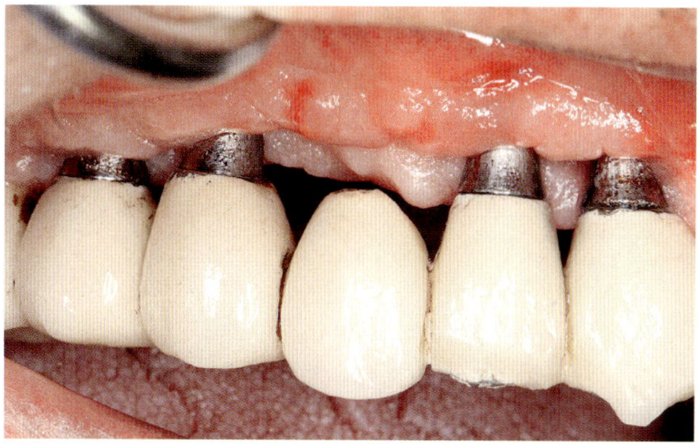

Fig 14-5t Two years after the operation, the result was stable. Although the implants were not successful, they survived. The low smile line makes the issue of esthetics irrelevant in this patient. Seven years after implant placement, peri-implantitis was diagnosed and recurred three times, despite previous and repeated surgical treatment. However, the implants have been maintained for a total of 14 years.

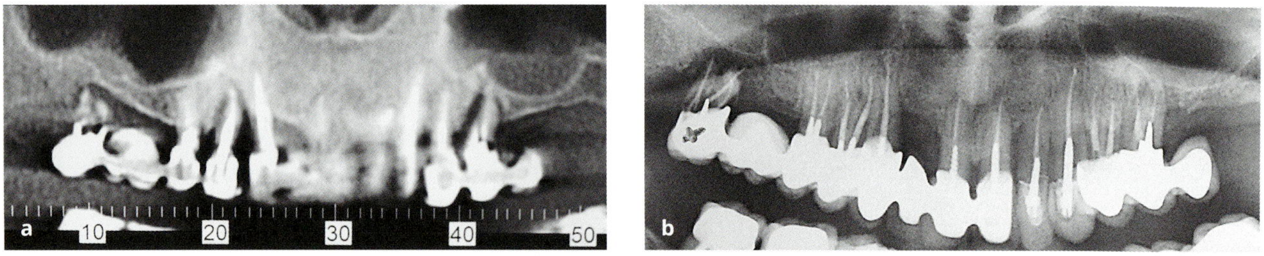

Figs 14-6a, b Panoramic imaging (computed tomography scan and panoramic radiograph) of the maxilla of a candidate for implant placement.

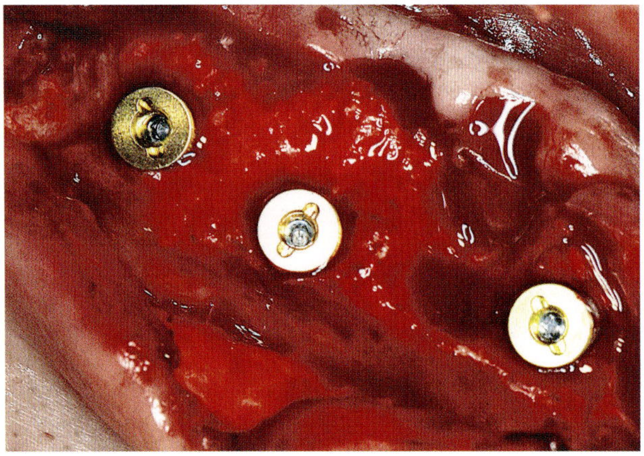

Fig 14-6c Three implants were placed in the first quadrant.

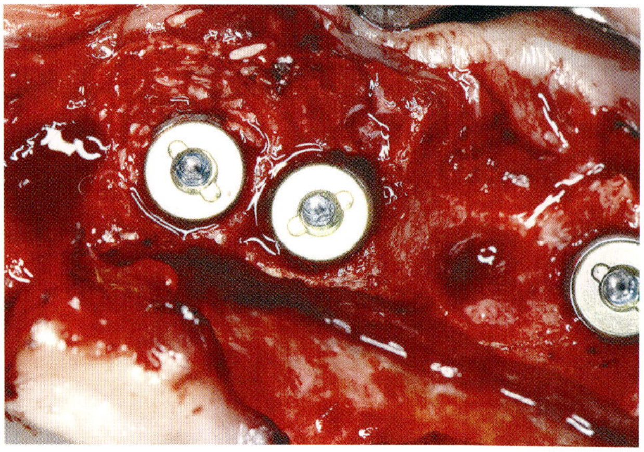

Fig 14-6d Three of the four implants placed in the second quadrant can be seen. Where necessary, surgery was performed to maintain the alveolar crest using guided bone regeneration, as well as transalveolar sinus elevation for implants nos. 15 and 25.

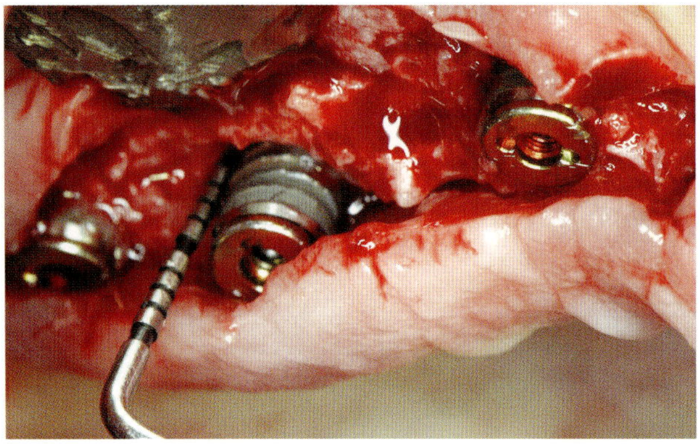

Fig 14-6e Six months after placement, the implants were uncovered. Some bone loss can be observed around implants nos. 12 and 15, while in implant no. 14 there is significant loss and intrabony defect. Therefore, implant no. 14 was removed.

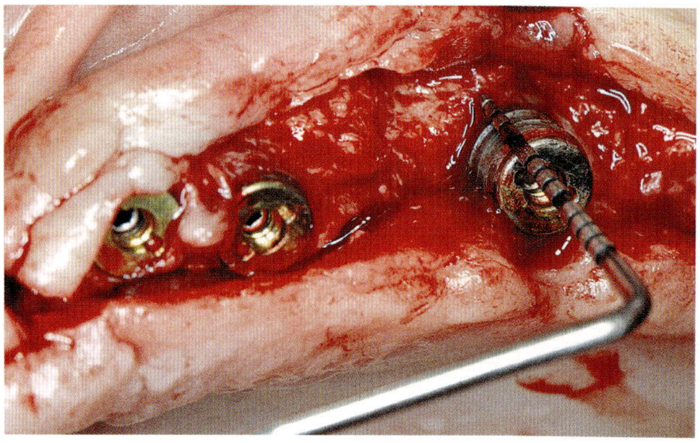

Fig 14-6f Bone loss of 5 mm can be observed at implant no. 25. It was decided that this implant should remain.

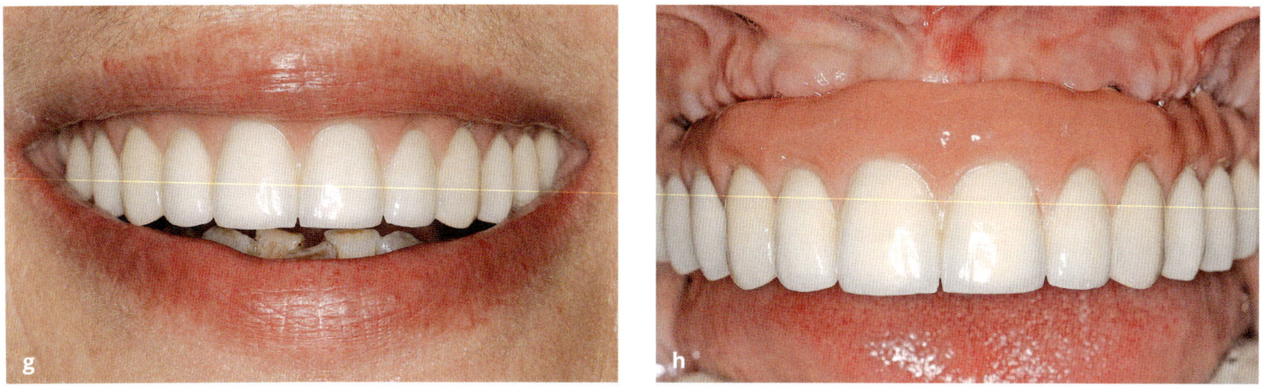

Figs 14-6g, h Clinical situation after the completion of rehabilitation with a hybrid prosthesis, 3 months after uncovering the implants.

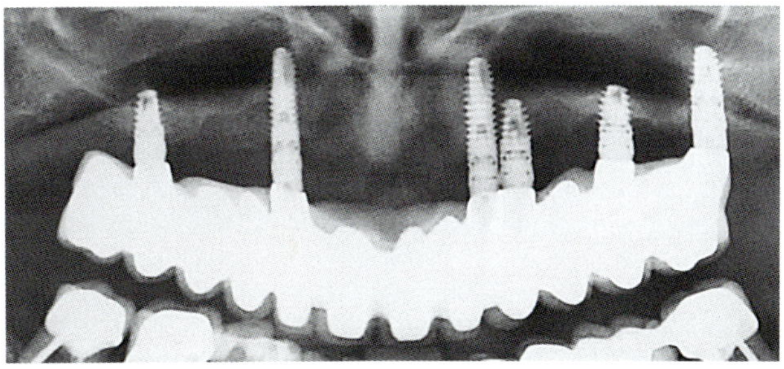

Fig 14-6i Panoramic radiograph showing the maxilla 2 years after implant placement. Significant bone loss can be seen at implant no. 25 and, to a lesser extent, at implants nos. 12, 22, and 23.

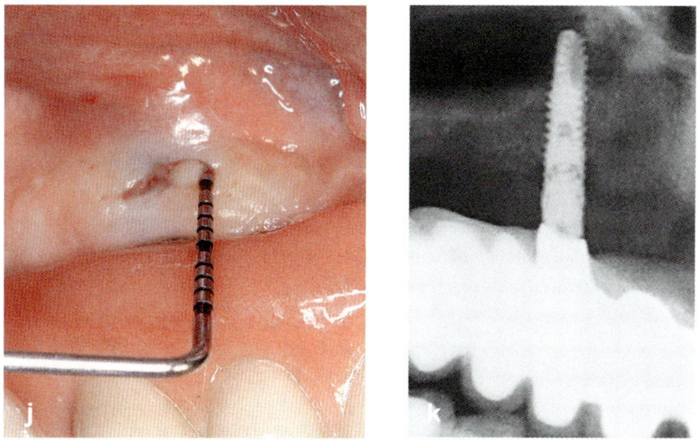

Fig 14-6j, k (j) Three years after implantation, soft tissue perforation can be observed at the border of the keratinized peri-implant mucosa at implant no. 12. **(k)** The radiographic image did not reveal severe bone loss. During this time, the patient responded consistently to quarterly supportive periodontal therapy after having applied steps A and B of the modified CIST protocol, with satisfactory effects.

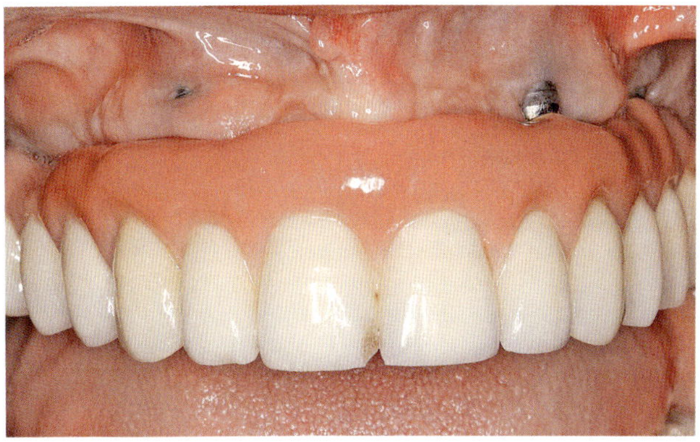

Fig 14-6l At the same time, at implant no. 22, recession was observed.

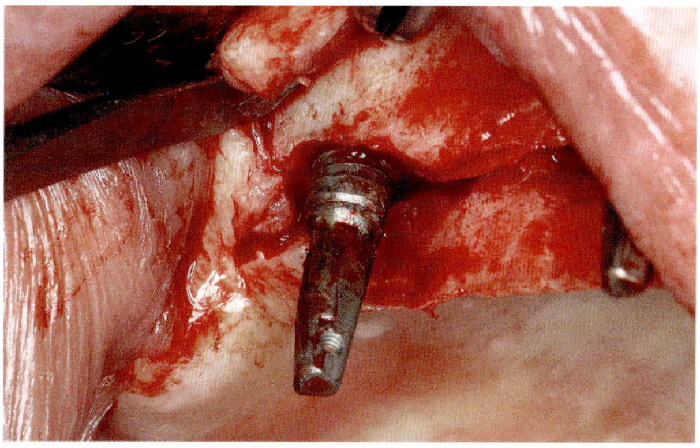

Fig 14-6m The modified CIST protocol was applied, specifically steps A, B, C, and D. At implant no. 15, three exposed threads are visible.

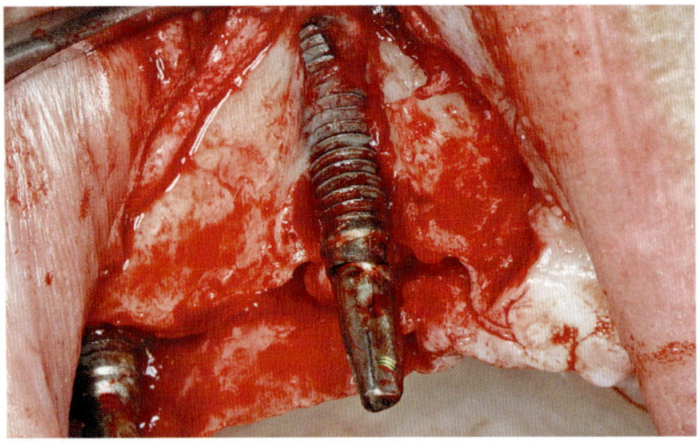

Fig 14-6n Implant no. 12 shows bone dehiscence, resulting in buccal exposure of the implant threads. This bone loss was not due to incorrect placement of the implant in a buccal position.

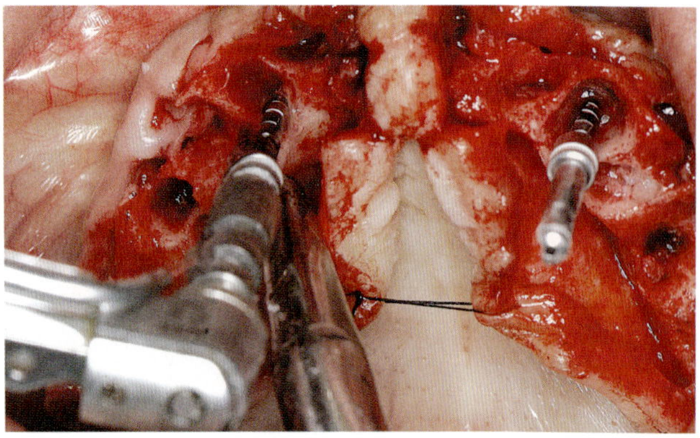

Fig 14-6o Photograph after implant placement surgery. Implant no. 12 was placed on the palatal side of the socket after extraction, followed by a bone graft (decalcified freeze-dried bone allograft) and collagen membrane for guided bone regeneration, the success of which was confirmed during re-entry.

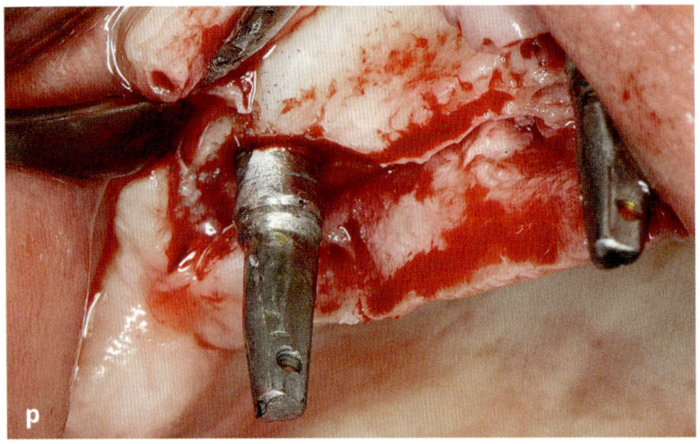

p

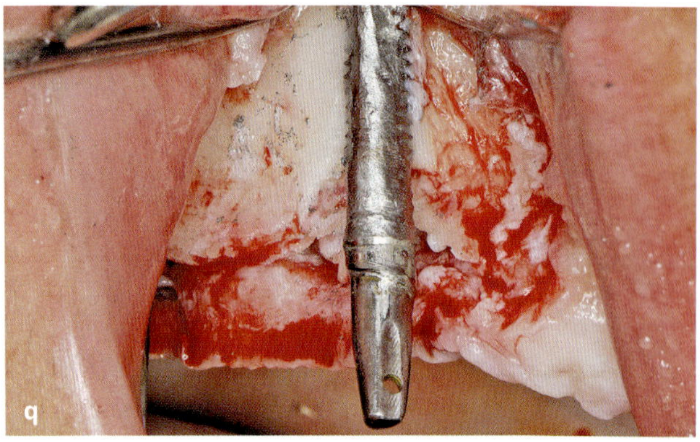

q

Figs 14-6p, q The two implants after mechanical removal of biofilms and smoothing of their threads.

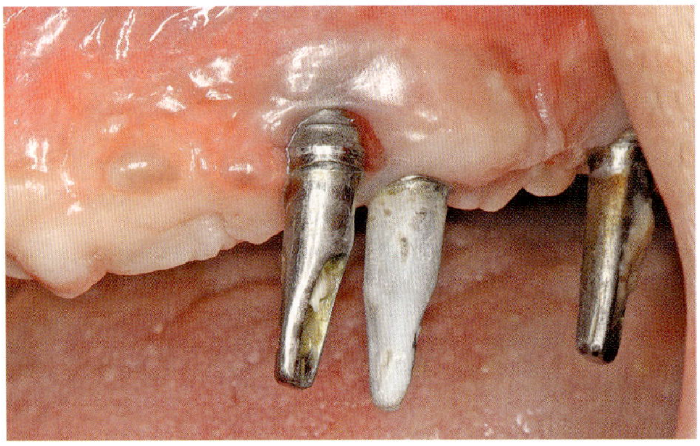

Fig 14-6r For 3 more years, the condition remained stable and the patient came into the clinic every 3 months; steps A and B of the modified CIST protocol were applied. However, 6 years after implant placement, inflammation and pockets were found in the area of implants nos. 22 and 23.

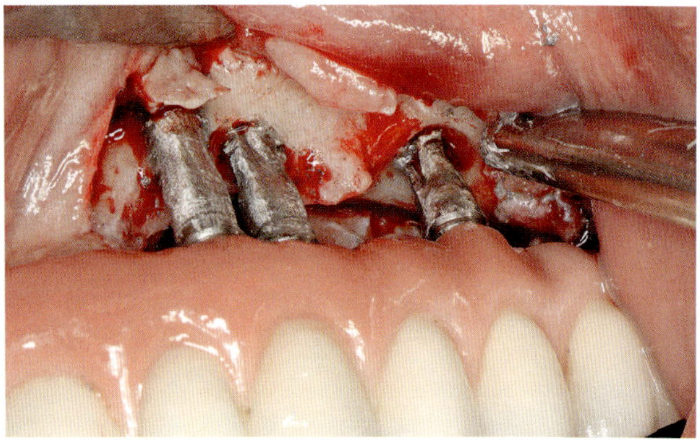

Fig 14-6s The modified CIST protocol was applied, namely steps A, B, C, and D. Flap elevation was performed and smoothing of the threads that were exposed in a pocket environment at implants nos. 22 and 23 was carried out, but also at implant no. 25, which had exposed threads from the time of uncovering.

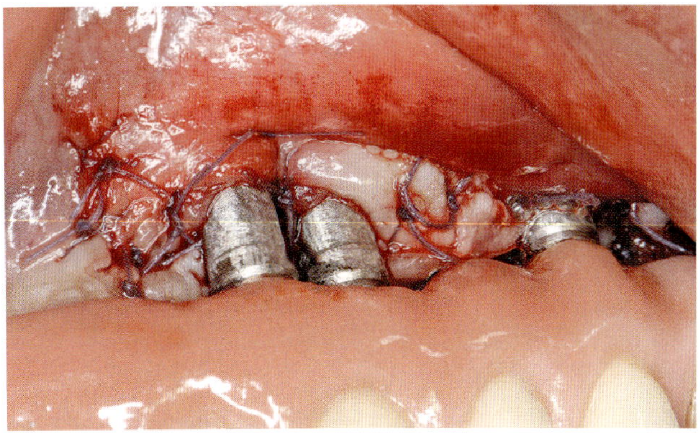

Fig 14-6t The result after apical displacement and suturing of the flap.

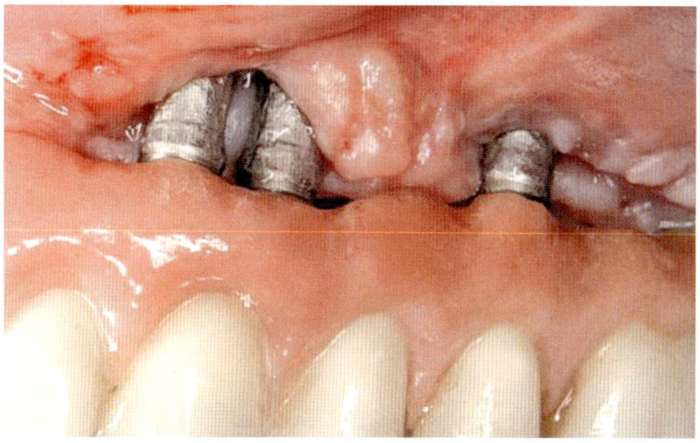

Fig 14-6u Clinical situation 10 days later, during suture removal.

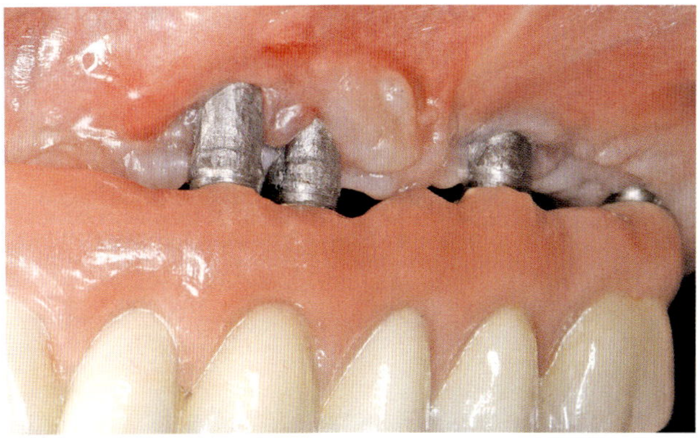

Fig 14-6v Clinical situation 1 month after surgery. Conditions that might facilitate oral hygiene practices were achieved.

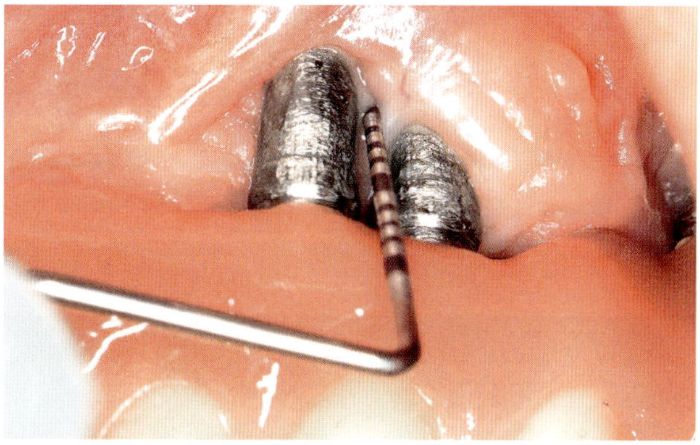

Fig 14-6w Seven years after placement and 1 year after surgery, a 4-mm pocket was observed during probing. On probing, pus exudation occurred. The relapse was addressed by applying steps A and B of the modified CIST protocol.

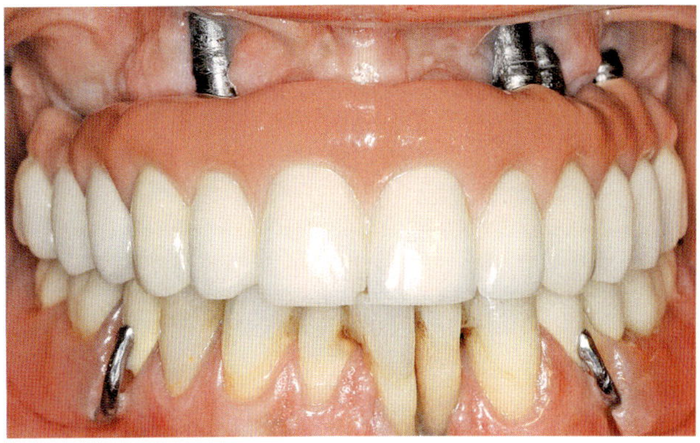

Fig 14-6x Clinical situation 9 years after implant placement. The patient attended the supportive periodontal therapy sessions every 2 months, and steps A and B of the modified CIST protocol were applied. Although the implants survived, the situation progressively deteriorated over the years.

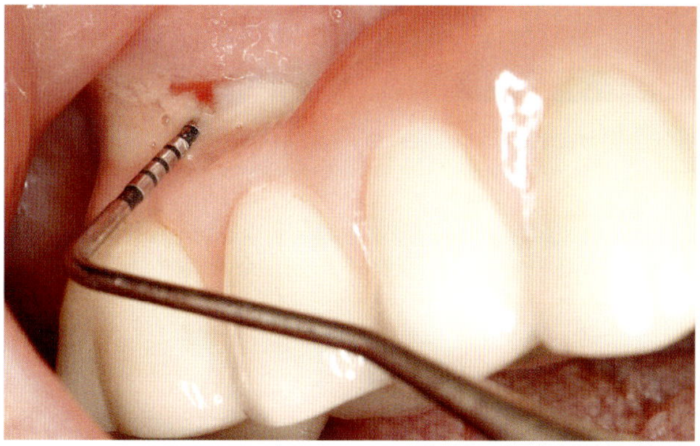

Fig 14-6y Ten years after the implants were placed, the patient presented with an abscess at implant no. 15, which was treated by applying steps A, B, and C of the modified CIST protocol. A complementary laser application for bactericidal control was also performed.

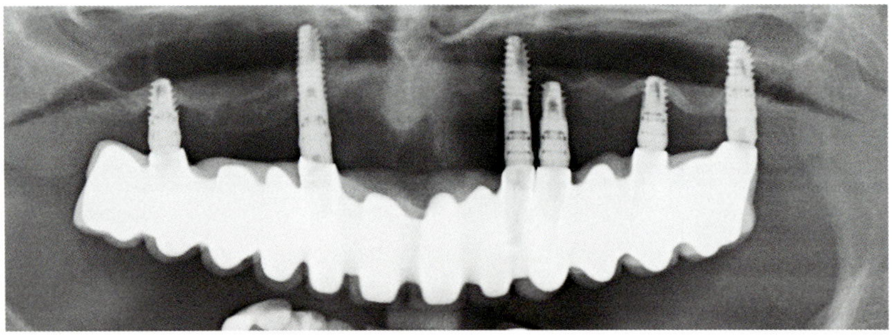

Fig 14-6z Panoramic radiograph taken 10 years after implant placement. Deterioration of the bone support of the implants is clear.

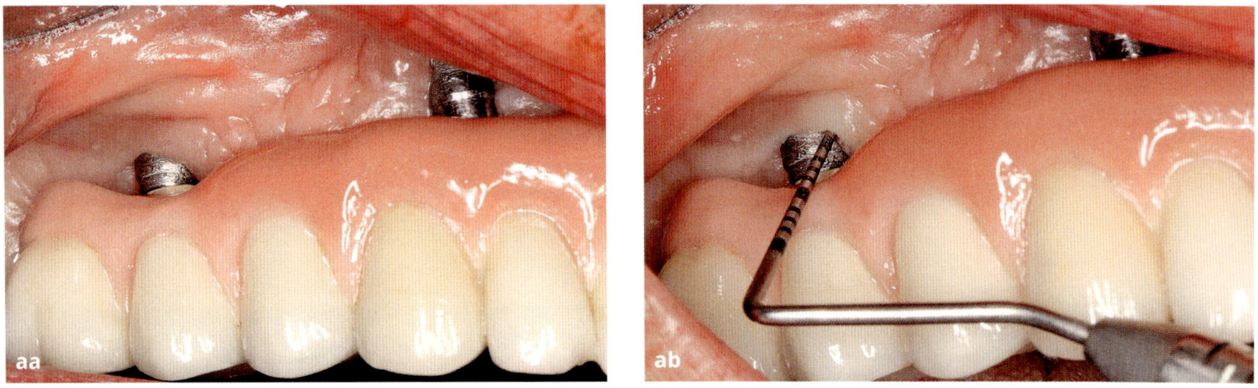

Figs 14-6aa, ab Two months later, the tissues were free of inflammation, while the periodontal probe penetrated the pocket of implant no. 15 with difficulty, without causing bleeding. The patient nevertheless complained of implant mobility.

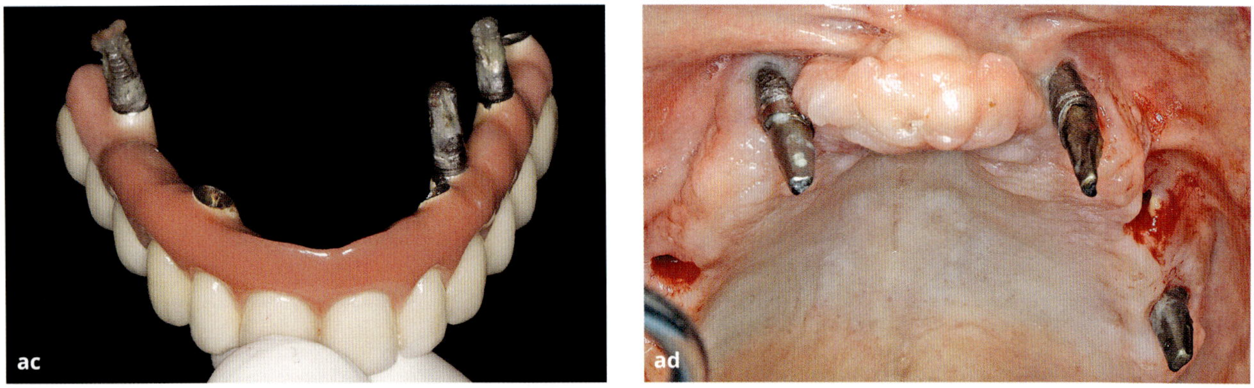

Figs 14-6ac, ad In an attempt to detach the partial denture, three implants were removed. This was a case in which, despite the efforts of both the clinician and patient, survival of the implants was extended. However, the implants were not maintained successfully.

References

1. Mombelli A, Lang NP. The diagnosis and treatment of peri-implantitis. Periodontol 2000 1998;17:63–76.
2. Renvert S, Roos-Jansåker AM, Claffey N. Non-surgical treatment of peri-implant mucositis and peri-implantitis: a literature review. J Clin Periodontol 2008;35:305–315.
3. Piacentini G, Spinoglio GL, Beltrami R, Silvestri M, Piacentini C. Non-surgical treatment of peri-implantitis: a systematic review of the literature. J Anesth Clin Res 2018;9:850.
4. Toledano M, Osorio MT, Vallecillo-Rivas M, et al. Efficacy of local antibiotic therapy in the treatment of peri-implantitis: a systematic review and meta-analysis. J Dent 2021;113,103790.
5. Gomi K, Matsushima Y, Ujiie Y, et al. Full-mouth scaling and root planing combined with azithromycin to treat peri-implantitis. Aus Dent J 2015;60:503–510.
6. Schwarz F, Bieling K, Bonsmann M, Latz T, Becker J. Nonsurgical treatment of moderate and advanced peri-implantitis lesions: a controlled clinical study. Clin Oral Investig 2006;10:279–288.
7. Heitz-Mayfield LJA, Mombelli A. The therapy of peri-implantitis: a systematic review. Int J Oral Maxillofacial Implants 2014;29:325–345.
8. Kotsovilis S, Karoussis IK, Trianti M, Fourmousis I. Therapy of peri-implantitis: a systematic review. J Clin Periodontol 2008;35:621–629.
9. Mombelli A, Moëne R, Décaillet F. Surgical treatments of peri-implantitis. Eur J Oral Implantol 2012;5(suppl):S61–S70.
10. Schwarz F, Sahm N, Schwarz K, Becker J. Impact of defect configuration on the clinical outcome following surgical regenerative therapy of peri-implantitis. J Clin Periodontol 2010;37:449–455.
11. Wiegner J-U, Klinsmann H, Kömmling T. Retrospective analysis of peri-fimplantitis therapy of 158 implants. J Oral Sci Rehabil 2017;3:32–42.
12. Heitz-Mayfield LJA, Salvi GE, Mombelli A, Faddy M, Lang NP. Anti-infective surgical therapy of peri-implantitis. A 12-month prospective clinical study. Clin Oral Implants Res 2012;23:205–210.
13. Charalampakis G, Rabe P, Leonhardt A, Dahlén G. A follow-up study of peri-implantitis cases after treatment. J Clin Periodontol 2011;38:864–871.
14. Esposito M, Grusovin M, Worthington HV. Treatment of peri-implantitis: what interventions are effective? A Cochrane systematic review. Eur J Oral Implantol 2012;5(suppl):S21–S41.
15. Adya N, Alam M, Ravindranath T, Mubeen A, Saluja B. Corrosion in titanium dental implants: literature review. J Indian Prosthodont Soc 2005;5:126–131.
16. Aparicio C, Gil FJ, Fonseca C, Barbosa M, Planell JA. Corrosion behaviour of commercially pure titanium shot blasted with different materials and sizes of shot particles for dental implant applications. Biomaterials 2003;24:263–273.
17. Bhola R, Bhola SM, Mishra B, Olson DL. Corrosion in Titanium Dental Implants/Prostheses—a review. Trends Biomater Artif Organs 2011;25:34–46.
18. Chaturvedi TP. An overview of the corrosion aspect of dental implants (titanium and its alloys). Indian J Dent Res 2009;20:91–98.
19. Noël JJ, Ebrahimi N, Shoesmith DW. Corrosion of titanium and titanium alloys. In: Wandelt K (ed). Encyclopedia of Interfacial Chemistry: Surface Science and Electrochemistry. Amsterdam: Elsevier, 2018:192–200.
20. Diamanti MV, Pedeferri MP. Effect of anodic oxidation parameters on the titanium oxides formation. Corros Sci 2007;49:939–948.
21. Heitz-Mayfield LJA. Peri-implant diseases: diagnosis and risk indicators. J Clin Periodontol 2008;35:292–304.

15 Explantation

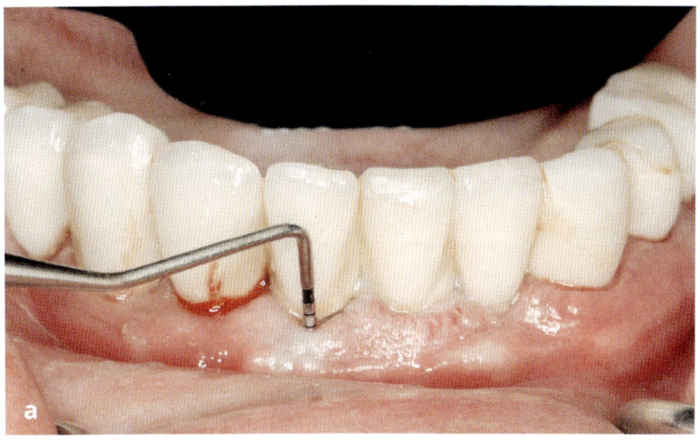
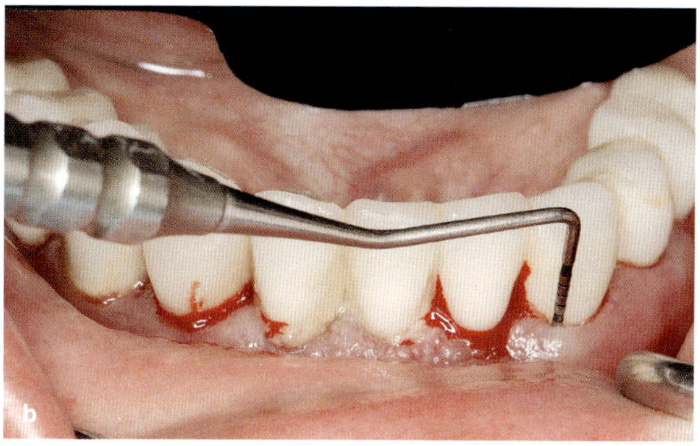

Figs 15-1a, b Implants placed 9 years prior in a patient who did not comply with the maintenance care program. The soft peri-implant tissues are red and swollen. Pockets with a depth of 14 mm and bleeding on probing are detected. This is a continuation of the case presented in Figs 7-1a–c.

The last treatment modality in the course of an implant with advanced bone destruction due to peri-implantitis is its removal. Removing or extracting one implant is often demanding because part of it remains osseointegrated; hence, it may still be stable despite extensive peri-implant bone loss. Removal of an implant is always performed surgically. The most common reasons for removing an implant are:[1,2]

- mobility: in this case, the process is simple because osseointegration is totally missing;
- fracture;
- when a faulty implant location makes reconstruction impossible;
- severe peri-implantitis;
- if the patient expresses psychological reasons to have it removed.

The clinician is especially attentive to a clinical situation where advanced peri-implant bone loss is present that may require explantation of the implant. The decision as to whether the implant will be removed or not depends on its strategic importance. If its removal does not affect the preservation of prosthetic devices, the decision is obvious. If the strategic value of the implant is crucial and preservation of the prosthesis is desirable, then treating peri-implantitis is preferred. A basic condition is that the implant is not mobile, as if it is, its rescue is impossible (Figs 15-1a–p).

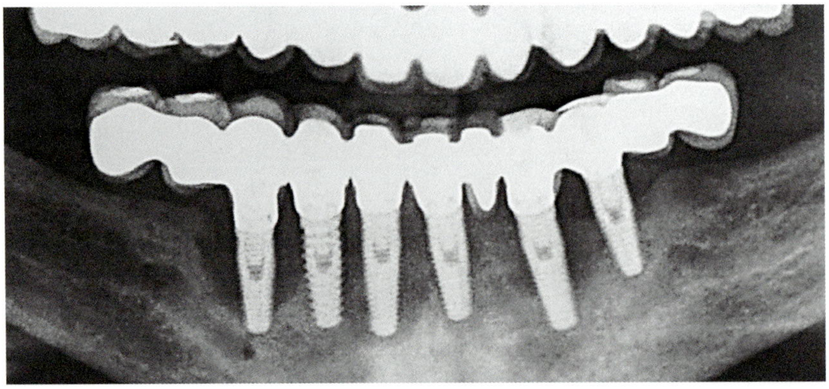

Fig 15-1c Radiograph revealing terminal bone destruction at implants nos. 41 and 43, as well as major bone damage at nos. 33, 32, 31, and 42. The dilemma arises as to whether all implants should be removed or if an effort should be made to maintain nos. 33, 32, 31, and 42.

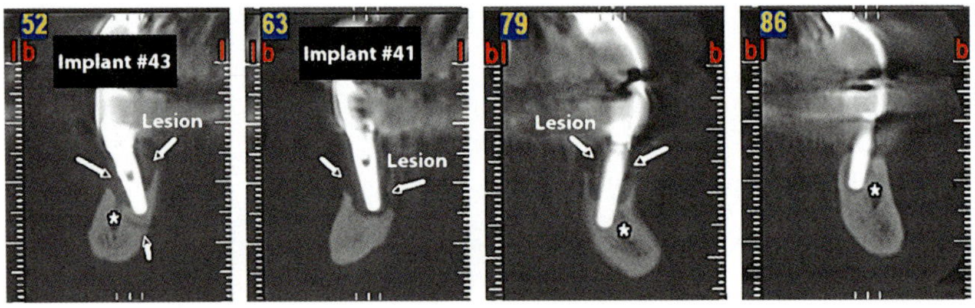

Fig 15-1d On computed tomography, the lesions are shown in 3D, confirming the extent of bone destruction and the poor prognosis of the implants, combined with the inability to maintain the existing prosthetic device because the implant in the strategic position no. 43 is about to be extracted. The decision was made to remove all the implants.

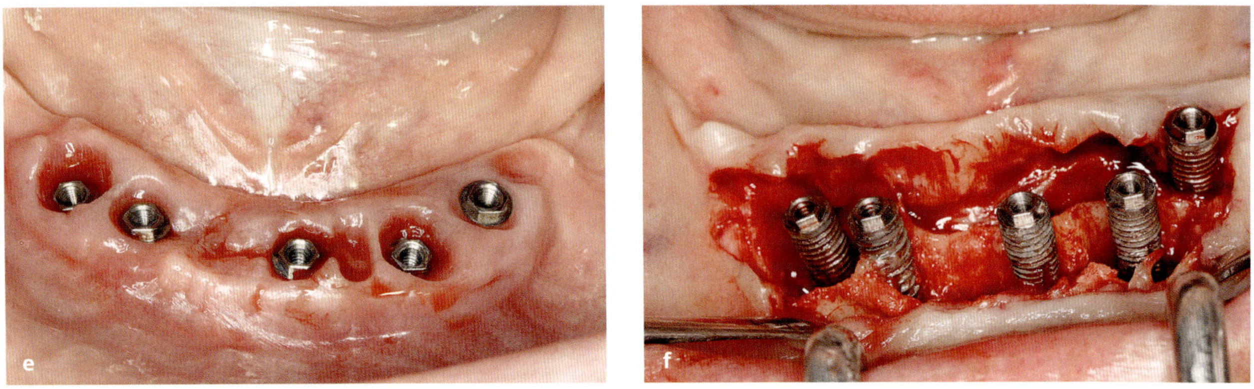

Figs 15-1e, f (e) The phase of inflammation control, with steps A and B, is always applied, even when it the decision has been made to remove the implants, to reduce bleeding but also to make incisions in less fragile soft tissues. As a provisional reconstruction, a complete denture was made. While unscrewing the prosthesis, implant no. 41 was removed on its own. **(f)** Flap elevation revealed the extent and degree of bone destruction.

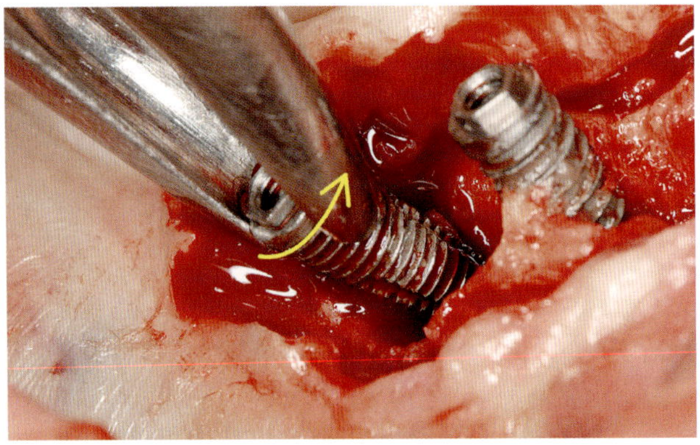

Fig 15-1 g The extraction of implants with forceps is always done by applying counterclockwise torque (yellow arrow) and never by traction or by buccolingual alternating force, as is done on a tooth, to avoid fracturing the jaw.

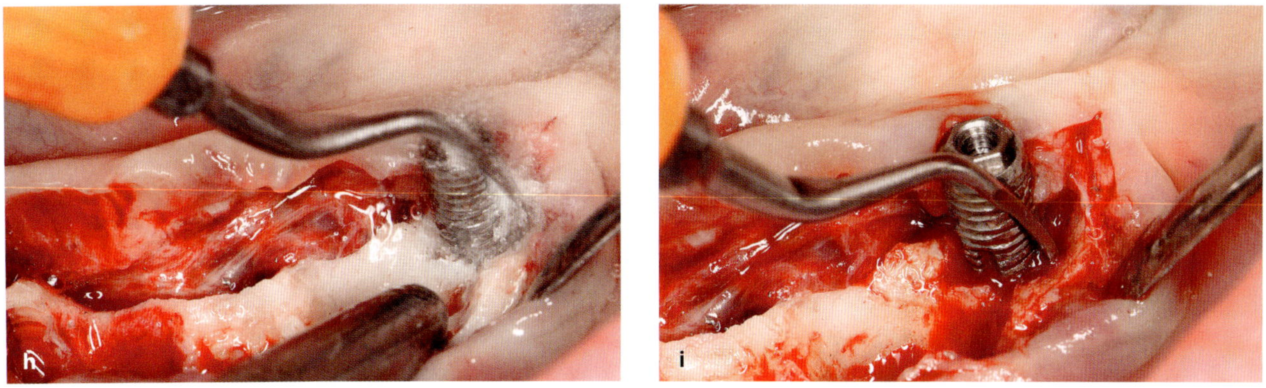

Figs 15-1h, i **(h)** Where removal of part of the supporting bone is necessary, a high-intensity ultrasonic tip may also be applied. **(i)** Removal of the peri-implant bone was performed carefully to maintain as much residual bone as possible.

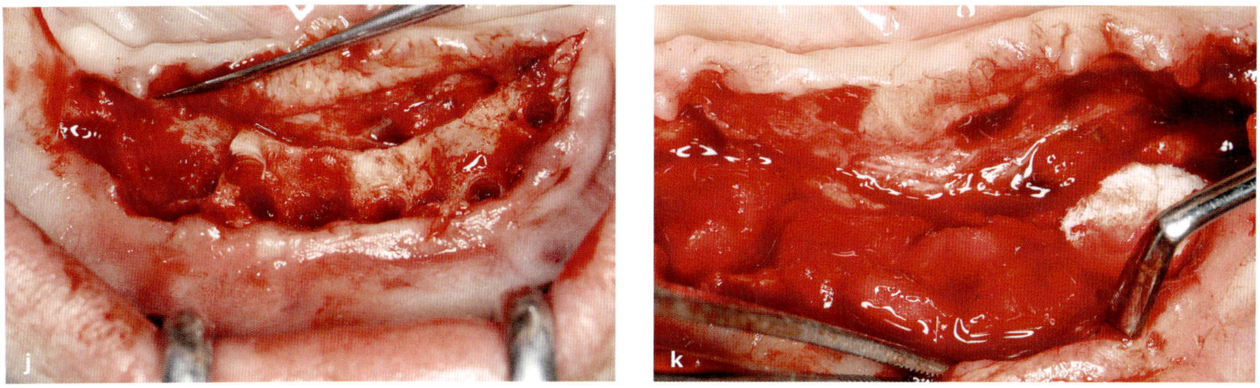

Figs 15-1j, k **(j)** After removal of all implants. **(k)** Placement of collagen graft to fill residual sockets and preserve the alveolar ridge.

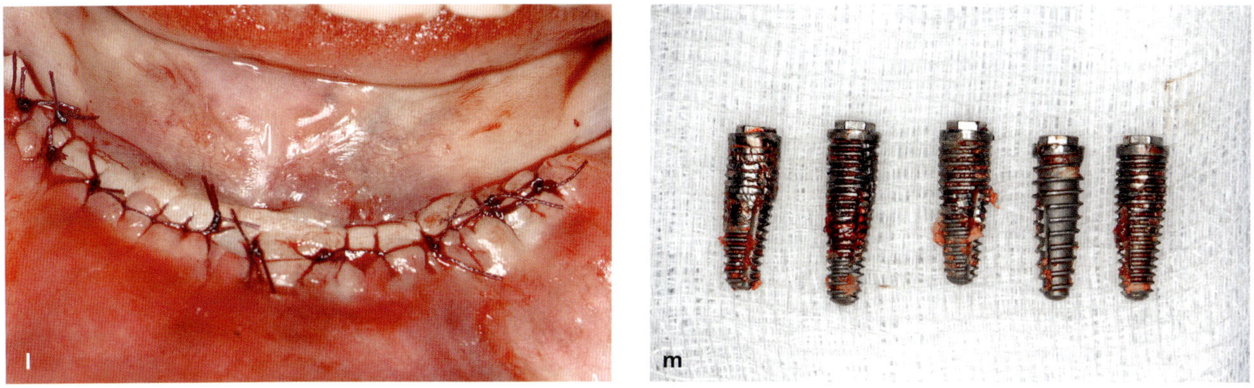

Figs 15-1l, m **(l)** Continuous suturing and primary healing. **(m)** The removed implants.

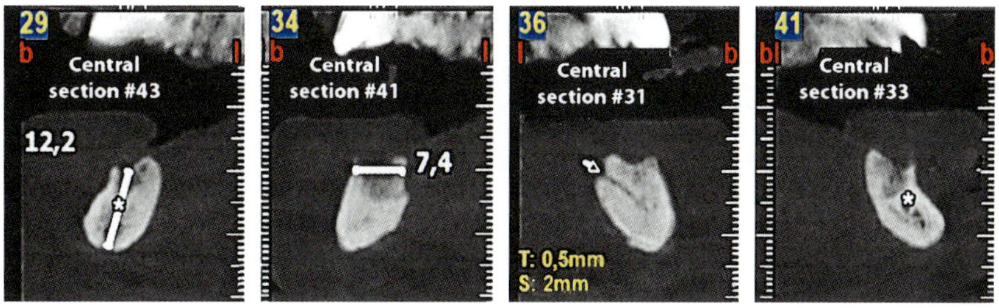

Fig 15-1n Four months after explantation and preservation of the alveolar ridge. The dimensions of the alveolar ridge were limited; however, they allowed the placement of new implants.

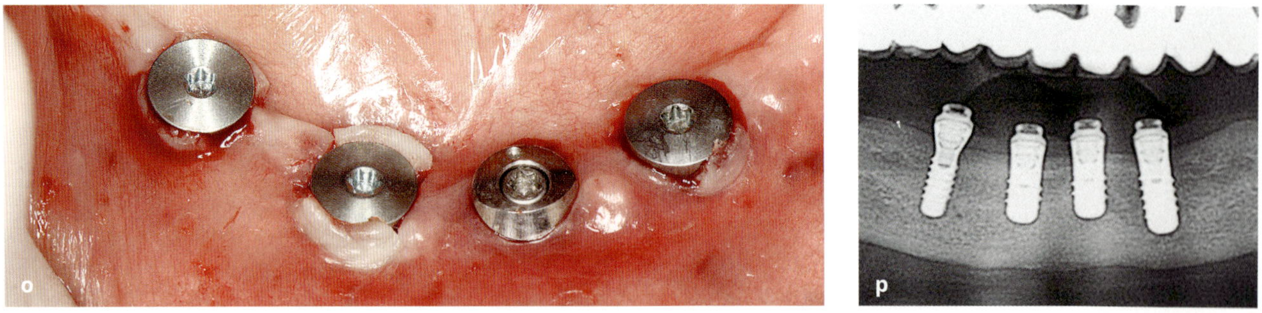

Figs 15-1o, p (o) After placement of four implants before the construction of an overdenture. **(p)** One-and-a-half years after placement of the implants, the patient attended a 3-month supportive periodontal therapy program. Stability of the therapeutic result was observed.

One prevailing view is that the implant must be removed if bone damage reaches 50% of its length; however, there is no scientific evidence for such a paradigm. Other factors to consider before taking a decision as to whether to retain or remove an implant are the total treatment time, the cost, and the number of interventions needed for preservation, as well as the wishes expressed by the patient. All individual details must be explained to the patient. Moreover, because treatment of peri-implantitis is often limited and accompanied by recurrence, this has to be mentioned to the patient.[3] If the decision for explantation is made, the technique of choice will be the one that will cause the least possible tissue loss, as well as the least difficulty for the patient and clinician.[2]

Various techniques for removing an implant have been described, including[4,5]:

- use of common forceps or forceps reinforced with diamond beads (Figs 15-2a-f to 15-4a–d);
- use of inverted screws that fit inside the inner thread and transmit torque through a ratchet. This method is the most conservative and is selected in cases where the implant has an internal connection that has been kept intact;
- hollow cylindrical trephines for implant removal together with part of the surrounding supporting bone. This technique is chosen for fractured, tissue-level, cylindrical, or thin-diameter implants.[6]

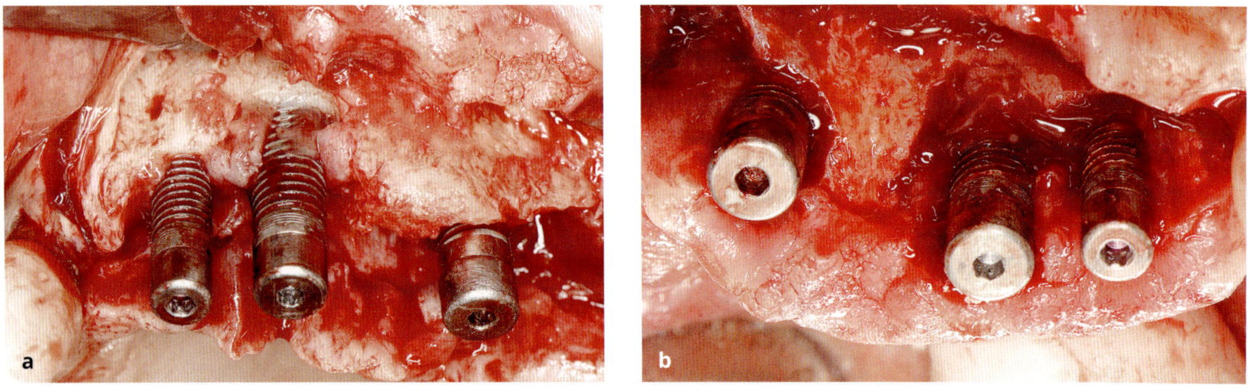

Figs 15-2a, b Advanced peri-implantitis. After control of inflammation, phased removal of the prosthetic appliances and flap elevation were carried out. The extent and degree of bone loss were assessed. A decision was made to remove the implants in the second quadrant.

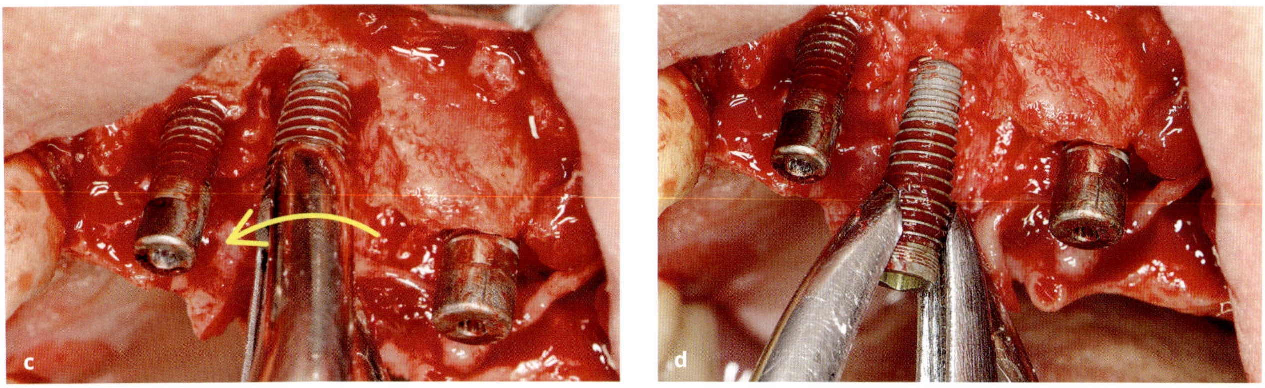

Figs 15-2c, d In the maxilla, removal of implants is a relatively simple procedure. The ease with which they can be removed with forceps is directly proportional to the degree of bone destruction.

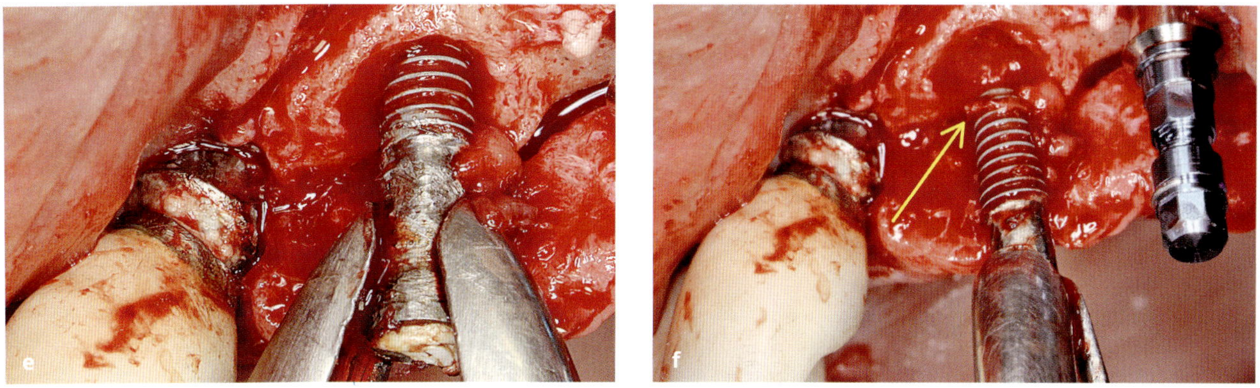

Figs 15-2e, f **(e)** Clinical picture of explantation using forceps. **(f)** Often, part of the bony tissue (yellow arrow) remains on the surface of the titanium, demonstrating the strength of osseointegration.

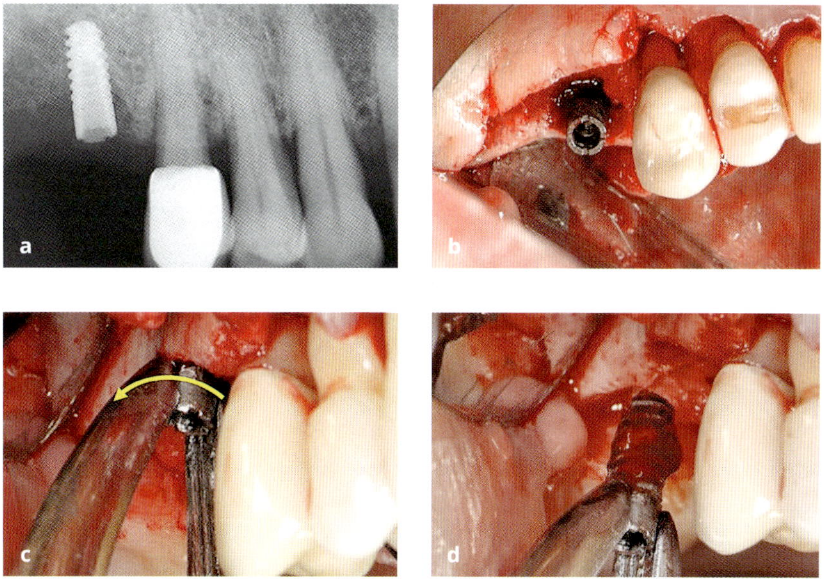

Figs 15-3a–d **(a)** Radiographic image of a fractured implant. Bone damage due to peri-implantitis sometimes leads to its rupture if the length of the implant located in the bone, the length of the lever, and mechanical strength are modified to the forces exerted on it. The crown on no. 15 was overcontoured. **(b)** After flap elevation. **(c)** In the posterior region of the maxilla, low bone density makes removal of the implant relatively easy. **(d)** After removal of implant no. 16.

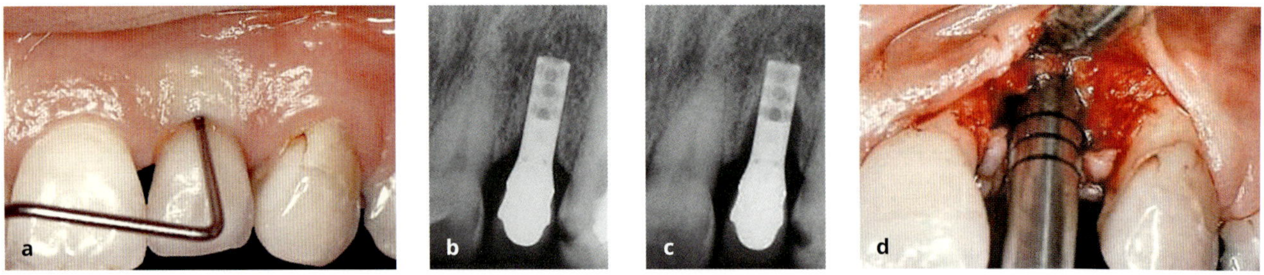

Figs 15-4a–d (a) Clinical picture of a 9-mm peri-implant pocket 10 years after placement of a hollow cylindrical implant. **(b and c)** Radiographs of the patient 1 year and 10 years after implant placement, respectively. **(d)** A trephine bur with calibrated sink depth lines at 8, 10, and 12 mm was used to remove the implant together with the surrounding bone.

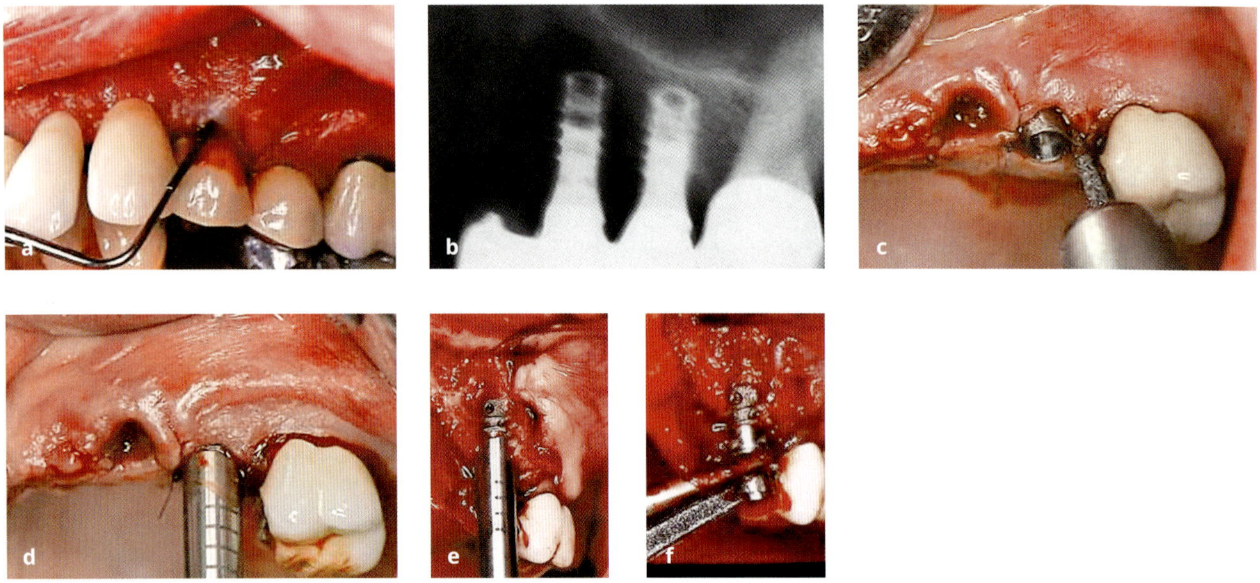

Figs 15-5a–f (a and b) Clinical and radiographic images of a patient with peri-implantitis and hollow screw-type implants, 11 years after their placement. **(c and d)** With removal of the partial denture, implant no. 24 was removed on its own. The implant in position no. 25, after a flap was raised and loss of support on its mesial surface was seen, was planned to be removed. The flap was temporarily sutured to sharpen the transgingival tulip-shaped part of the implant to prevent dispersion of titanium particles in the surgical field and to enable the use of a trephine bur of the smallest possible diameter to remove the implant. **(e and f)** After using the bur, the implant together with the surrounding bone may be removed with forceps.

Removal of the implant with part of its surrounding bone leaves an open implant bed that is minimally traumatized and has a diameter that may allow immediate placement of a larger-diameter implant specifically in the posterior region. The explantation trephine must be sharp. The existence of trephines of different diameters allows selection of the appropriate size depending on the diameter of the implant to be removed. The speed of trephines indicated by the manufacturer is between 1,200 and 1,500 rpm. Continuous water cooling has to be used (Figs 15-4a–d, 15-5a–f, 15-6, and 15-7a–j):

- Tips for ultrasonic use in piezosurgical systems, that is, powerful ultrasonic devices for bone surgery, under saline irrigation. This technique is time-consuming; despite being effective, it is not the clinician's first choice due to ergonomic reasons (Figs 15-1h, i).

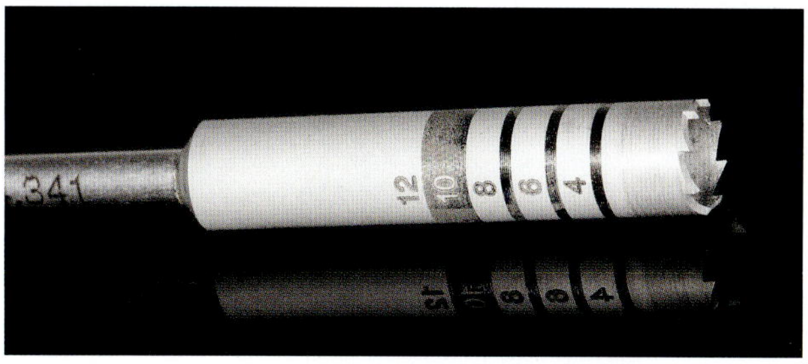

Fig 15-6 Trephine bur with calibrated sink depth lines for implant removal.

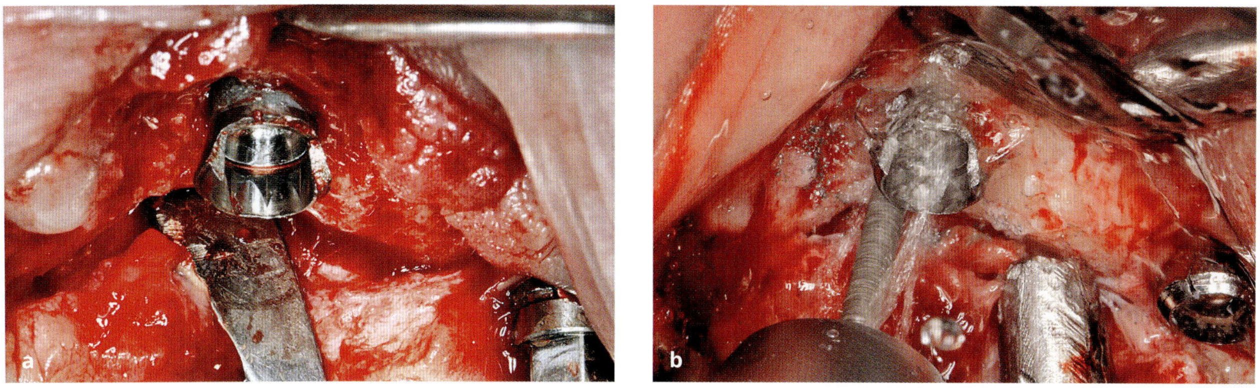

Figs 15-7a, b **(a)** Implant broken in the neck area. This is the same case as in Figs 7-13a–d. **(b)** The transgingival part of the tulip-shaped implant must be prepared so that the special trephine bur can be used.

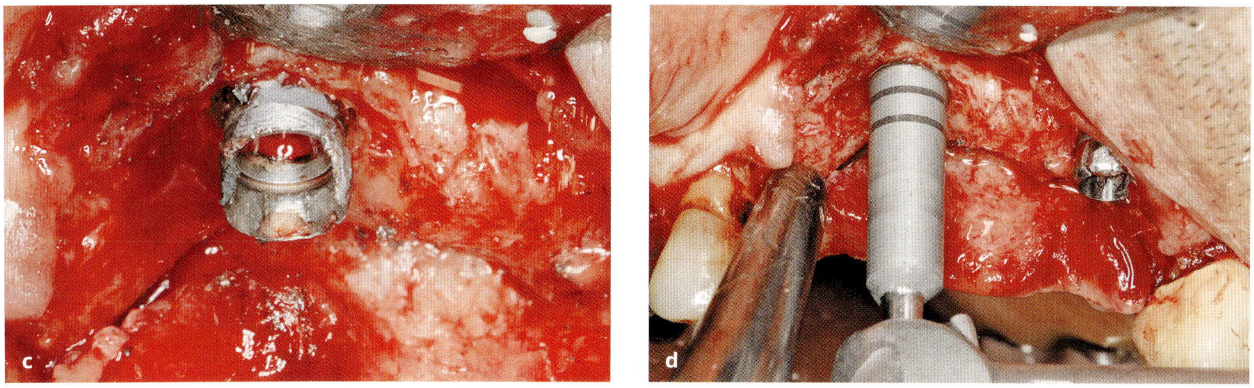

Figs 15-7c, d **(c)** After reducing the diameter of the neck of the implant. **(d)** The trephine bur enters the desired depth as determined by the implant length.

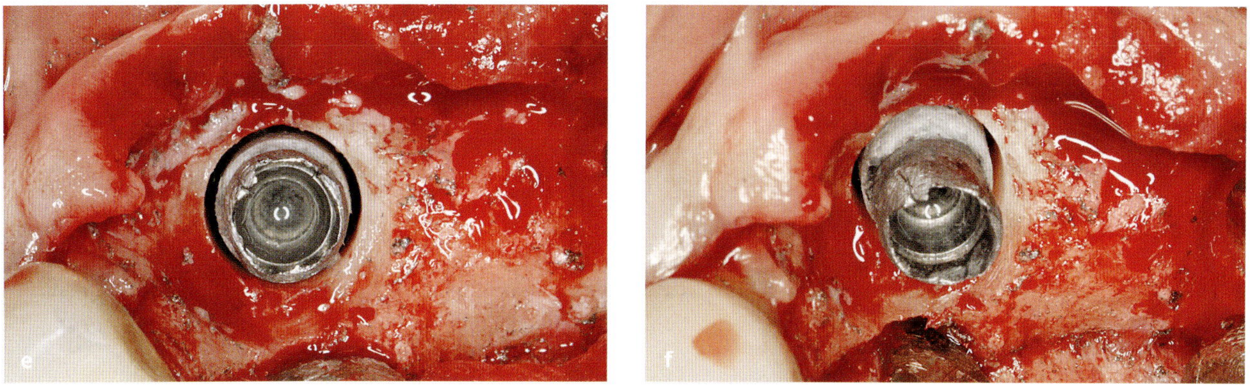

Figs 15-7e, f **(e)** Preparation with the trephine leaves a space around the implant and detaches the implant from the surrounding bone. **(f)** With a thin lever or elevator, the apical part of the bone is removed and so too is the implant with the surrounding bone sheath.

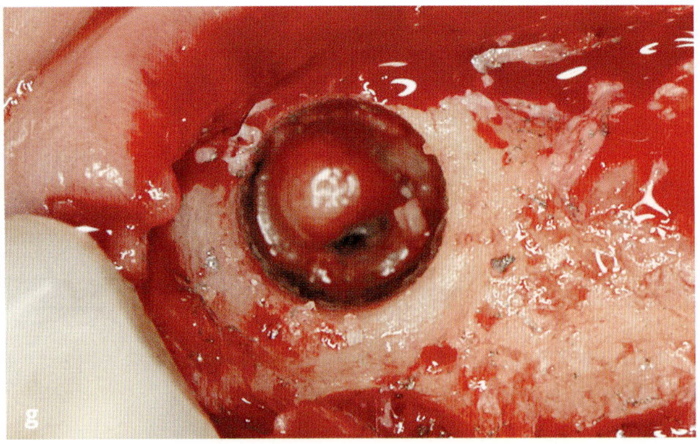

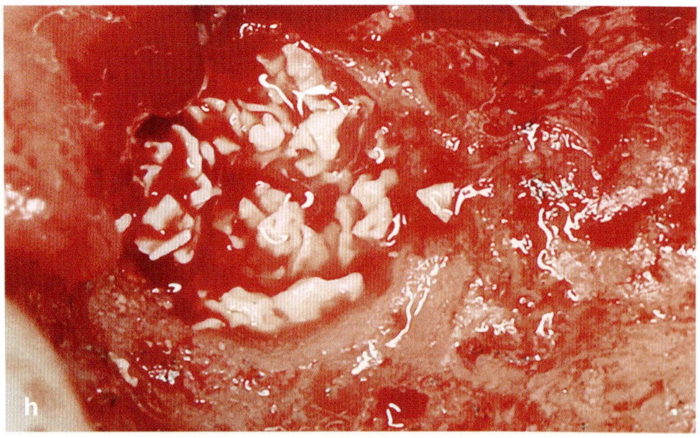

Figs 15-7g, h **(g)** The socket that is left has a larger diameter than that of the implant. **(h)** Filling the socket with xenograft for guided bone regeneration.

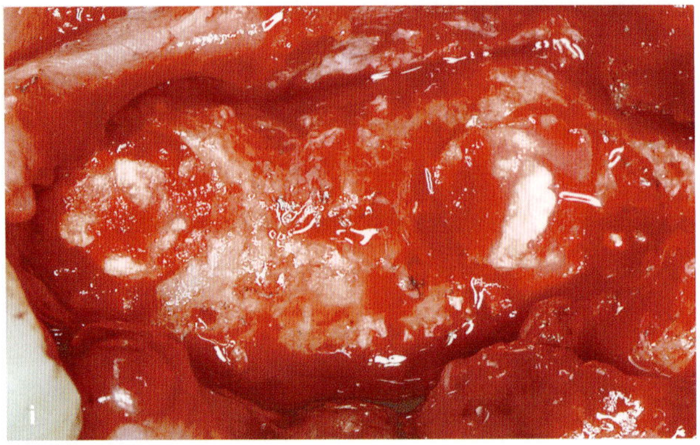

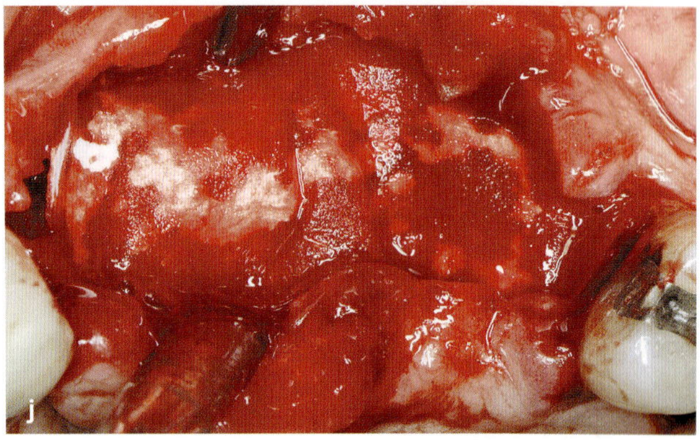

Figs 15-7i, j **(i)** Condensation of the graft with collagen before placement of the membrane. **(j)** Placement of a collagen membrane to achieve guided bone regeneration.

- Special explantation kits with shafts and screws that can anchor in a steel screw. Anchoring of the steel screw engages into the softer titanium; then, using a ratchet, it may exercise high torques that unscrew the implant after the osseointegration is fractured in the apical part of the implant.[7] This technique may be preferred because shafts and screws are designed to unscrew the implants with minimal damage to the surrounding tissues (Figs 15-8a–f).
- If the removal torque exceeds 200 Ncm^2 when unscrewing the implant to be removed, explantation may be chosen as one of a combination of methods. First, part of the surrounding bone may be removed with Piezosurgery or a trephine bur. Then, a torque explantation kit may be used. Care must be taken with all explantation techniques not to exercise too much torque to avoid trauma to the jawbone.

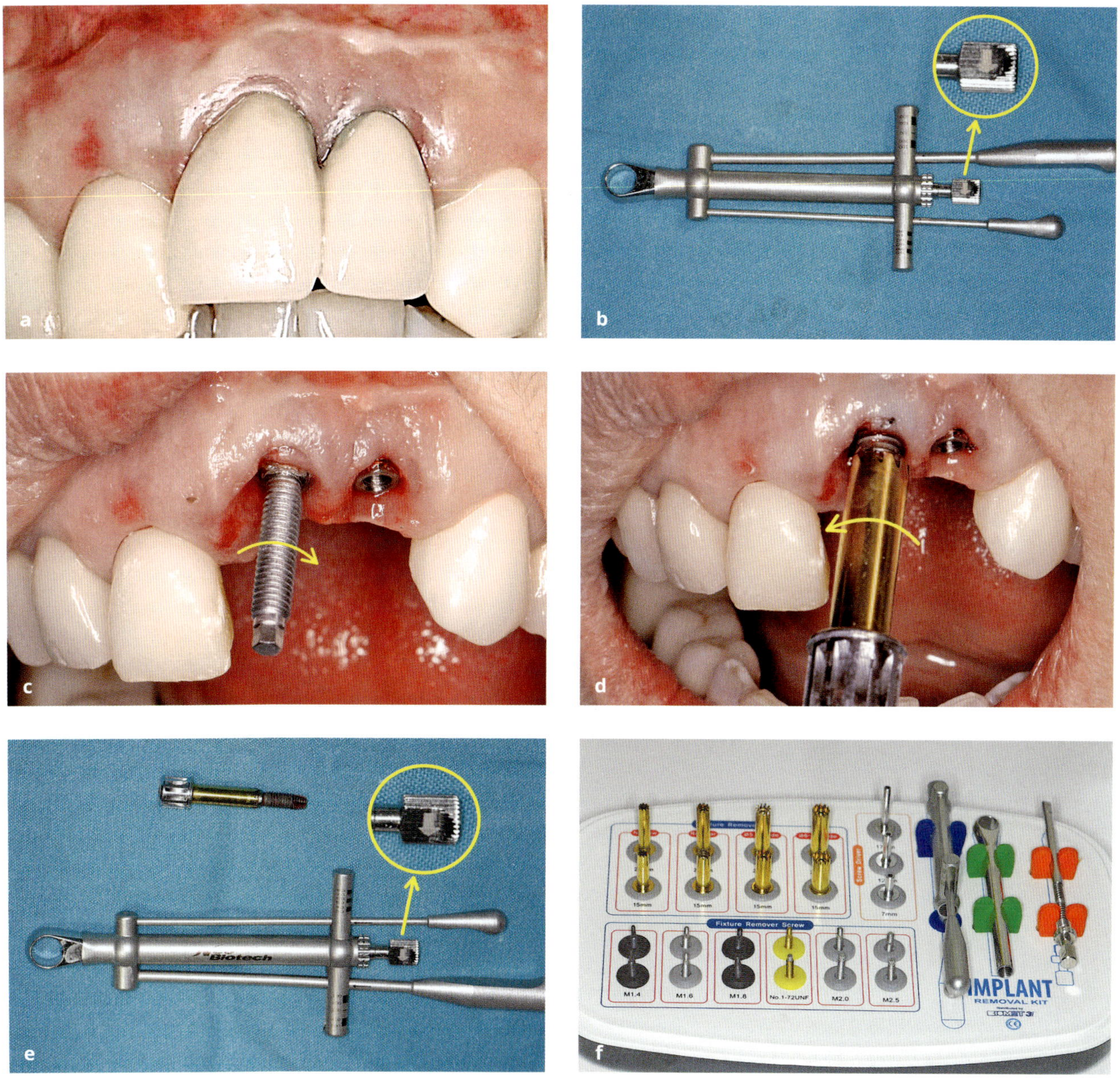

Fig 15-8a–f Clinical situation of implants to be removed. This is not a peri-implantitis case, but it reveals the ability of the system to remove implants, even with full bony support, with relatively limited trauma **(a)**. Locking of the ratchet in the small stem function before the ratchet is fitted to the driver transfer tool in a clockwise direction **(b)**. Positioning of the guide, which is screwed clockwise to stabilize the internal thread of the implant with torques up to 50 Ncm^2 **(c)**. Installation of the special implant removal tool, which is screwed counterclockwise on the neck of the implant, initially by the clinician's hand **(d)**. The ratchet is locked into the function of the large stem. This applies to the implant removal tool; a torque of up to 500 Ncm^2 may be applied. Using a counterclockwise torque, the implant surface is detached from the bone tangent to it, at which point the implant is unscrewed **(e)**. Explantation kit. This technique may only be applied to implants that have a screw design and shape **(f)** (case courtesy of Dr George Vilos).

References

1. Roy M, Loutan L, Garavaglia G, Hashim D. Removal of osseointegrated dental implants: a systematic review of explantation techniques. Clin Oral Investig 2020;24:47–60.
2. Levin L. Dealing with dental implant failures. J Appl Oral Sci 2008;16:171–175.
3. Goodacre CJ, Kan JY, Rungscharassaeng K. Clinical complications of osseointegrated implants. J Prosthet Dent 1999;81:537–552.
4. Solderer A, Al-Jazrawi A, Sahrmann P, Jung R, Attin T, Schmidlin PR. Removal of failed dental implants revisited: questions and answers. Clin Exp Dent Res 2019;5:712–724.
5. Young L, Brown T. Lamont TJ. A comparison of techniques for the explantation of osseointegrated dental implants. Evid Based Dent 2020;21:126–127.
6. Dvorak G, Franz A, Pommer B, Tangl S, Cvikl B. Explantation techniques for fractured dental implants. Int J Stomat Occ Med 2012;5:143–146.
7. Carlsson L, Röstlund T, Albrektsson B, Albrektsson T. Removal torques for polished and rough titanium implants. Int J Oral Maxillofac Implants 1988;3:21–24.

16 Maintenance Care in Implant Patients

A successful treatment outcome in patients with periodontitis or peri-implantitis depends on the fulfillment of three conditions:

- optimal design and thorough implementation of appropriate treatment, drawing on current knowledge and the capabilities of periodontology;
- application of effective oral hygiene daily using mechanical means by the patient;
- consistent implementation of an individualized maintenance care program (supportive periodontal therapy [SPT]).

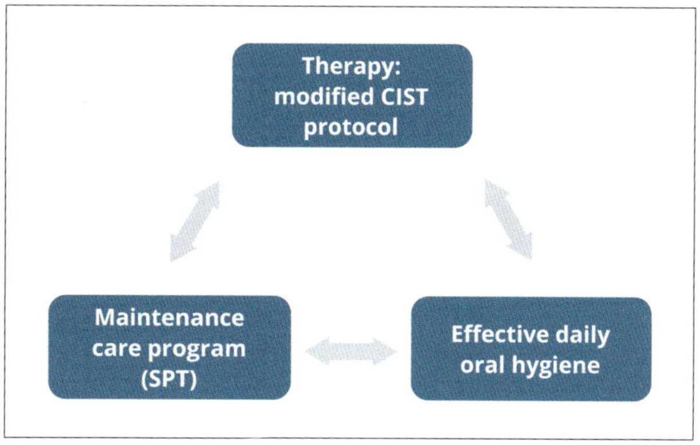

Fig 16-1 The tripod of success for any periodontal or peri-implant treatment. CIST, cumulative interceptive supportive therapy; SPT, supportive periodontal therapy.

Each of these important steps plays an equally crucial role. If one of these conditions is not met, the long-term outcome of therapy will not be successful. The patient should be informed of this during the very first session, when presenting the treatment plan to them. An easy-to-understand way to present this concept to the patient is to describe it as a tripod. To be stable, a chair needs at least three legs (Fig 16-1).[1]

Patients should be enrolled in an individualized maintenance care program for secondary disease prevention. The word "recall", which has been used to describe communication between dental practitioners and patients, is correct because it relates to the recall process.

Patients may understand the value of being monitored by their physician when they have a medical problem, but they do not tend to have the same view for the dental office.[2] Whenever the dental practitioner explains the importance of preventing peri-implantitis, the difficulties managing it, and the possible complications that may occur, patients tend to ignore this information because they are confident that these pathologies will not occur in their oral cavity. Hence, the need for a preventive SPT program must be reiterated at every possible opportunity. Only with acceptance of and meticulous compliance with an SPT protocol can therapy begin. Even in the long term, both natural dentition and implants are maintained with regular supervision and compliance with an organized recall system (Figs 16-2a–b).[3,4]

When treatment of peri-implant mucositis is not performed in a timely fashion, a higher incidence of peri-implantitis is expected. Moreover, difficulties in treating peri-implantitis result in high recurrence

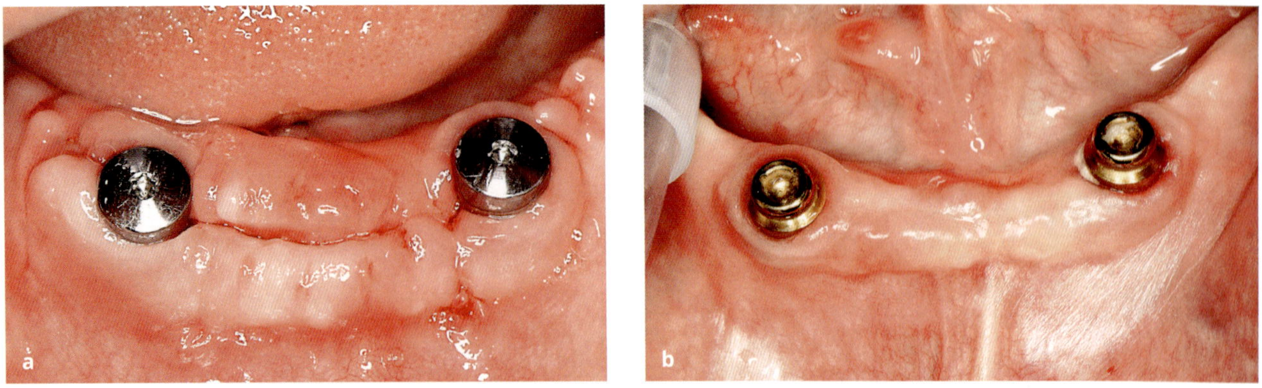

Figs 16-2a, b (a) Clinical picture of a patient after suture removal, performed 8 days after implant placement. (b) Photograph of the area 10 years later when the patient came in for SPT. Minor calculus deposits can be observed but the peri-implant condition is stable. The patient was practicing effective oral hygiene and attending SPT every 4 months.

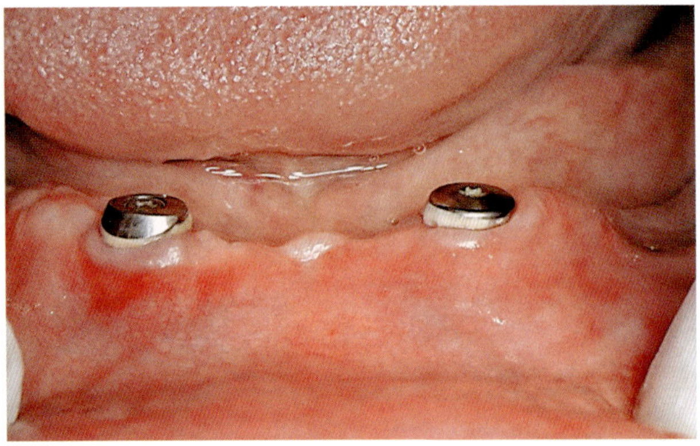

Fig 16-3 SPT begins immediately after implant placement. This image shows mineralized biofilm 6 weeks after implant placement.

rates, even with adherence to SPT programs. It is therefore clear that patients must be enrolled in a maintenance care program, and it is important that the program begins on the day of implant placement and not after completion of prosthetic rehabilitation (Fig 16-3).

However, for the practitioner, removal of the local causative factors, that is, dental biofilms from the peri-implant sulcus, or even from the peri-implant pockets, is a particularly demanding procedure.[5] The difficulty of removing deposits effectively is related to the different anatomy of the peri-implant situation, with morphologic variations in many implant suprastructures. The emergence profile of an implant from the soft tissues as well as the shape of implant restorations may differ from the usual contours encountered at the gingiva around teeth. This may create conditions that require detailed instruction for administration of oral hygiene and use of appropriate cleansing devices for daily home care (Figs 16-4a, b). The inability of a patient to learn how to administer and practice effective daily oral hygiene is a contraindication for the placement of dental implants.

16.1 Configuration of the recall program in implant patients

The maintenance phase is the logical and necessary continuation of inflammation control or the corrective phase (or both). It aims to[6]:

- control the risk factors that cause periodontal and peri-implant diseases;
- diagnose inflammation or its recurrence early;
- treat peri-implant diseases effectively at an early stage.

The patient is recalled at regular intervals that are dependent on their oral health and the standard of their oral hygiene. A crucial component in maintaining oral health is the complete removal of biofilms.

A patient with dental implants should be treated like one who has been treated for chronic periodontitis. Therefore, they should be reexamined at least every 3 months for the first 1.5 years. Subsequently, depending on the risk of presenting a peri-implant

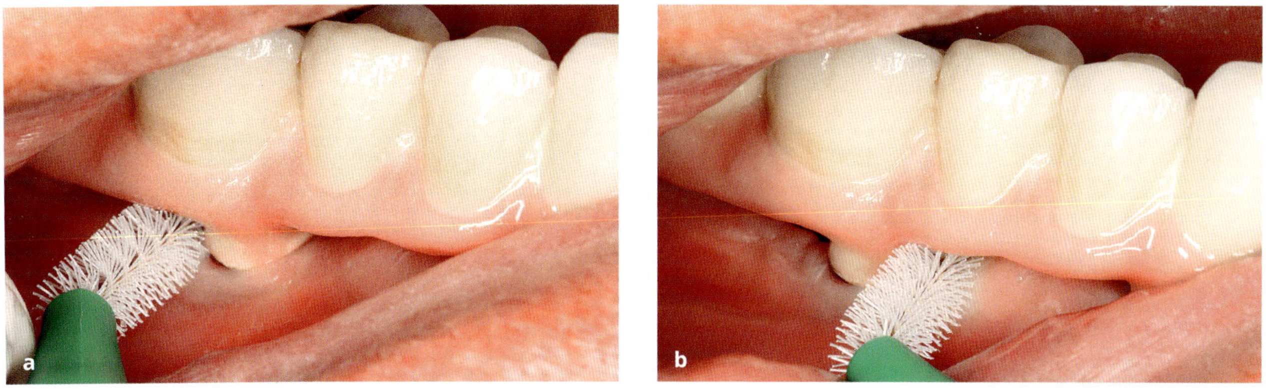

Figs 16-4a, b It is essential to check the effectiveness of oral hygiene and individualize the recommendations, especially where the morphology and anatomy of the area have changed.

pathology, the interval between consecutive examinations is determined by the clinician and ranges from 2 to 6 months. Studies in human behavior argue that it takes about 18 months to establish a new habit or get rid of an old one. The establishment of oral hygiene habits in a morphologically variable dentition must be supported. The patient's ability to apply cleaning techniques effectively should be closely monitored. At the same time, the condition of the peri-implant tissues and occlusion are evaluated. Patients with effective oral hygiene do not need to attend recall visits as frequently as patients with dental biofilm scores greater than 15%. Important factors to consider are a history of periodontitis, the complexity of prosthetic rehabilitation, the presence of teeth with questionable prognosis, smoking habits, and the presence of systemic diseases.[7,8] Occlusal abnormalities and parafunctional habits should also be observed because they may contribute to mechanical complications in implant restorations.

Patients with a history of peri-implantitis or implant loss (or both) are at an increased risk for further peri-implant pathology.[9] Thus, the decision on the time interval between SPT sessions is based on an assessment of the following factors[10,11]:

- existence of risk factors for the development of peri-implantitis (see Chapter 4);
- age of the patient: young age combined with any risk factor makes the need for regular follow-up even greater;
- history and severity of previous periodontal diseases;
- periodontal status at the time of completion of the active phase of periodontal treatment;
- presence of teeth with questionable prognosis;
- history of previous peri-implant pathology;
- presence of implants with questionable prognosis;
- tendency for dental caries;
- type and complexity of prosthetic restorations;
- effectiveness of daily oral hygiene administered by the patient using mechanical means;
- smoking habit.

16.2 Points of interest during maintenance care in implant patients

In each maintenance care session, clinicians should be informed about the patient's medical and dental history so they can identify any changes that could affect the prognosis, such as the emergence of uncontrolled diabetes mellitus, the administration of antiosteolytic medicines, and the development of diseases associated with movement disorders that will affect oral hygiene practices. At the same time, smoking cessation should be recommended, and its negative contribution to the occurrence and progression of periodontal and peri-implant diseases should be reiterated. Finally, special attention should be given to devoting sufficient time to allow the patient to express any questions and concerns about their oral condition.

In every reexamination of the periodontal patient, the clinician evaluates and records the same parameters as in the initial examination:

- evaluation of medical and dental history in relation to the previous reexamination;
- clinical examination of extraoral and intraoral anatomic areas;
- clinical examination of teeth and implants:
  - dental caries;
  - status of existing prosthetic restorations and screening for any technical complications;
  - tooth and implant mobility.
- clinical examination of peri-implant and periodontal tissues[12]:
  - presence of microbial biofilms;
  - presence of bleeding on probing (BOP) or suppuration;
  - presence of calculus;
  - probing pocket depths;
  - clinical attachment loss;
  - presence of rough implant surfaces exposed to the oral environment;
  - presence and adequate thickness and width of keratinized peri-implant mucosa;
  - recessions and other mucogingival deformities;
  - presence of root furcation involvement;
  - radiologic reexamination when and if necessary due to the appearance of signs suggesting the presence or recurrence of peri-implantitis (probing pocket depth of at least 6 mm).
- assessment of the condition of the periodontal and peri-implant tissues. It is possible to find that there is a manifestation of pathology;
- evaluation of the degree of patient compliance, categorizing it as positive, neutral, moderate, or negative;
- recording the patient's therapeutic needs;
- planning for the next recall session;
- evaluating the presence and amount of dental biofilms. Unless microbial biofilm is made visible through disclosure, incomplete biofilm removal will result.

Implants with rough surfaces are not more prone to peri-implantitis; exposure of rough surfaces to the pocket environment is the result rather than the cause of bone loss (see Chapter 11).

However, once peri-implantitis occurs and the rough surface is exposed to microbial colonization, bacterial accumulation is greater than that on a smooth surface; hence, their removal is more difficult.[13] Exposure of rough surfaces in the oral environment is an important factor when planning SPT sessions.

Probing of the peri-implant sulcus or pocket should be performed at each SPT session, and recorded to facilitate comparative evaluation. Changes in probing pocket depth usually favor the presence of inflammation of peri-implant soft tissues or even peri-implant bone loss. The peri-implant mucosa is more susceptible than the gingiva around teeth; therefore, application of a small force is recommended during probing (0.15 N). However, even this gentle probing may separate epithelial adhesion from the implant surface. Nevertheless, this does not extend to the connective tissue; 3 to 5 days after clinical examination, the implant–mucosa unit is restored without endangering health.[14]

The presence of BOP is a prognostic factor of limited sensitivity for the development of peri-implant disease, whereas its absence assures implant stability and health.

Production of pus or exudate from the peri-implant sulcus or pocket is usually observed after probing. Although the role of suppuration as an indicator of the manifestation or progression of peri-implant disease has not yet been fully elucidated, it is an indication of an active destructive inflammatory process. Pus as a product of tissue destruction is composed of dead bacteria and polymorphonuclear neutrophils, whereas the presence of exudate indicates a high concentration of inflammatory cells in the peri-implant tissues (Figs 16-5a, b).

To check the stability of an implant and correctly evaluate any presence of mobility, the implant restoration may have to be removed, if feasible. In cases of extensive implant reconstructions, removal of the prosthesis is a prerequisite to allow all implants to be examined separately. This test is performed either manually or with the help of specialized equipment to record implant stability.

Removing the prosthetic restoration during every SPT session is a time consuming and non-ergonomic process; hence, it is not done frequently. Disinfection via guided biofilm therapy provides the required efficacy without needing to remove the prosthesis in each session.

An implant may have extensive bone loss and yet remain stable, without any mobility, remaining osseointegrated, even at a level of 1 to 2 mm.[15]

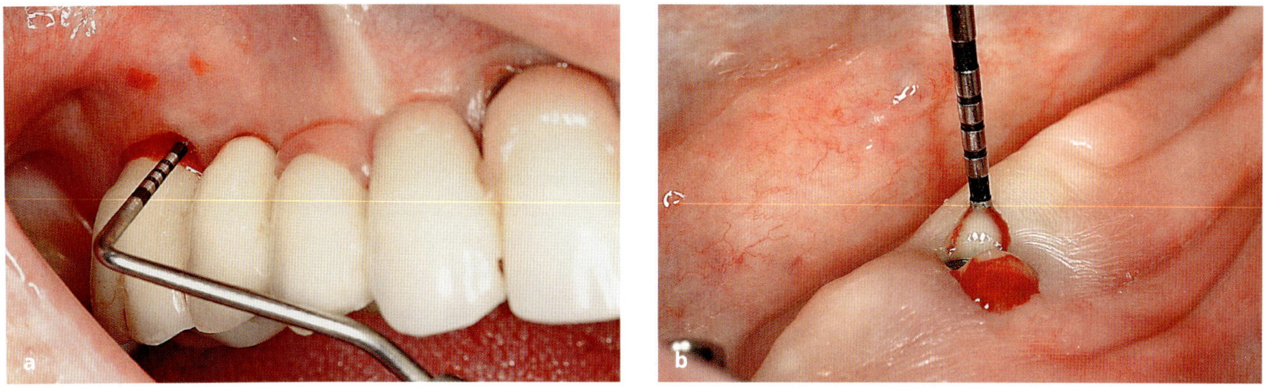

Figs 16-5a, b Bleeding and pus formation on probing are signs of inflammation and tissue damage, respectively.

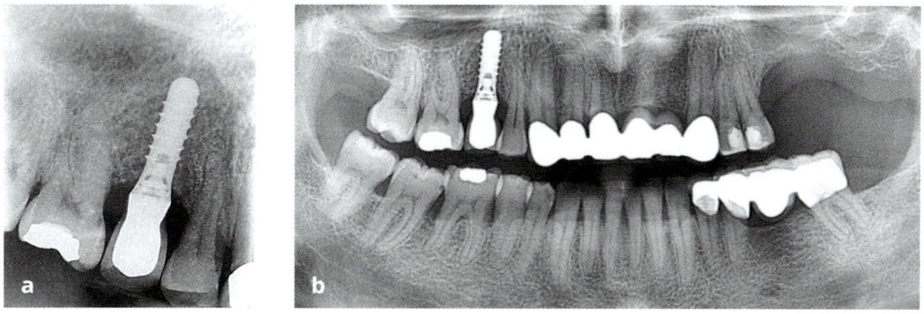

Figs 16-6a, b (a) Periapical radiograph 1 year after placement of the implant restoration in site no. 15. **(b)** Panoramic radiograph 8 years after implant placement in site no. 15.

However, implant mobility is evidence of complete loss of osseointegration. The presence of mobility indicates failure of the implant, meaning it has to be explanted.

Periapical radiography is a valuable diagnostic tool to assess the status of implants and peri-implant tissues. Radiographs are often used where limited space or insufficient accessibility makes probing impossible. Obtaining periapical radiographs and archiving the corresponding record is considered extremely important as it allows the comparison of bone levels over time (Fig 16-6).

An ideal protocol for SPT is one that ensures effective removal of biofilms and calculus, while creating the least discomfort for the patient and providing optimal ergonomics for the clinician.

From the outset, the cumulative interceptive supportive therapy (CIST) protocol was designed to be applied during the maintenance phase in such a way as to guide the clinician in providing appropriate treatment, depending on the clinical and radiographic data available when either the patient arrives for a scheduled session or a new patient attends for their first visit.

In both instances, the CIST protocol offers step-by-step preventive and therapeutic interventions, depending on the severity of any condition seen in each patient. The modifications proposed in Chapter 8 emerged as a necessity to increase the effectiveness of therapeutic or supportive interventions.[16]

Before presenting the guided biofilm therapy (GBT) protocol, it is worth mentioning the means, instruments, and devices used for the mechanical removal of deposits (Figs 9-7 and 9-8).

16.3 Instruments and devices used for mechanical removal of biofilms during SPT

Several mechanical means have been proposed and implemented to remove the local causative factors from the surface of dental implants without causing damage, namely:

- plastic instruments;
- rubber cups;

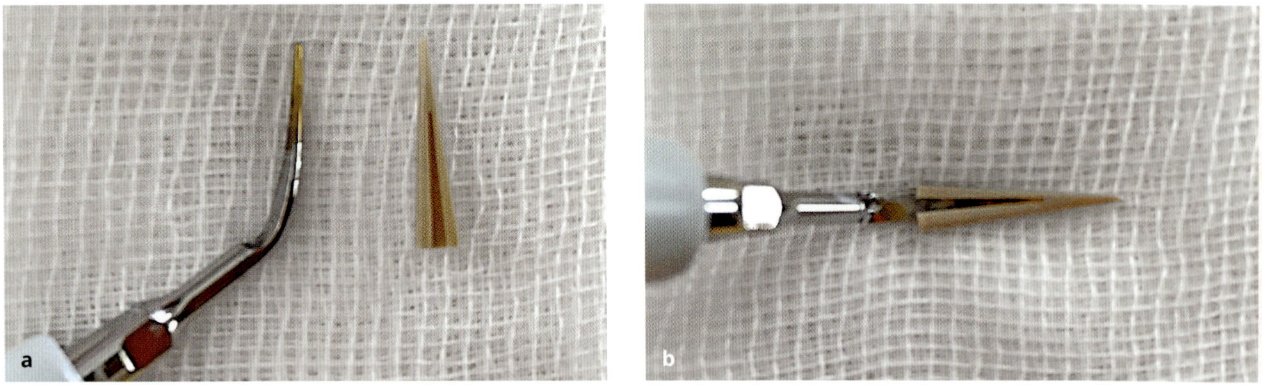

Figs 16-7a, b Plastic-coated system adapted to a special ultrasonic tip for mechanical removal of biofilms from peri-implant pockets or sulci. Its size precludes placement between chewing elements.

- polishing pastes;
- carbon fiber or titanium instruments;
- instruments for ultrasonic devices made of synthetic materials or carbon fiber or aluminum or polyetheretherketone (PEEK);
- irrigation devices with granules of various sizes.

Instruments made of carbon fiber, Teflon, or titanium may be used, but they are large in size. Instruments made of carbon fiber have limited bending strength. Instruments made of hard materials (titanium or aluminum) can be inserted into the peri-implant sulcus and may remove the local causative factors; however, they can damage the surface of the restorative materials and titanium.[17]

The use of conventional metallic ultrasonic tips leads to the scraping of the surface of titanium implants, thereby contributing to higher rates of microbial biofilm retention. In an attempt to address this, ultrasonic tips made of PEEK or other synthetic materials have been developed to effectively remove deposits. They cause significantly less damage to the implant surface. The coated tips easily remove mineralized deposits without the risk of breakage. However, due to the metal plate around the soft material, the instrument is inflexible. This makes it difficult to enter the peri-implant sulcus (Figs 16-7a, b).

In the past, sodium bicarbonate irrigation devices were used. In recent years, however, water spray devices with glycine or erythritol granules have been favored due to their better biologic behavior. Irrigation systems are high-pressure jet spray devices that apply a mixture of air, powder, and water. However, because not only the size but also the type of powder is essential, powders have been improved. Today, erythritol with a very small grain size (14 μm) is generally preferred.[18] Recently, the GBT protocol has been implemented successfully for implant surface disinfection (Figs 16-8a–d).[16]

Removal of dental biofilms from the surfaces of dental implants using a rubber cup with a polishing paste, or a gauze strip with tin oxide, has been suggested. Based on current scientific data, it is known that rubber cups used with micromotor handpieces, usually in combination with polishing paste, cannot remove biofilms from the peri-implant sulci, interdental areas, or pockets.[19] Moreover, the increasing temperature may cause patient discomfort. Furthermore, the polishing paste must contain extremely fine granules because the friction of larger-diameter granules leads to wear, leaving scratches on the surface of the restorative materials. Biofilm removal with rubber cups has therefore been replaced by AIRFLOW (EMS Dental, Nyon, Switzerland) (Figs 16-9 and 16-10a–e).[20]

The result of using different means or instruments on smooth titanium surfaces is presented in Figs 16-11a–f, 16-12a–f, and 16-13a–f.

As mentioned in Chapter 9, titanium surface scratches and detachment of titanium particles, restorative materials, or the instrument used to mechanically remove deposits are undesirable conditions that have been implicated in the accumulation of larger amounts of biofilms and mechanical irritation (Figs 9-14a–d to 9-18a–d).

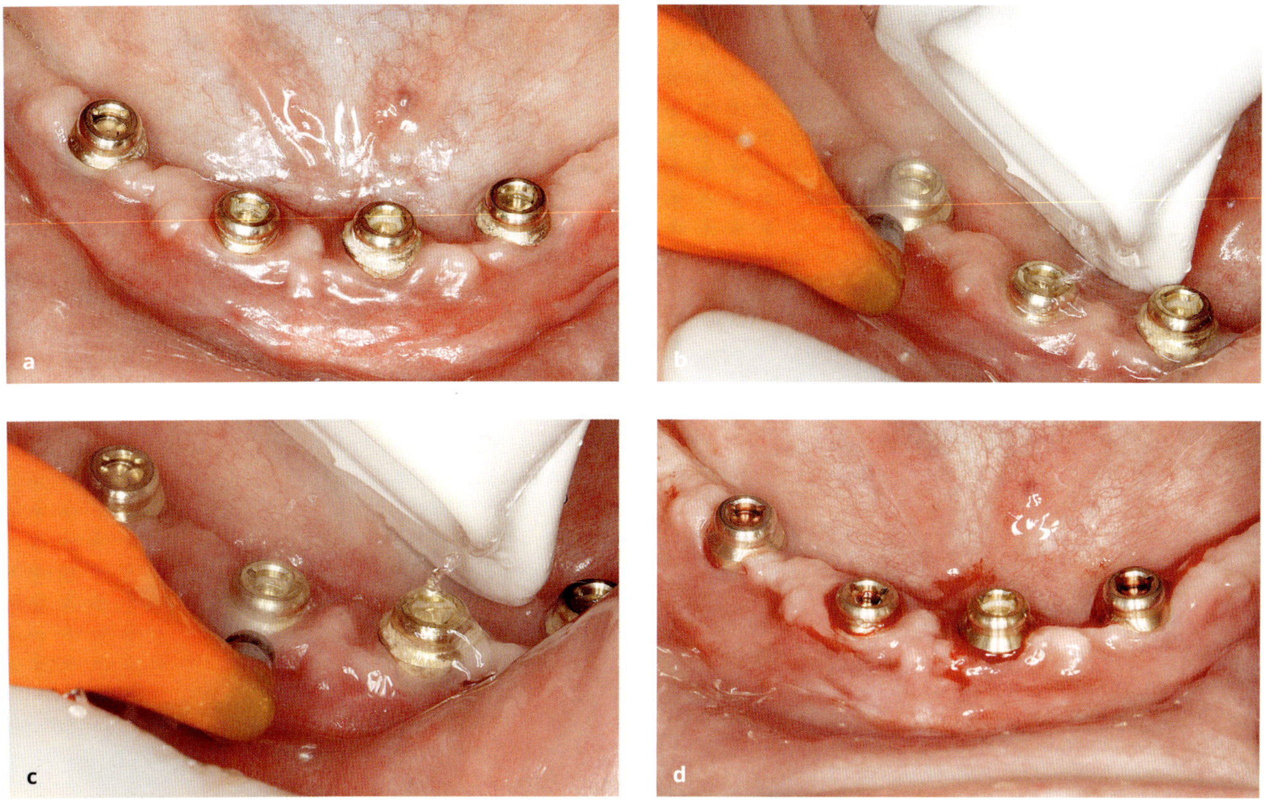

Figs 16-8a–d Application of erythritol spray for the painless removal of soft and partially mineralized biofilms from the surfaces of transmucosal abutments. Disinfection of the peri-implant sulcus to a depth of 4 mm was achieved. In areas where inflammation was established, minor bleeding was present.

16.4 GBT in implant patients

GBT was designed based on the recommendations of the 11th European Workshop on Periodontology of the European Academy of Periodontology. The key to the prevention of caries, and periodontal and peri-implant diseases is effective daily oral hygiene combined with a frequent recall system for the patient to maintain oral health.[21]

The protocol consists of the following eight steps:

1. Assessment.
2. Disclosure of dental biofilms.
3. Education and motivation of the patient.
4. Removal of dental biofilms with theAIRFLOW system in sulci and pockets up to 4 mm.
5. Removal of dental biofilm with the PERIOFLOW irrigation system (EMS Dental) and a nozzle in pockets of 5 mm or deeper.
6. Removal of calculus with PIEZON ultrasonic devices (EMS Dental) and the PI tip, which is specially designed for implants, covered with PEEK.
7. Evaluation of deposit removal.
8. Planning the future recall interval to maintain the therapeutic result. Before the start of each session, mouth rinsing with chlorhexidine digluconate is recommended because this reduces the dispersion of bacteria in aerosols in the dental clinic.

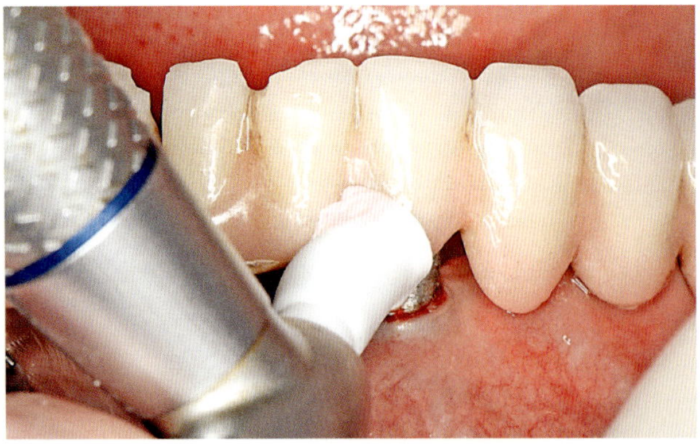

Fig 16-9 Rubber cup and polishing paste with low abrasion. Its use requires caution to avoid damaging the mucosa, and is restricted to supramucosal surfaces.

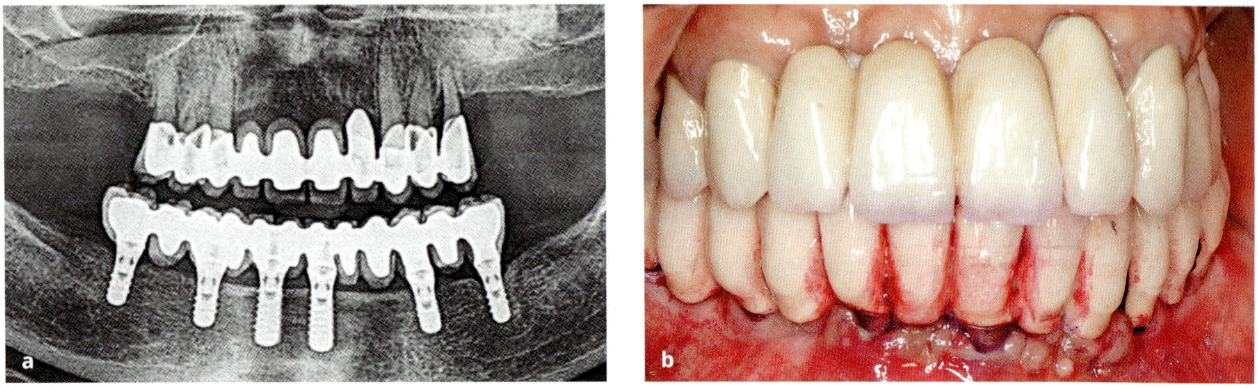

Figs 16-10a, b **(a)** Radiographic image of a patient presenting for SPT. **(b)** Disclosing the biofilm both educates the patient about oral hygiene and removes deposits.

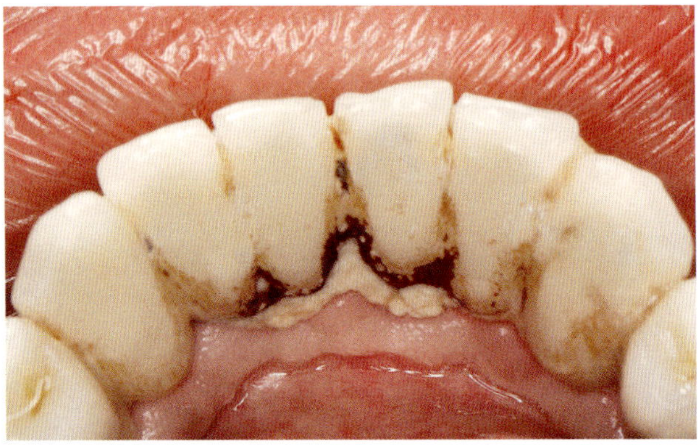

Fig 16-10c Note the concentration of stains, dental biofilm, and calculus.

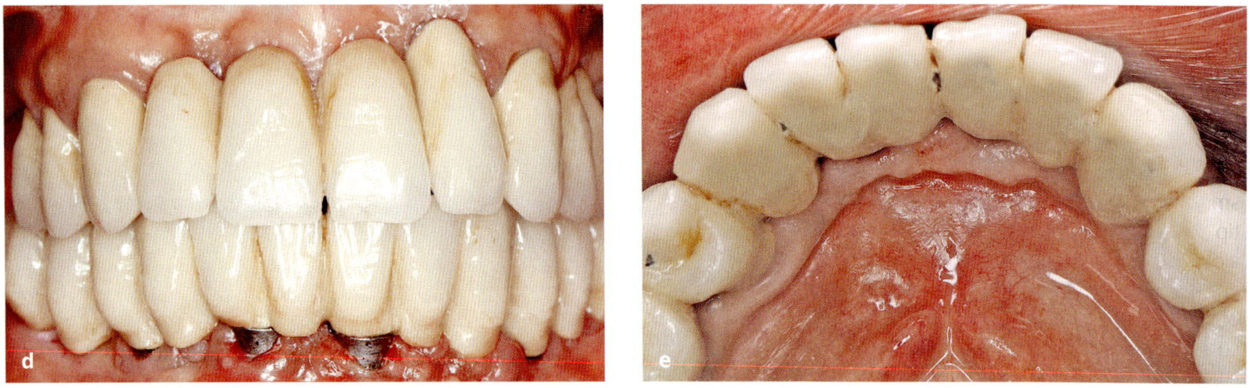

Figs 16-10d, e After completion of the GBT protocol.

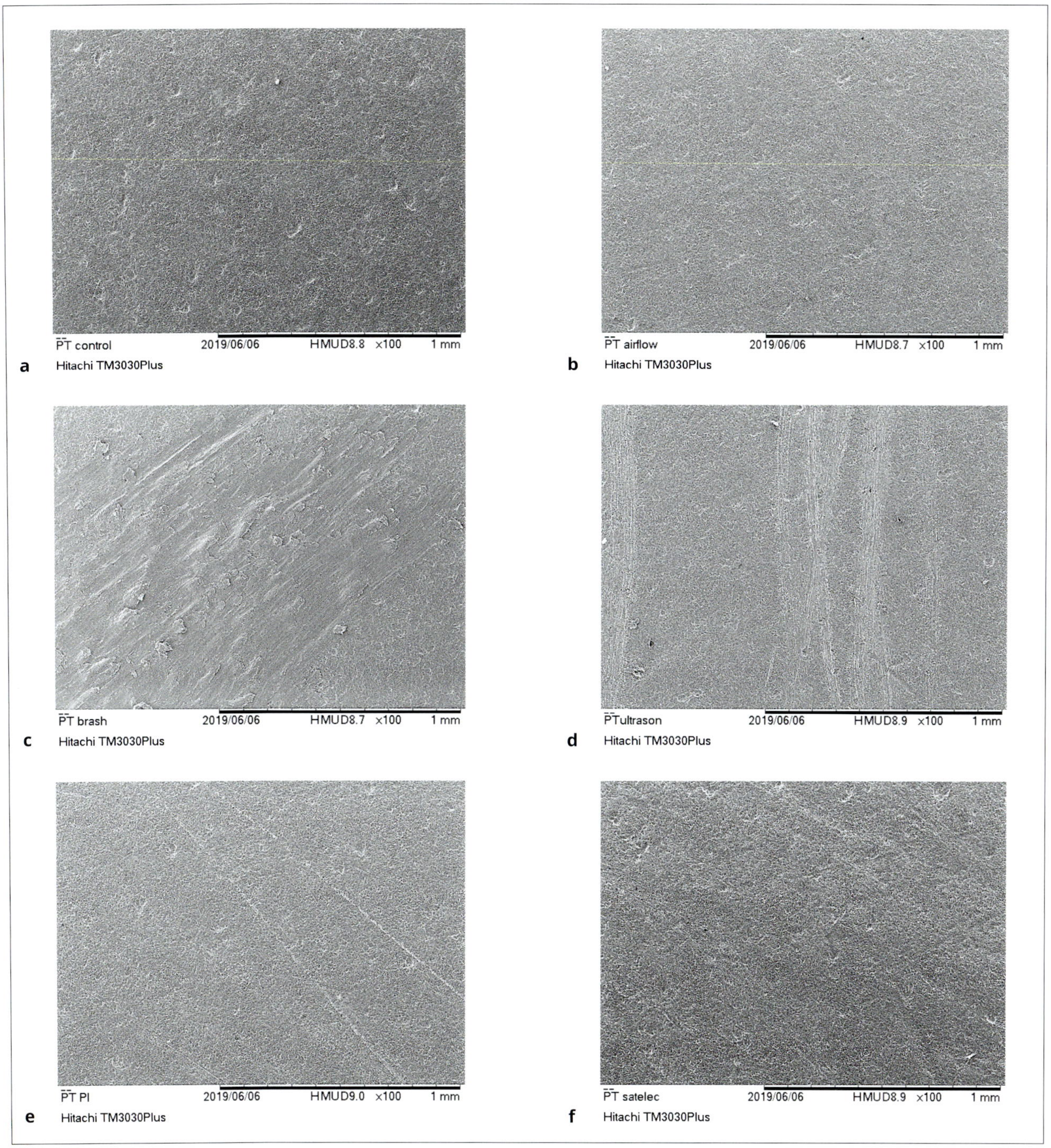

Figs 16-11a–f Comparative evaluation of various methods used in the SPT phase to remove dental biofilms in implant patients. The micrographs were taken using a scanning electron microscope at a magnification of ×100. **(a)** Polished titanium surface where no treatment has been carried out; this is used as a control. **(b)** The effect of AIRFLOW application with erythritol on a smooth polished titanium surface. This magnification shows no change in the surface. **(c)** The effect of applying a titanium brush on a smooth polished titanium surface. Destruction of the surface morphology is evident. **(d)** The effect of applying a metallic ultrasonic tip (SATELEC, Merignac, France) on a smooth polished titanium surface. Linear lesions can be observed, that is, scratches that run along the entire surface. It appears that the tip touched it during its movement, which was done along a flat line. **(e)** The effect of application of a PEEK tip (EMS Dental) on a smooth polished titanium surface. Thin lines with light-colored material on the surface of the titanium can be seen. **(f)** The effect of applying a synthetic ultrasonic tip (NSK, Tokyo, Japan) on a smooth polished titanium surface. Thin colored zones alternate with dark colored zones on the titanium surface.

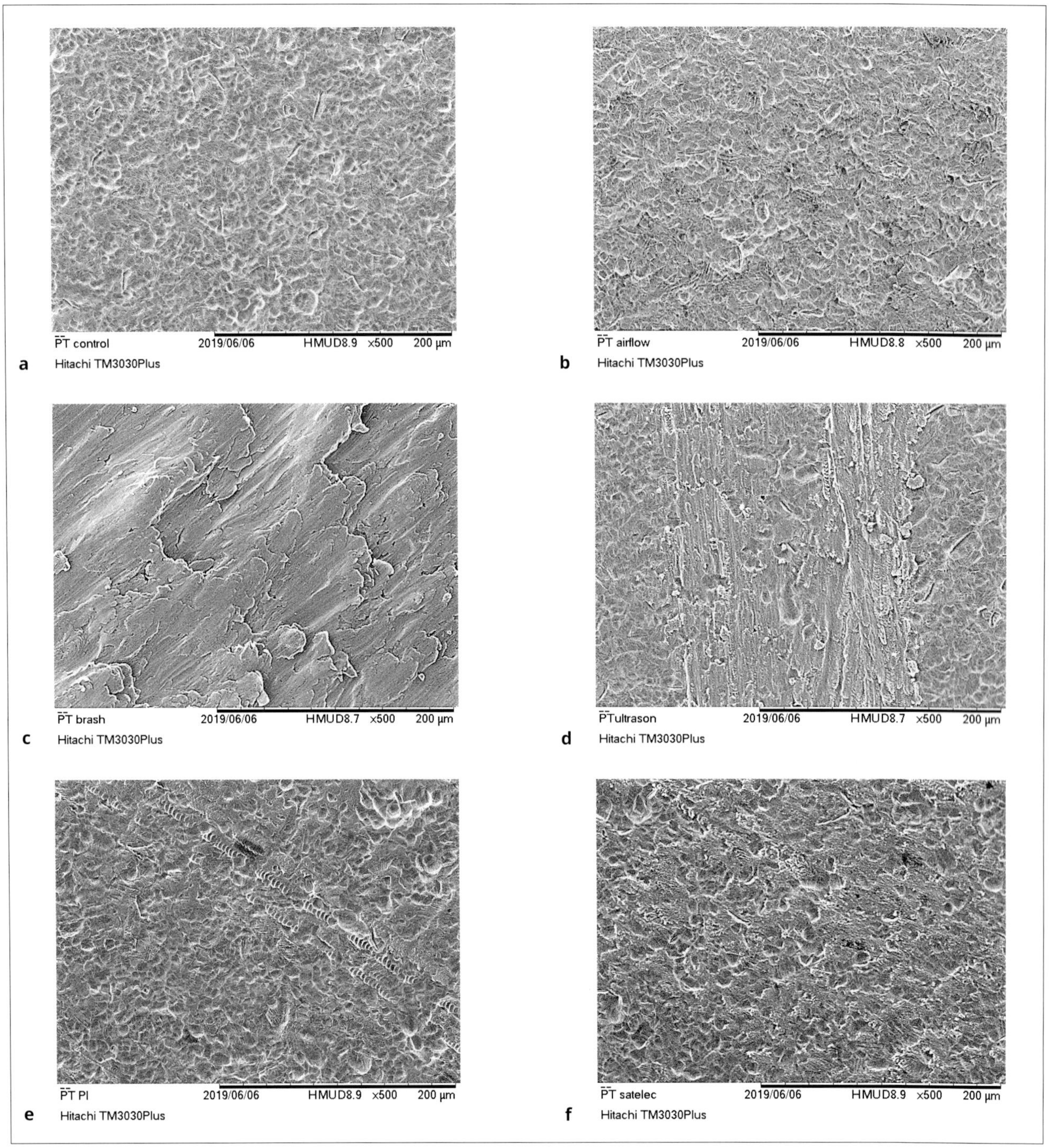

Figs 16-12a–f Comparative evaluation of several methods used in the maintenance phase to remove dental biofilms from implants. The micrographs were taken using a scanning electron microscope at ×500 magnification. **(a)** A polished titanium surface; this is the control. **(b)** The effect of AIRFLOW application with erythritol on a smooth polished titanium surface. At this greater magnification, no change on the titanium surface is observed. **(c)** The effect of applying a titanium brush on a polished titanium surface. The damage to the surface of the titanium is evident. It looks as if the titanium has melted superficially and leaked in one direction, with pieces ready to detach. **(d)** The effect of application of a metallic ultrasonic tip (SATELEC) on a polished titanium surface. At this magnification, the detrimental effect of the metallic tip on the surface of titanium is evident; however, it is smaller than that of the titanium brush. **(e)** The effect of application of a PEEK ultrasonic tip (EMS Dental) on a polished titanium surface. Small semicircular lines appear parallel to each other, forming two parallel columns. It represents deposition of the tip's coating material because the surface has not been scratched or damaged. **(f)** The effect of applying synthetic material (NSK tip) on a polished titanium surface. Throughout the surface, minor deposits of light-colored material can be seen, while the texture of the titanium surface has changed, albeit not significantly.

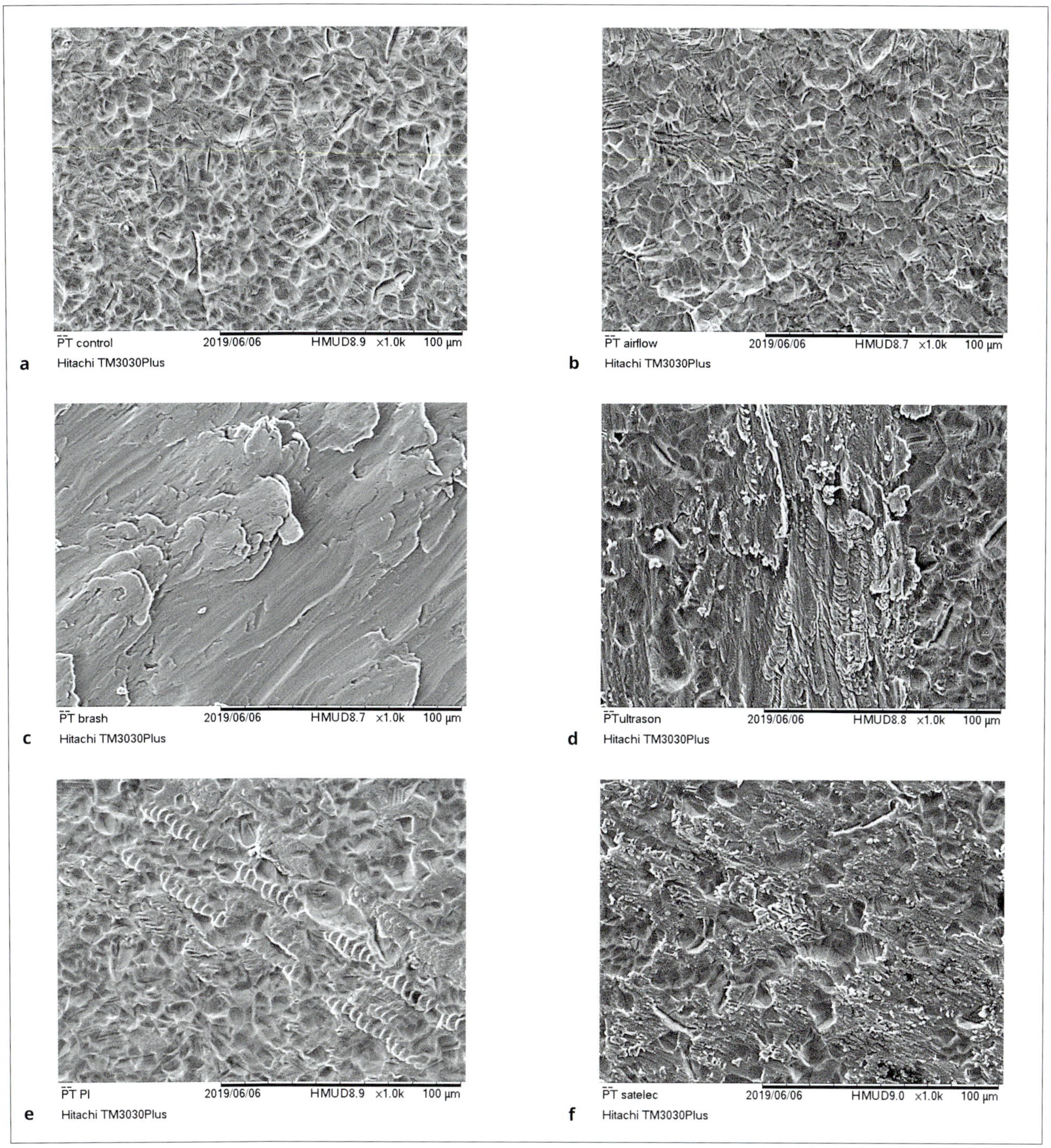

Figs 16-13a–f Comparative evaluation of various methods used in the maintenance phase to remove dental biofilms from implants. The micrographs were taken using a scanning electron microscope at ×1,000 magnification. **(a)** A polished titanium surface; this is the control surface. **(b)** The effect of AIRFLOW with erythritol application on a smooth polished titanium surface. AIRFLOW with erythritol did not cause damage to the titanium surface. **(c)** The effect of applying a titanium brush on a polished titanium surface. The smooth surface of the titanium is substantially altered. **(d)** The effect of applying a metallic ultrasonic tip (SATELEC) to a polished titanium surface. At this magnification, the surface damage caused by the metallic instrument is evident, as well as detachment of titanium particles. **(e)** The effect of applying a polyetheretherketone ultrasonic tip (EMS Dental) on a polished titanium surface. The two columns shown correspond to traces extracted from the coating material, but without causing damage to the smooth surface. **(f)** The effect of applying synthetic material (NSK tip) on a polished titanium surface. Note the considerable wear of the implant surface and many pieces of synthetic material that have been removed and remained on the titanium surface .

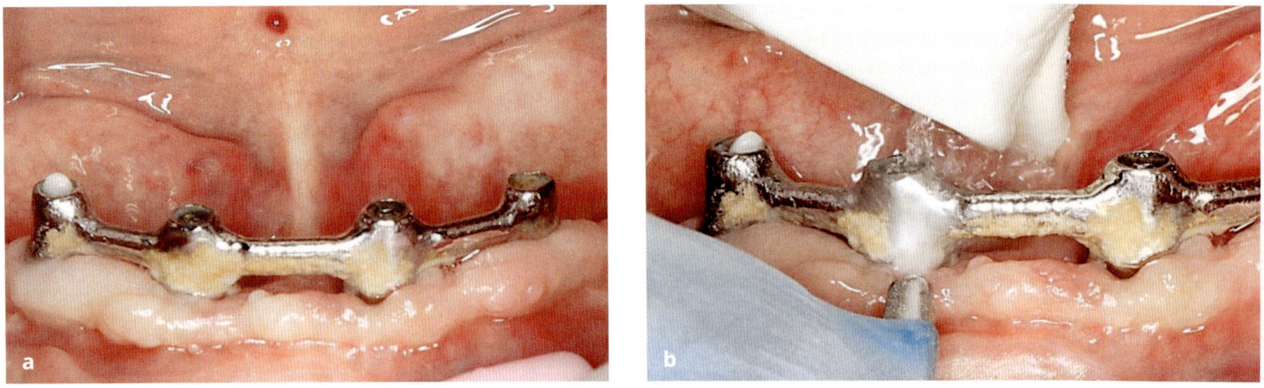

Figs 16-14a, b **(a)** Implant rehabilitation and overdenture 12 years prior. The patient did not apply effective oral hygiene but attended their maintenance care sessopms every 3 months throughout the aforementioned period. **(b)** After implementing the modified CIST protocol, AIRFLOW with erythritol was applied at each supportive periodontal therapy session. Guided biofilm therapy removed not only soft but also early mineralized deposits.

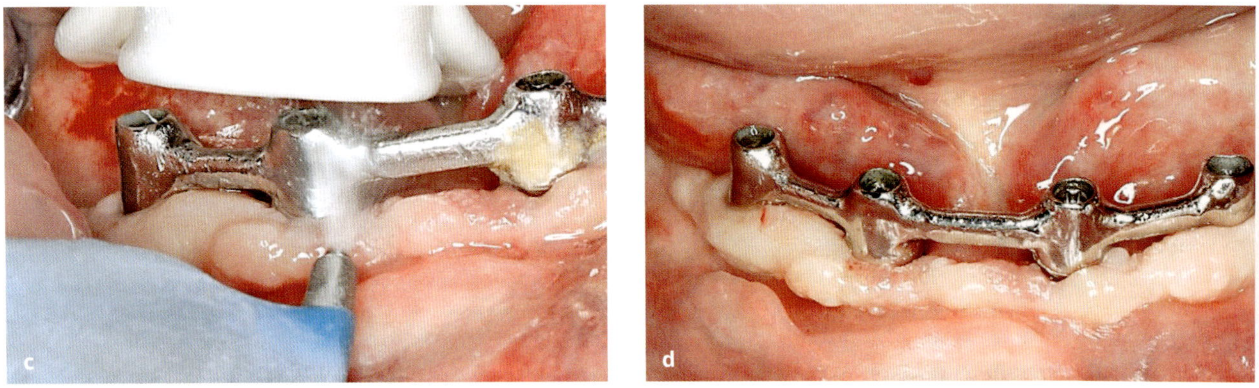

Figs 16-14c, d **(c)** The procedure is quick and effective and does not cause any discomfort to the patient. **(d)** Most of the biofilms were removed from the prosthetic reconstruction (bar).

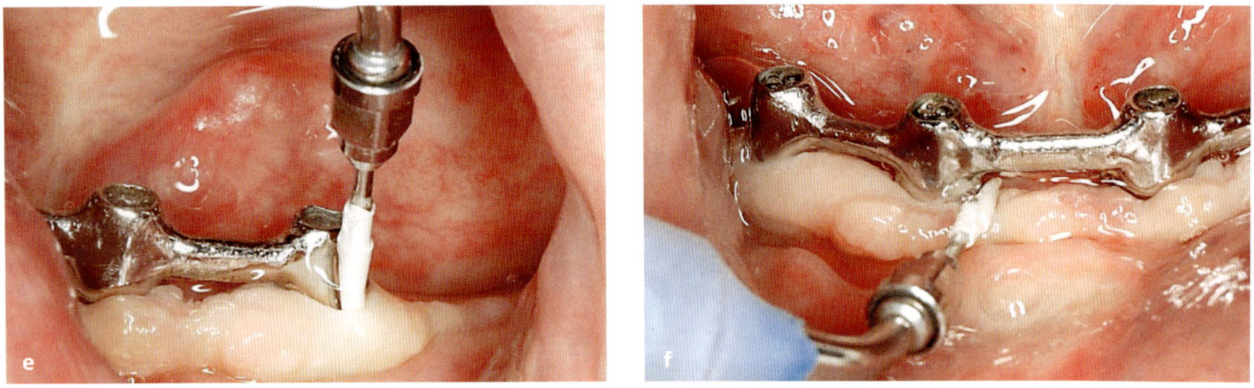

Figs 16-14e, f Subsequently, the PI tip was used to remove any mineralized biofilms that were not eradicated using AIRFLOW.

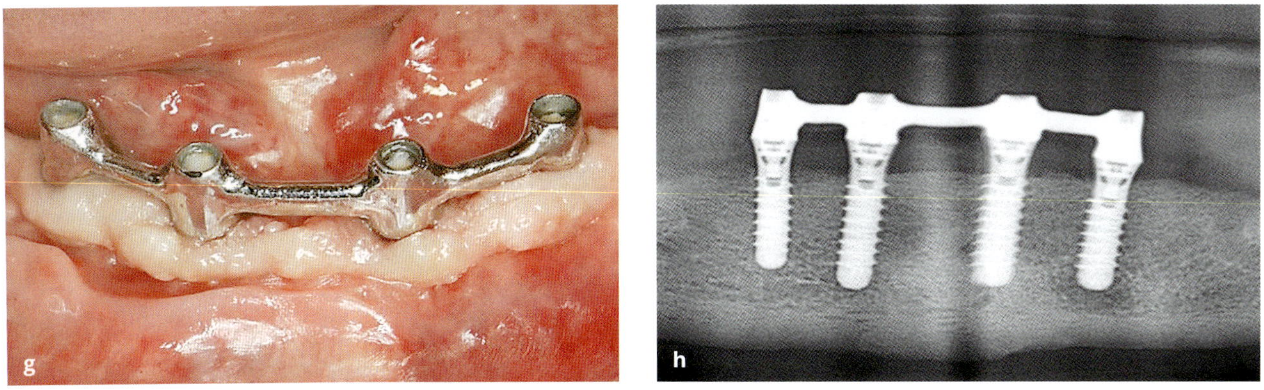

Figs 16-14g, h (g) Prosthetic restoration 3 months after its completion. **(h)** The radiograph taken 12 years after implant placement shows a well-preserved implant–bone contact.

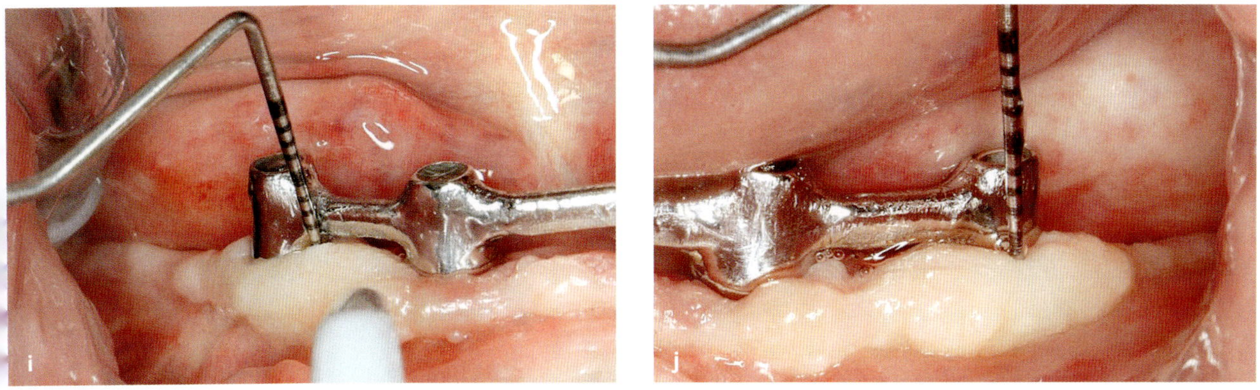

Figs 16-14i, j Stability of clinical measurements confirming peri-implant sulci and absence of pockets.

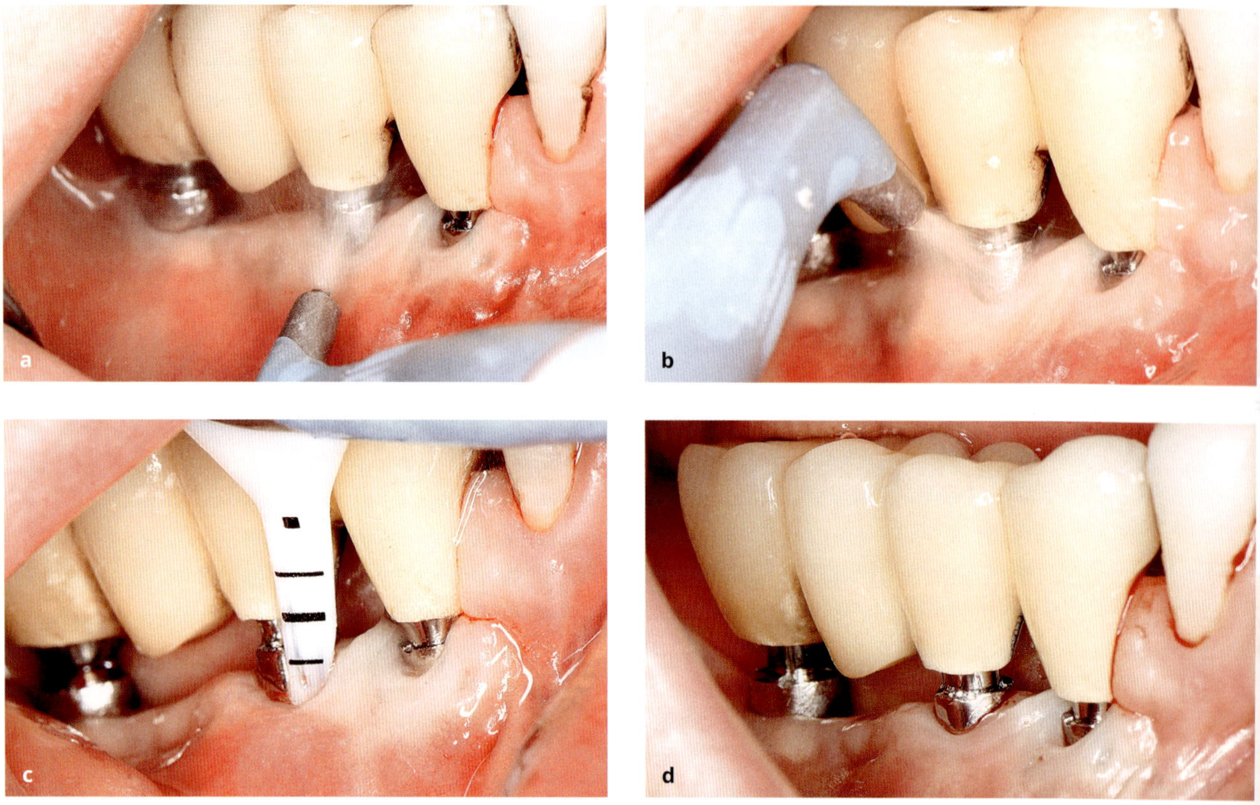

Figs 16-15a–d AIRFLOW application with erythritol. Six years after completion of the peri-implantitis treatment, health was maintained. This is a continuation of the clinical case presented in Figs 11-17a–f. **(a)** Most of the time, AIRFLOW was directed coronally, aiming to remove the microbial load located supramucosally. **(b)** The handpiece was then directed to the peri-implant sulcus to remove deposits up to a depth of 4 mm. **(c)** Application of the PERIOFLOW nozzle followed, which aimed to remove deposits from pockets with a depth greater than 4 mm. **(d)** After the procedure was completed, the surfaces of the implants and restorations were left clean, with no harm having been done to the soft tissues.

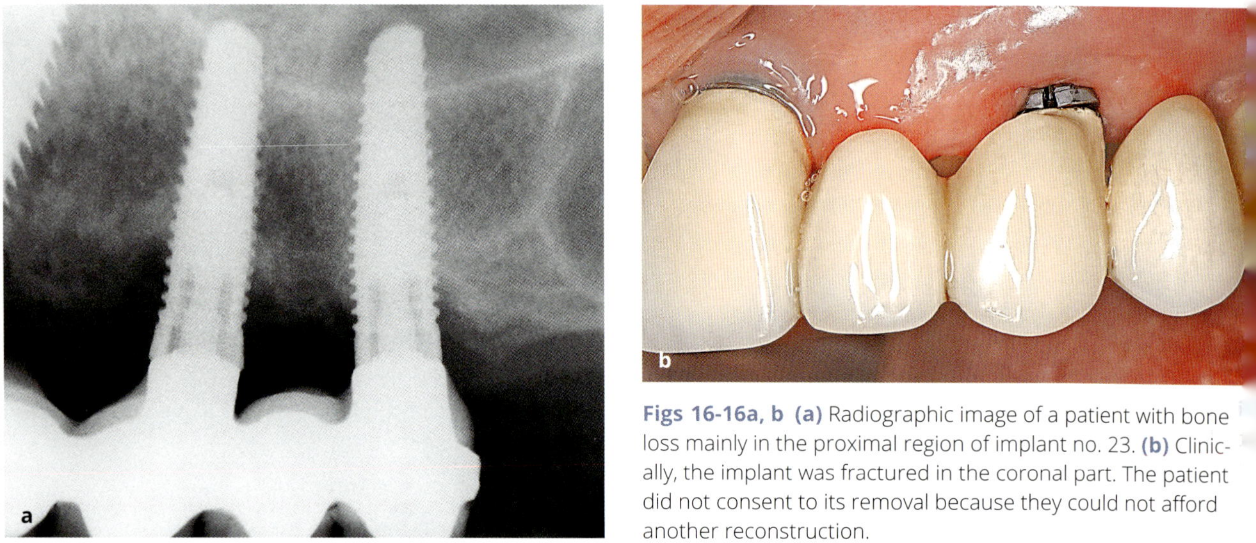

Figs 16-16a, b **(a)** Radiographic image of a patient with bone loss mainly in the proximal region of implant no. 23. **(b)** Clinically, the implant was fractured in the coronal part. The patient did not consent to its removal because they could not afford another reconstruction.

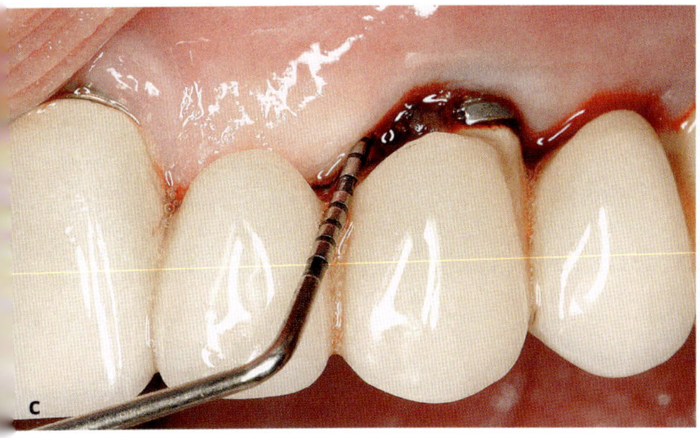

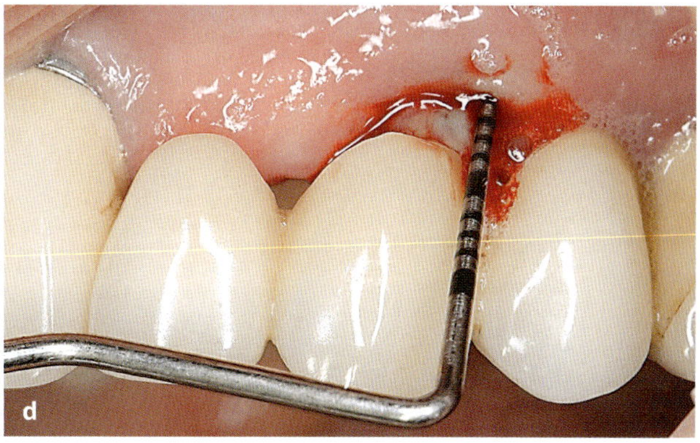

Figs 16-16c, d Peri-implant pockets were observed, as well as profuse BOP and pus formation.

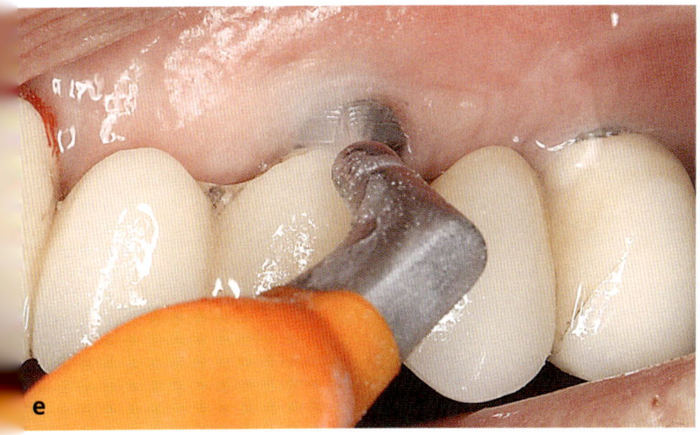

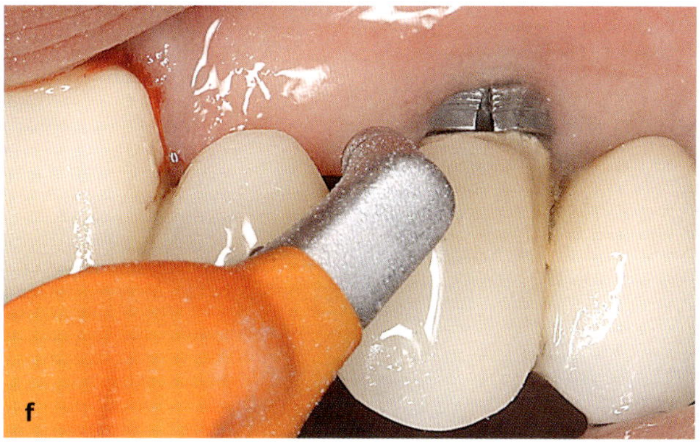

Figs 16-16e, f (e) As a result of consistent patient attendance every 3 months for SPT with AIRFLOW and effective oral hygiene, 2 years after diagnosis, the peri-implant status was stable and free of inflammation. (f) Immediately after discontinuation of AIRFLOW application, no bleeding was observed.

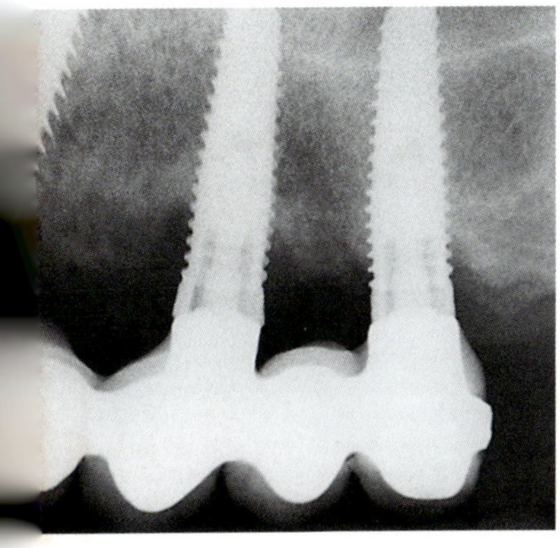

Fig 16-16 g Radiograph showing a stable level of bone–implant contact, without further bone loss for 2 years.

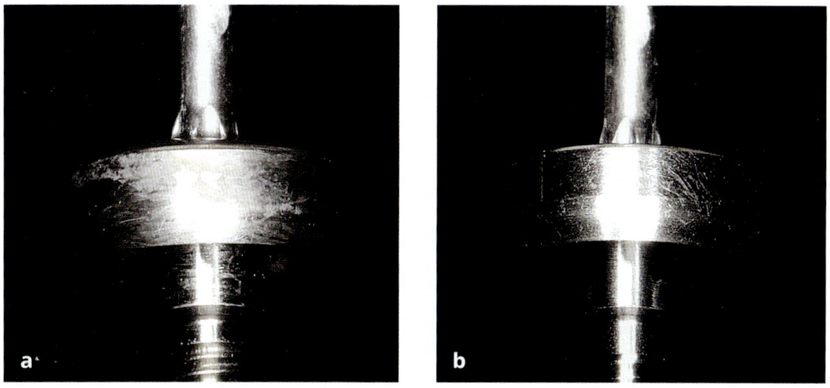

Figs 16-17a, b (a) Biofilm on the healing abutment. (b) After its removal using AIRFLOW with erythritol.

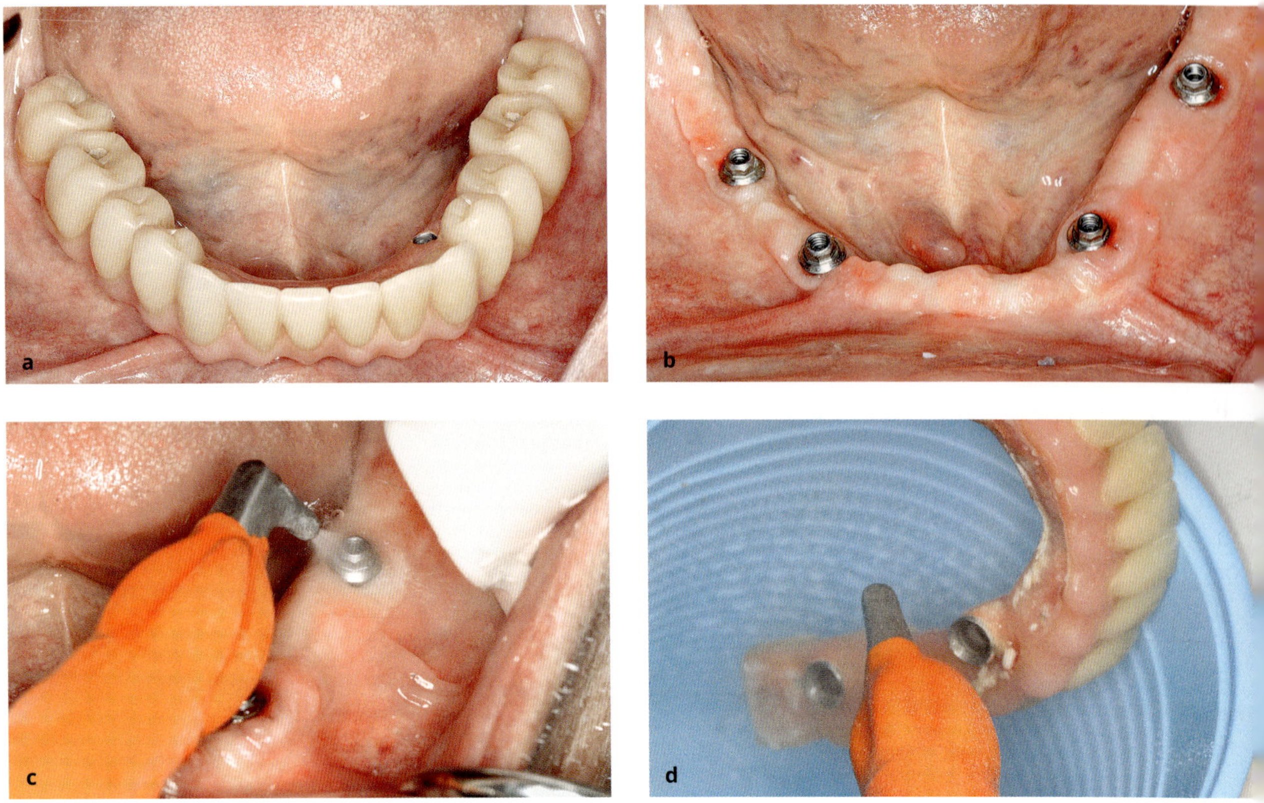

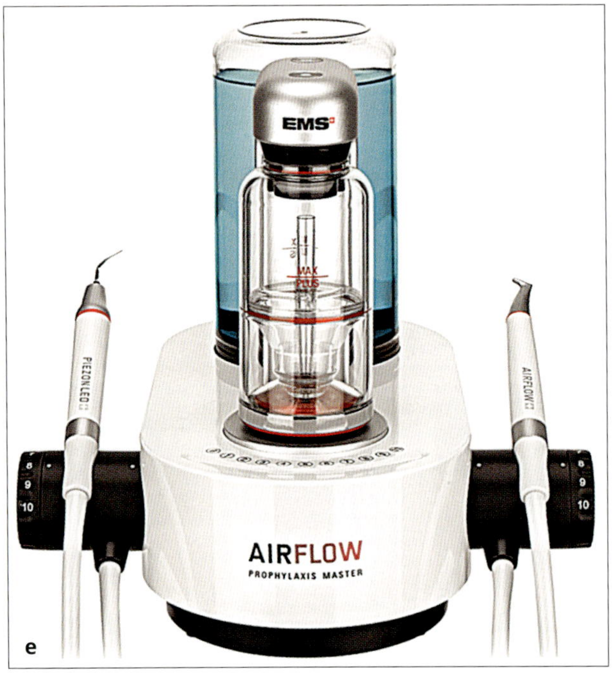

Figs 16-18a–e **(a to c)** During the maintenance phase, the prosthetic restoration may have to be removed and biofilm disruption by AIRFLOW and erythritol polishing may be performed. **(d)** The procedure may also be applied to remove soft and hard deposits from the prosthesis. **(e)** The Prophylaxis Master device (EMS Dental) was used to apply the GBT protocol.

16.4.1 Assessment

Patient assessment is particularly important. Once the patient's medical and dental history have been evaluated, extraoral and intraoral clinical examinations are performed, as well as examination of periodontal and peri-implant tissues. A periodontal chart is recorded, a radiologic examination may be performed where necessary, and the case diagnosis is made.

16.4.2 Disclosure of dental biofilms

In an attempt to maintain or restore health in periodontal and peri-implant tissues, education and motivation of the patient in administering effective oral hygiene on a daily basis is crucial. This is both a preventive and therapeutic measure for periodontal and peri-implant diseases. However, the process is demanding as hygiene administration needs to be individualized to suit the patient, and is therefore time-consuming and the patient may require a degree of persuasion in order to comply with it. Additionally, the patient's difficulty in understanding both the method to be used and the time required to remove the dental biofilm is increased because the color of dental biofilm is similar to that of the teeth. The extent of the biofilm may be revealed using disclosing agents, such as erythrosine, fuchsin, Bismarck brown, and fluorescein.

16.4.3 Education and motivation of the patient

It is necessary to inform the patient of the importance of prevention and the role of oral hygiene. Dental biofilm disclosure contributes to patient motivation.

After motivation, education regarding and practicing of oral hygiene procedures follows using a mirror, toothbrush, and interdental cleaning devices. Then, the patient should realize that simply using a toothbrush or interdental devices may not be enough to remove the disclosed dental biofilm. The practitioner needs to explain to them that the biofilm takes time to be removed.[21]

The means of oral hygiene are selected by the practitioner based on the skills and anatomical characteristics of each patient. Motivating the patient is an integral part of treatment and contributes to the development of a relationship of trust with the clinician. Professional removal of dental biofilm is of little value if applied alone without educating the patient in how to administer oral hygiene (Figs 16-14a–j).

16.4.4 Removal of dental biofilm with the AIRFLOW air-powered system in sulci and pockets up to 4 mm deep

The specially designed AIRFLOW handpiece applying 14 µm of erythritol powder is used to remove the dental biofilm not only above the margin of the peri-implant mucosa but also below it to a depth of up to 4 mm. Its use is safe for implants, natural dentition, and prosthetic restorations. Air polishing with AIRFLOW removes stains, dental biofilm, and early (soft) calculus. The handpiece is placed inclined in relation to the tooth axis at a distance of 3 to 5 mm and at an angle of 30 to 60 degrees, with continuous movement, always using surgical suction to prevent aerosols from escaping into the atmosphere of the dental office. Biofilms should be removed even from the surface of the tongue and palate. Their removal is not only effective but also painless for the patient.

16.4.5 Removal of dental biofilm with the PERIOFLOW irrigation system in pockets of 5 mm or deeper

Application of the PERIOFLOW handpiece and nozzle, exclusively with erythritol powder, is the solution to remove biofilms from deep peri-implant sulci and pockets. The plastic, flexible disposable nozzle inserted in the handpiece allows access to peri-implant pockets deeper than 5 mm. The nozzle is moved in a coronoapical direction for 5 seconds at each position (eg, mesiobuccal, middle of the buccal surface, and distobuccal). According to research, the irrigated mixture sprayed from this special nozzle results in spinning, thereby also removing the dental biofilm from the apical surfaces of the threads of the implants exposed in a pocket environment due to bone destruction.

16.4.6 Removal of calculus, with PIEZON ultrasonic devices and the PI tip

Application of air polishing using the AIRFLOW handpiece usually removes the calculus deposited on the titanium or restorative surfaces, especially if the patient is compliant with the recall program. However, if some calculus deposits remain after air polishing, their removal with the specially designed PI tip (EMS Dental) follows. For the implants, special PI tips covered with PEEK polymer are used so as not to scratch the titanium surface.

It is useful for the clinician that, after removal of the dental biofilm through air polishing, calculus is very visible; therefore, it takes less time for it to be removed (Figs 16-14a–j).

16.4.7 Evaluation of biofilm removal

Checking the effective removal of soft and hard biofilms follows to confirm the success of the session. The final check may be performed using a specific probe and optical magnification.

16.4.8 Planning of future recall visits to maintain the therapeutic result

Recall frequency is individualized for each patient and is determined by evaluating the aforementioned factors.

The next recall session is scheduled at the end of the visit, and the clinician is responsible for reminding the patient to attend. This may be done by phone, text messagie, or email. Maintaining the therapeutic result prevents the reccurrence of periodontal and peri-implant diseases. The success of the recall program is directly related to factors such as the perception of pain, fear, anxiety, noise, and vibration, which, although not identical to pain, is an unpleasant sensation for the patient.

16.4.9 Advantages

GBT offers a number of benefits. It is desirable for all techniques to remove biofilm and calculus effectively from tooth and implant surfaces (Figs 16-15a–d and 16-16a–g).

Compared to other methods implemented to maintain peri-implant health, GBT is a minimally invasive method that is effective in removing biofilms without damaging the surface of the implants, teeth, and restorations. It does not cause any unpleasant sensations to the patient, nor fatigue to the clinician (Figs 16-17a, b and 16-18a–e).

Considering the factors of speed, safety, and tolerability for the patient, this protocol is advantageous over anything other that has been proposed thus far.

16.4.10 Contraindications

Contraindications are infections of the upper respiratory tract, unstable asthma, bronchitis, and allergy to flavoring additives. In patients following a low-salt diet, it is possible to apply GBT only with glycine and erythritol powders. GBT is not indicated when there are peri-implant abscesses or peri-implant pockets with suppuration. This is mentioned in the protocol to prevent emphysema. However, if AIRFLOW is used in an apical-coronal direction and the PERIOFLOW device is placed at a short distance from the apical part of the pocket, the risk of emphysema is extremely low.

From the clinician's perspective, the protocol offers effective and safe removal of biofilms, reduces fatigue, saves time, and results in high performance for all the steps of the CIST protocol. From the patient's perspective, the protocol guarantees a feeling of comfort, as well as minimizing the vibrations caused by ultrasonic drills. Thus, a trusting relationship between the clinician and the patient, which is necessary for patient compliance in a maintenance program and for long-term health maintenance, is established (Figs 16-19a–h).

For all the aforementioned reasons, GBT is always step A of the modified CIST protocol,[22] which is applied to each session during the maintenance care program.

When no bone loss is present, compared to previous examinations (health confirmed or no recurrence after peri-implantitis treatment), GBT will be performed (step A). However, if there is inflammation that is, peri-implant mucositis for the preservation of the integrity of the peri-implant bone or in cases of treated peri-implantitis, in addition to GBT (step A, step B, that is, the use of chlorhexidine, will be applied (Fig 16-20).

If bone loss is detected after radiologic examination in any session during the SPT phase, GBT will be performed, that is, steps B, C, and D will be added to step A (Fig 16-21).

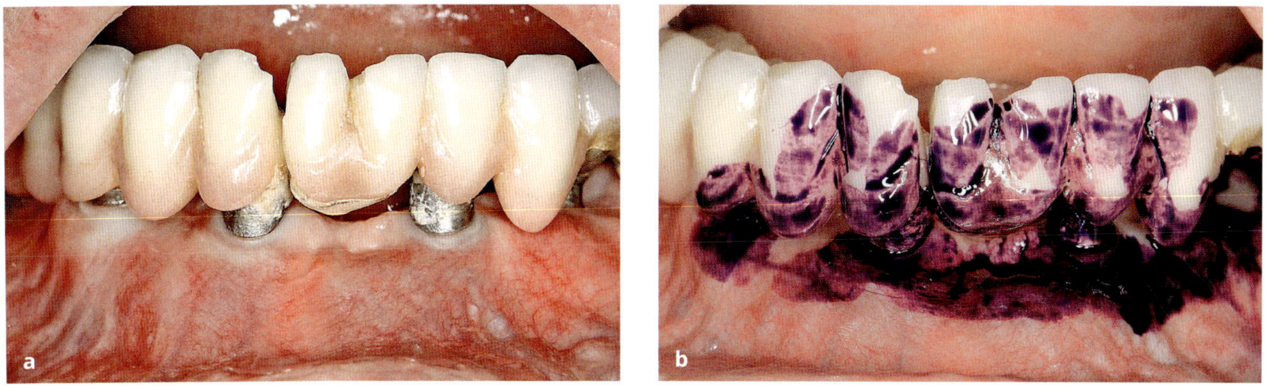

Figs 16-19a, b (a) Clinical picture of a patient who underwent peri-implantitis treatment 10 years prior (this is the clinical case presented in Fig 11-21). Following the adoption of rhe modified CIST protocol and thereafter, the GBT protocol was applied every 3 months. **(b)** Application of a disclosing agent to reveal dental biofilms.

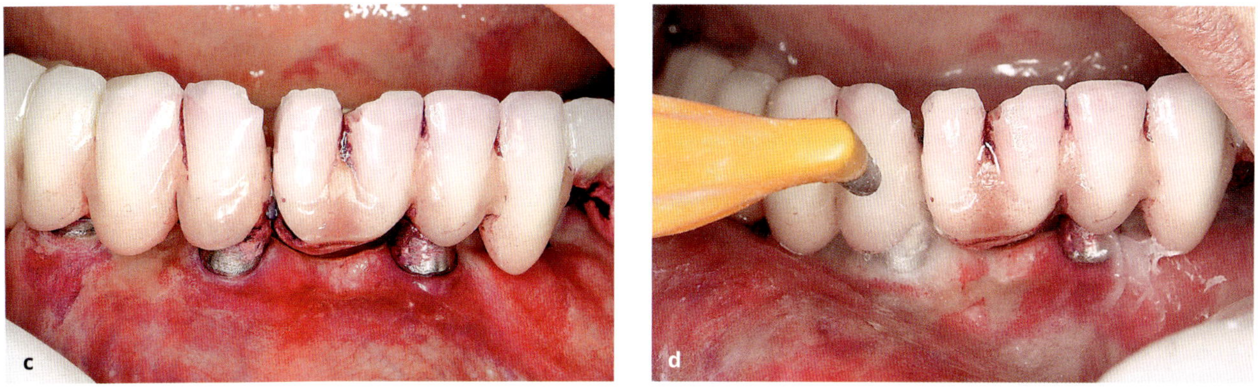

Figs 16-19c, d (c) After rinsing the disclosing agent using strong surgical suction to avoid aerosols in the dental office, but not to sputter the container as happens when the patient performs rinsing alone. **(d)** AIRFLOW application. The disclosing agent that remained on the implant surfaces guides the clinician to direct AIRFLOW to the specific area and for the amount of time needed to remove all the deposits.

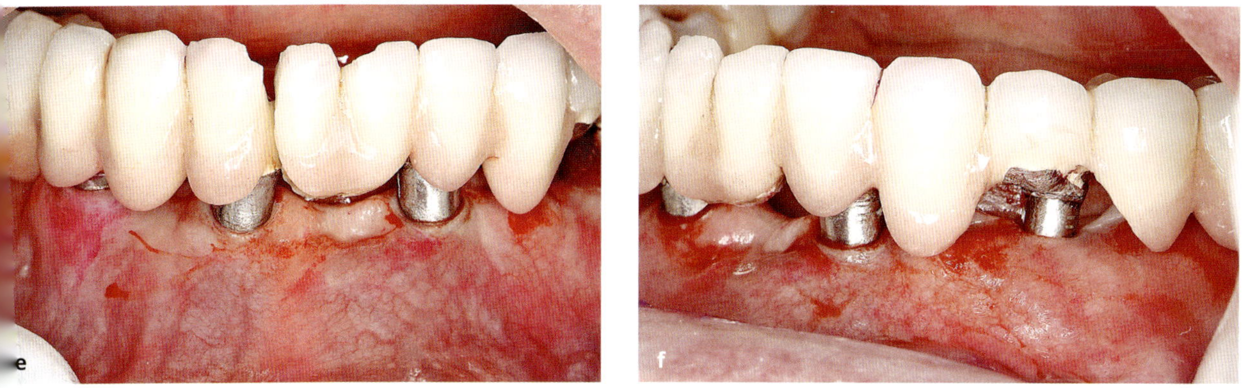

gs 16-19e, f After completion of AIRFLOW application, slight bleeding was observed, indicating a low degree of inflammation. ıere was no need to employ a PI tip in the ultrasonic device because the use of an AIRFLOW mat removed the biofilms.

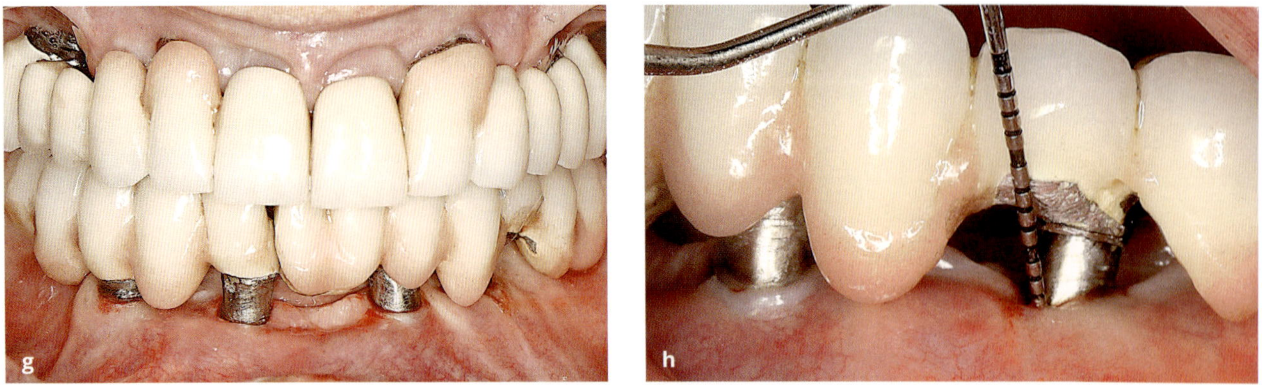

Figs 16-19g, h Despite the frequent occurrence of inflammation in the peri-implant mucosa over the years, the patient's compliance with the SPT program and the efficacy of their oral hygiene administration, combined with the application of the CIST protocol, kept the implants free of peri-implant pockets greater than 5 mm and further bone loss.

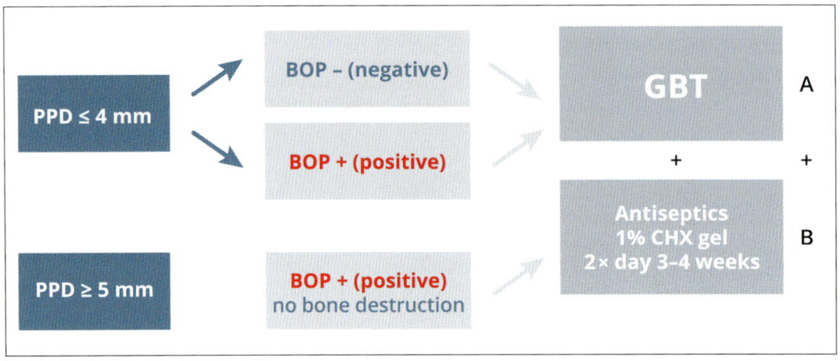

Fig 16-20 Modified CIST protocol in peri-implant health or in cases with peri-implant mucositis, as well as in cases of peri-implant mucositis in patients previously treated for peri-implantitis. CHX, chlorhexidine; PPD, probing pocket depth.

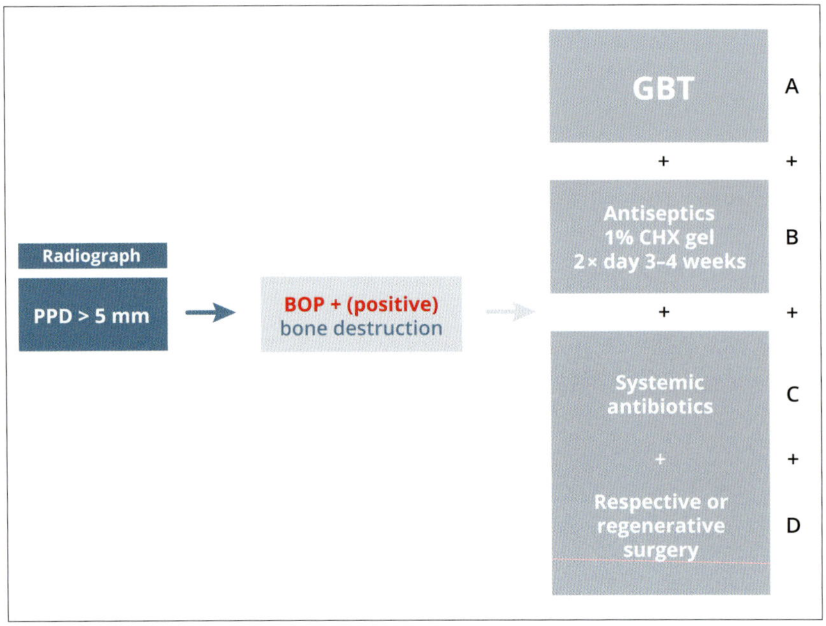

Fig 16-21 Modified CIST protocol for peri-implantitis or recurrence of it. CHX, chlorhexidine; PPD, probing pocket depth.

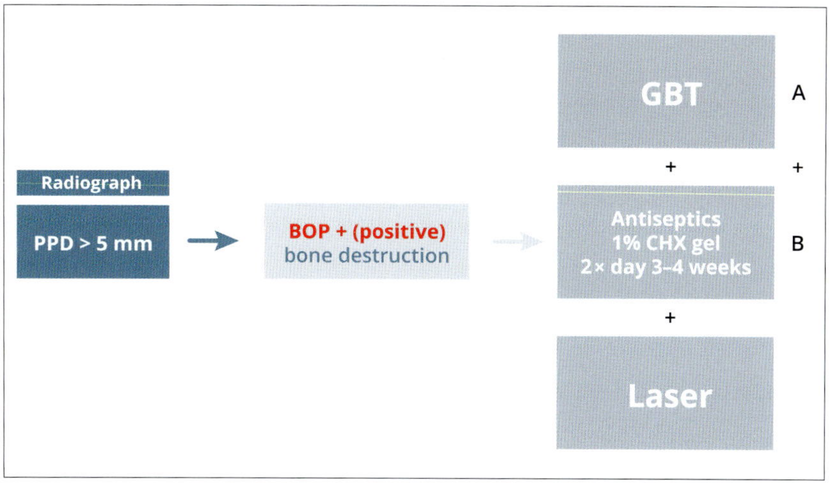

Fig 16-22 Modified CIST protocol for peri-implantitis or its recurrence if laser application is needed. CHX, chlorhexidine; PPD, probing pocket depth.

If the clinician selects to apply supplementary laser protocols to manage recurrence in any session during the SPT phase, GBT will precede this (Fig 16-22). Then, all the selected steps of the modified CIST protocol may be applied in the same session. This is clearly advantageous in terms of ergonomics and treatment immediacy.

References

1. Vrotsos IA, Karoussis IK. Peridodontology-Implantology. Athens: BETA Publications, 2016.
2. Wilson TG Jr, Glover ME, Schoen J, Baus C, Jacobs T. Compliance with maintenance therapy in a private periodontal practice. J Periodontol 1984;55:468–473.
3. Costa FO, Takenaka-Martinez S, Cota LO, Ferreira SD, Silva GL, Costa JE. Peri-implant disease in subjects with and without preventive maintenance: a 5-year follow-up. J Clin Periodontol 2012;39:173–181.
4. Pjetursson BE, Helbling C, Weber H-P, et al. Peri-implantitis susceptibility as it relates to periodontal therapy and supportive care. Clin Oral Implants Res 2012;23:888–894.

Rudeejaraswan A, Pisarnturakit PP, Mattheos N, Pimkhaokham A, Subbalekha K. Dentists' attitudes toward dental implant maintenance in Thailand. JDR Clin Trans Res 2021;23800844211049405.

Humphrey S. Implant maintenance. Dent Clin North Am 2006;50:463–478.

Lang NP, Nyman SR. Supportive maintenance care for patients with implants and advanced restorative therapy. Periodontol 2000 1994;4:119–126.

Schwarz F, Alcoforado G, Guerrero A, et al. Peri-implantitis: summary and consensus statements of group 3. The 6th EAO Consensus Conference 2021. Clin Oral Implants Res 2021;32(suppl 21):245–253.

9. Mombelli A. Maintenance therapy for teeth and implants. Periodontol 2000 2019;79:190–199.
10. Wilson TG Jr. A typical maintenance visit for patients with dental implants. Periodontol 2000 1996;12:29–32.
11. Wilson TG. A typical implant maintenance visit. In: Wilson T Jr, Harrel S (eds). Dental Implant Failure. Cham: Springer, 2019.
12. Bauman GR, Mills M, Rapley JW, Hallmon WH. Clinical parameters of evaluation during implant maintenance. Int J Oral Maxillofac Implants 1992;7:220–227.
13. Duarte PM, Reis AF, de Freitas PM, Ota-Tsuzuki C. Bacterial adhesion on smooth and rough titanium surfaces after treatment with different instruments. J Periodontol 2009;80:1824–1832.
14. Lang NP, Wetzel AC, Stich H, Caffesse RG. Histologic probe penetration in healthy and inflamed peri-implant tissues. Clin Oral Implants Res 1994;5:191–201.
15. Albrektsson T. On long-term maintenance of the osseointegrated response. Aust Prosthodont J 1993;7(suppl):15–24.
16. Chernysheva A, Fourmousis I, Karoussis I, Vrotsos I. Guided Biofilm Therapy. An innovative approach. Odont Prog 2018;72:60–71.
17. Fox SC, Moriarty JD, Kusy RP. The effects of scaling a titanium implant surface with metal and plastic instruments: an in-vitro study. J Periodontol 1990;61:485–490.
18. Amate-Fernández P, Figueiredo R, Blanc V, Àlvarez G, León R, Valmaseda-Castellón E. Erythritol-enriched powder and oral biofilm regrowth on dental implants: an in vitro study. Med Oral Patol Oral Cir Bucal 2021;26:e602–e610.
19. Patil SS, Rakhewar PS, Limaye PS, Chaudhari NP. A comparative evaluation of plaque-removing efficacy of air polishing and rubber-cup, bristle brush with paste polishing on oral hygiene status: a clinical study. J Int Soc Prev Community Dent 2015;5:457–462.

20. Wennström J, Dahlén G, Ramberg P. Subgingival debridement of periodontal pockets by air polishing in comparison with ultrasonic instrumentation during maintenance therapy. J Clin Periodontol 2011;38:820–827.

21. Silverstein L, Kurtzman G. Oral hygiene and maintenance of dental implants. Dent Today 2006;25:70–75.

22. Lang NP, Lindhe J. Clinical Periodontology and Implant Dentistry, vol 2. Hoboken, NJ: John Wiley & Sons, 2015.